Treating
Cancer *with*
HERBS

An Integrative Approach

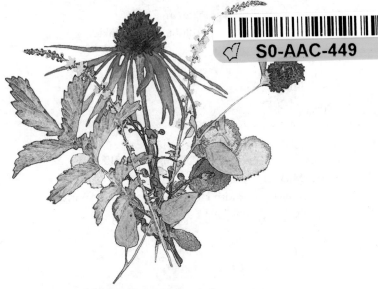

S0-AAC-449

Dr. Michael Tierra
L.Ac., N.D., AHG

LOTUS
PRESS

P.O. Box 325, Twin Lakes, Wisconsin 53181

This book is a reference work not intended to treat, diagnose or prescribe. The information contained herein is in no way to be considered as a substitute for a consultation with a duly licensed health-care professional.

Cover design and execution: Susan Tinkle
Book design and page composition: Susan Tinkle

First Edition 2003
Reprinted 2012
Printed in the United States of America

Library of Congress Control Number : 2003100487
Tierra, Michael,
    Treating Cancer with Herbs: An Integrative Approach
    ISBN: 978-0-9149-5593-1

Published by
Lotus Press, P.O. Box 325, Twin Lakes, Wisconsin 53181
email: lotuspress@lotuspress.com
website: www.lotuspress.com
1 (800) 824-6396

CONTENTS

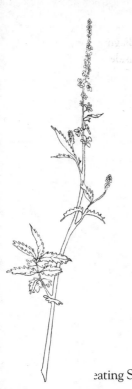

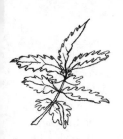

ACKNOWLEDGMENTS

I offer heartfelt gratitude to the many cancer patients that have passed through my care, for their faith, trust and for sharing the intimacy of their hopes and fears. I honor them for their courage in the face of a great battle. While it may be "better to give than to receive," this lesson seems more for the caregiver. For cancer patients, the many lessons include the strangely difficult one of being able to accept and receive unconditional love from others. How strange it is that for some a crisis is needed to help us recognize the extent to which our survival is dependent upon the invisible web of universal love that abounds everywhere—and that all we need do is acknowledge it.

Deep thanks and gratitude to Lesley Tierra, my beloved wife and life partner, for sustaining me through times of self-doubt and for reading the manuscript and making suggestions that hopefully will result in a better book.

Thanks and gratitude to the publisher of Lotus Press, Santosh Krinsky, who has given me more than one reason to believe that his primary motivation is uncommonly not the bottom line as it is with most who are in the publishing business, but in the use of considerable talents and resources to serve the higher good. I wish him the very best in all of his endeavors and that this and other books of mine that he has published will be worthy of his faith and trust.

Others that I need to express my thanks to include Donald Yance, AHG, whose personal work with cancer patients and his book *Herbal Medicine Healing & Cancer* (published by Keats) and personal teaching are amongst the finest today, Ralph Moss, whose books on cancer, especially *Questioning Chemotherapy* and the *Moss Reports* (available on the Internet) on individual cancers should be the first steps anyone with cancer should take in pursuing a course of treatment. Also, Jeanne M. Wallace, PhD, CNC (certified nutritionist) for her review of the supplements chapter, Richard Goldberg, friend and frontline health food store guru who is always encouraging and effective for the hundreds of people who visit him at Felton's New Leaf Market.

With all this supportive and loving assistance, I am responsible for the content of this book and may it go forth and be of some assistance, great or small, to others.

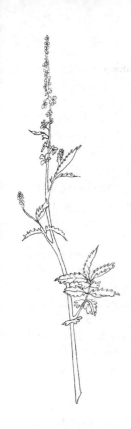

INTRODUCTION

One of my most amazing cancer cases involved a Croatian man named Anthony. At the time of our first meeting he was in his early 70's. Originally raised on a farm in rural Yugoslavia, Anthony was the respected patriarch of a large extended family living in the Northern California Bay Area. His family brought him to me out of desperation when he received a diagnosis of pancreatic cancer at Stanford Hospital. The doctors proposed a resectioning of his bile duct to alleviate pain and gave him three or four months to live. Although Anthony could not speak English, he understood enough to reply "Thank you, but no thank you."

After explaining the situation to me, the family presented their father with the request that anything I could do to help him would be appreciated. Respecting Anthony's decision to not undergo a strenuous and at best palliative surgical procedure, I proposed that since conventional medicine had nothing to offer, we forget about the pancreatic cancer and focus on treating whatever was apparent. At that time it was pain in the liver area, extending towards the epigastria.

In view of other diagnostic assessments, I gave Anthony an herbal liver formula[1] in tablet form along with a strong daily decoction of dandelion root tea. I also recommended a strict diet with no alcohol (he was a winemaker), no sugar and plenty of wholesome foods, especially green vegetables.

Over the course of three months Anthony's liver pain disappeared and we both forgot that he was supposed to be dead within four months from pancreatic cancer. For the next two years, I saw him fairly regularly, on the average of twice a month, for acupuncture, dietary and health maintenance.

I gradually came to realize that Anthony viewed me like one of the country village shamans from his youth in rural Croatia. Several times he'd grab my arm and imploringly say, "Help me, I think of you all the time." A few times, thinking that I had the power to dispel subtle negative energy, he asked for a protective amulet on behalf of himself or members of his family.

I believe Anthony's faith played a significant role in his recovery because he seemed to derive benefit from everything I prescribed for him, though I must say that a good herbal liver formula is often the best to consider when treating any chronic disease such as cancer. In time I noticed a hard lump near his liver which seemed to vary in dimension over time. Suspecting a gallstone or gall bladder obstruction, I sent him back to Stanford medical clinic for examination. They confirmed that he had an obstructive lump in his gall bladder, but most amazing of all they found no evidence of active pancreatic cancer.

* * *

As we can see from this case, treating the underlying cause of liver dysfunction ultimately proved to be more effective than trying to treat a known 'incurable' pancreatic cancer. Herbs are, after all, only a minor aspect of a cancer patient's diet and nutritional program. Usually alone they are unable to make the metabolic changes necessary to sufficiently shift the body from a self destructive mode to one of healing. In the following case the combination of diet, acupuncture and herbs made the difference in a patient's long-term survival from bone cancer.

* * *

Dick, a 48 year old man, was diagnosed with bone marrow cancer. He sought treatment at a metabolic clinic where he had followed a strict carrot juice fast for a couple of weeks. When he came to see me, his body was jaundiced and stiff, and he could barely move without excruciating pain. I decided that the carrot juice had exerted its beneficial influence and it was time to switch to a more balanced ongoing macrobiotic diet.

After a few weeks of bi-weekly acupuncture treatments, a macrobiotic diet and herbs, Dick moved freely with no pain. He was supposed to have only

---

[1] Planetary Formula's Bupleurum Liver Cleanse.

six months to a year to live; therefore, despite the fact that he felt more vital and alive than he had in decades, Dick returned for another biopsy upon my recommendation after six months of treatment.

You can imagine our elation when no sign of bone marrow cancer was found in any of the tests. For two years he continued to see me and take his herbs, yet over time his visits tapered off. I warned that he needed to follow the diet strictly (or at least 80% of the time) for the rest of his life. I saw him less and less frequently and his concerned wife occasionally called to say that Dick increasingly veered off track from the prescribed whole foods diet. Four and a half years after I first saw him, his cancer returned and eventually led to his demise.

* * *

In this second case, herbs helped but diet was the key to Dick's survival. As he ultimately ignored his healing process, the cancer reasserted itself.

As with many adverse situations in life, cancer may be seen as a purely negative event or as an opportunity. If and when we are able to come to terms with our mortality, it is possible to discover deeper meaning and joy in the simpler, more spiritual aspects of life. This awareness may include or transcend conventional religious beliefs, and ultimately becomes a powerful healing ally for our survival. For many, cancer is an end-stage disease and while it is not always possible to save someone from their appointment with destiny, cancer may be beneficially used as a wake-up call to better realize our innate life potential. By so doing, we are able to recharge our immune systems and naturally deepen and prolong the quality and expanse of our lives.

In a third case we see how, although cancer could not be overcome, a change in attitude and lifestyle significantly enhanced this patient's remaining life.

* * *

By the time Joan came to me, tumors were spread throughout her body. She had already undergone a mastectomy and the doctors gave her two months to live.

Upon first beginning her treatment of cancer with me, Joan divested herself of all things that were burdensome and of little meaning. Eventually this led to her not having a place to call her own. Consequently she became a welcome guest in many people's homes because, despite her metastasized breast cancer, she maintained such a positive survival outlook on life that others derived inspiration by just being in her presence.

Joan's treatment plan included weekly acupuncture, a reasonable non-fanatic macrobiotic diet based on whole grains, beans and organic vegetables, and a comprehensive herbal protocol. The objective was to enhance her wellness and strengthen her immune system in order to slow the progress of the cancer.

During the course of our visits, Joan shared stories of her life, and I also listened to her dreams. Often I or others would see her determinedly walking back from the local natural foods market with a grocery bag full of foods, such as brown rice, miso, shiitake mushrooms, organic carrots, broccoli, spinach, kale and other types of green vegetables, azuki beans, mung beans, black beans, tofu, tempeh, miso paste, seaweed and seasonal fruits. (All these foods have been thoroughly documented and researched as to their positive anticancer properties.)

To Joan, cancer served as a personal awakening, a call to life. Having experienced the mutilation of surgery, radiation and chemotherapy, she realized that these had nothing more to offer and dedicated herself to her own guided self treatment with which I was honored to offer assistance. After six months on her new life-enhancing program, it appeared that tumor growth had slowed and her pain greatly reduced.

Having outlived the time allotted to her by doctors, Joan decided to return to the local community college to realize her lifelong dream of completing her degree as a counselor. At the same time she cultivated her spiritual awareness by attending growth seminars on meditation and death and dying with Stephen and Ondrea Levine.

Joan continued in this wonderfully unique and positive approach to life, but after two and a half years, she realized that her time for passing was near. She was then in an early stage of cachexia (cancer weight loss). True to her newly evolved self, she invited a number of select friends for a special 'moving on' ceremony in a living room in the California Santa Cruz mountains. About 75 or so of us sat in a circle on the floor of a large living room as Joan expressed her personal gratitude to all of us in turn. Eventually this was reciprocated by each of us in honor of this wonderful, gentle soul who, by rising above her own personal adversity, managed to serve as an inspiration to so many.

The ceremony ended with Joan giving each of us a special gift, either from her remaining few possessions, or something special that she acquired. My gift was a transparent glass candle with a wick immersed in clear fuel. Its bright clarity symbolized what Joan had become to me over the previous two years: a clear light shining in the darkness.

* * *

Few of us may have the opportunity to end our lives with such sweet surrender and dignity. By living each moment of the day with dedication, intension and focus we achieve more value and meaning in a short period of time than many who live for decades. If we approach the healing of cancer in such high spirits, there can be no failure. By that we may not be able to affect a complete cure or remission, but there is still plenty of opportunity for true healing. To achieve this goal, we need to do everything in our power to rise beyond our natural fears.

The natural approach to treating cancer should be the first, not the last, method of treatment. Cancer patients are always confronted by seemingly impossible dilemma's where the available choices seem less than optimal. The tendency is to put one's faith in an outer authority, such as an oncologist or even a natural healer. However, the first order of business is to realize that these people are only allies, and that ultimately we must take responsibility and charge of our own decisions. To do this requires a certain amount of soul searching solitude.

If at all possible, providing there is a window of time and opportunity, embark on a natural treatment approach before committing to heroic measures such as surgery, chemo-therapy and radiation. The reason is that these latter injure the body's immune healing capabilities and may impair any opportunity for natural healing to occur. Furthermore, one needs to weigh carefully the question of life extension versus life quality.

I usually direct patients to get a balanced perspective on things by availing themselves of quality alternative resources, such as books by Ralph Moss, Donald Yance, Patrick Quinlin and others mentioned in the Bibliography. Next, I caution against becoming overly intimidated by statistical prognosis. These usually represent only a portion of the population and do not represent individuals who have chosen alternative diet, herbs and lifestyle.

Of the many times I publicly speak about alternative cancer treatment, I begin by asking how many know of someone who was medically diagnosed with cancer, chose to not follow the conventional medical treatment, and outlived the 5 year survival rate held by some to be a standard of cure for cancer. The response of these audiences, numbering from a few to over a hundred, has consistently averaged from forty to sixty percent. This is, of course, highly unscientific but it does at least prove that there is a sizable percentage of diagnosed cancer patients who are beating the odds without conventional medical intervention.

Patients are often told to be wary of alternative cancer therapies that have not passed the gold standard of being subjected to double blind, placebo controlled studies. However, what is overlooked in this argument is that 50% of the drugs in common use have not been subjected to such studies, and medical doctors unwittingly continue to prescribe them simply because they work.

Are herbs effective in the treatment of cancer? In a word, yes. Further, as we shall see, herbs have varied and important roles to play in the treatment, management and prevention of all types of cancers.

At least two herbs have yielded powerful anticancer compounds that have been integrated as part of the protocol of conventional Western cancer treatment. Taxol, a compound originally derived from the Yew tree and only recently synthesized, is considered one of the most important anti-cancer compounds of the past three decades. It is currently used to treat ovarian, breast and lung cancers, and has been effective against Kaposi's sarcoma, a cancer associated with AIDS. Chemicals from the leaves of the Madagascar Rosy Periwinkle (Apocynaceae Catharanthus roseus) also yields two important anti-cancer drugs, vincristine for the treatment of childhood leukemia, and vinblastine for the treatment of Hodgkin's disease.

One important thing to realize, however, is that the discovery of active anticancer compounds from herbs begins with the use of the whole herb by traditional herbalists. Because drug companies are unable to patent whole herbs, such as the common plants dandelion and honeysuckle flowers, these along with thousands of other herbs that have a considerable body of research attesting to their anticancer properties, will never find their way into the pharmaceutical marketplace. Considering the average cost of hundreds of millions of dollars needed to bring a drug to market, if a pharmaceutical company cannot own an exclusive patent based on identified active compounds, there is no economic incentive to pursue serious research.

Further, considering that a single herb may have literally thousands of chemical compounds, it may be difficult, if not impossible, to isolate a single active compound. According to many herbalists, the whole herb is always greater than the sum of its parts, so that compounds found in plants often need to work in concert with each other to achieve therapeutic goals. These are just a few among many reasons that thus far only the constituents from a very few plants have achieved scientific acceptance as anticancer drugs.

The U.S. National Cancer Institute has identified 3000 plants that are active against cancer cells. 70% of these plants are found in the rainforest.[2] Ethnobotanists, who have extensively researched plants used for the treatment of cancer and other so called incurable diseases by natives of the vast Amazon Rain Forest, are disappointed when pharmaceutical companies are unable to develop them as medicine.

This entire issue becomes even more complex as we realize that herbalists seldom use herbs for named diseases, but to activate innate organic processes that assist the body's ability to overcome disease. Usually this is done in complex formulas with several plants combined together according to individual patient requirements. Most herbalists would argue that herbs are exponentially more powerful in complex formulas than they are as single agents. This stretches the limits of modern pharmacy that tends to be based on the 'magic bullet' concept.

---

[2] Rain Forest Action Network; http://www.ran.org/info_center/factsheets/05f.html

This book is primarily intended to provide a systematic integrated approach for the creation of individual complex formulas using whole herbs and based on a model that is commonly followed in Mainland China. It also endorses an integrative approach of herbs with Western medicine in treating cancer. For too long our culture has supported a polarity between conventional and alternative medicine. Western doctors discredit alternatives as unsubstantiated by scientific proof while alternative practitioners are caught up in a negative reactionary mode to conventional techniques. Yet both paradigms are valid, have something important to offer, and are particularly effective when combined in a complementary way together. Many people are now ready to go beyond defined healing modalities known as "alternative," "conventional," "Western," "Eastern," "complementary," or "holistic" and are moving toward a truly integrative medicine. It's an exciting time, reflecting our readiness to bring together seemingly opposing forces and tailor treatment plans to the unique values and priorities of each individual patient.

Take the example of my friend Shannon. At the tender age of twenty, she was diagnosed with one of the most potentially deadly cancers, malignant melanoma. Doctors performed emergency surgery on her leg. However, they underestimated the size of her cancer. She had to undergo a second operation where they cut nearly to the bone, leaving a hole an inch deep on the inside of her calf. This time, all the cancer was removed.

In the aftermath of this traumatic experience, Shannon began an internal quest, exploring the various emotional and spiritual factors that had contributed to her illness. She enhanced her immune system with acupuncture, herbs, bodywork, whole foods, meditation and prayer. Today, she is much healthier than before the cancer, and has herself become a practitioner of Chinese medicine. From time to time, Shannon helped out in my clinic. Her presence served as a reminder that good medicine can both save lives, and change them.

There is, however, still another dimension to this story. Because it is often impossible to prove what causes a particular cancer, Shannon has wondered whether the huge amount of antibiotics and antihistamines given to her as a child compromised her immune system so that it was unable to produce the necessary antibodies created in our bodies on a daily basis that destroy cancer cells. If she had originally been given herbs, such as honeysuckle blossoms or burdock seeds for minor colds and coughs (both being herbs with anticancer properties) instead of immune suppressive drugs, perhaps Shannon would have had the ability to resist the development of cancer.

Like so many similar conjectures, we may never know. The fact remains, however, that with the increasing incidence of cancer in Western society, there is still little will to take an aggressive stand for prevention. Perhaps it is simple laziness, but a less happy thought is that such a stand might lead to an all-out confrontation with the two largest worldwide industries involved in the multibillion dollar cancer industry, the petroleum and the pharmaceutical industry.

There are many levels of understanding not considered in current medical practice: Why did the cancer arise in the first place? How can we strengthen the body's systems to prevent a cancer's recurrence? Alternative therapies generally address these issues and emphasize things we can do, such as diet and lifestyle changes and therapies to enhance immunity and improve vitality. These are all vital to any integrated program for health, and to the standard healthcare of every person in this country.

It is at least to this end that I offer this book – as a powerful approach to treat and prevent cancer through an integrated dietary, lifestyle and herbal approach. Generally all of these integrate with the protocols of various professional health practitioners, such as oncologists, herbalists, chiropractors and naturopaths. As gifts of Divine Providence for suffering humanity, herbs have always been and remain the first medicine. I wish that all cancer patients will feel empowered to experience their many positive benefits.

Michael Tierra
East West Herb and Acupuncture Clinic
Santa Cruz, California

Part One

THEN & NOW

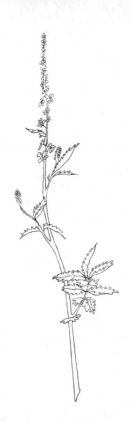

CHAPTER ONE

THEN & NOW

C ancer is not a twentieth-century disease. Archeologists discovered tumors on dinosaur skeletons and Egyptian mummies. While recorded attempts to treat cancer go back as far as 1600 B.C., scientific study in the West is often dated to 1775, when the English doctor, Percival Pott noticed repeated cases of testicular cancer in chimney sweeps. Chimney soot, then identified as a cancer-causing agent, led to a new understanding of the carcinogens potentially present in our environment. What in the 1700's was considered a serious carcinogen, chimney soot, has in our own time erupted into a Pandora's box of pollution and carcinogenic agents that have regrettably become nearly accepted byproducts of modern Western civilization.

With the dawn of the new millennium, cancer has surpassed heart disease as the leading cause of death in the United States while according to Dr. John Mendelssohn, president of the M.D. Anderson Cancer Center in Houston, at the turn of the 20th century it was only 8[th.]

Despite the 1970's declared war on cancer, 42% of all males and 39% of all females are expected to develop cancer during their lifetime. Studies show that the incidence of cancer is 44% higher today with overall mortality 3% greater than it was 40 years ago.

After a quarter of a century in the U.S. of spending two and now three billion dollars a year on cancer research, the results unequivocally show that conventional cancer treatment, including surgery, radiation and chemotherapy have not been able to cure, significantly prolong or otherwise improve the life of the vast majority of patients with various forms of cancer.

According to World Health Organization statistics it is estimated that there are about 10 million cancer cases reported annually around the world of which 6 million people die. In the U.S. over one million patients are diagnosed annually with cancer. Only half of these receive surgery, radiotherapy or chemotherapy and are cured of the disease based upon a survival rate of five years. The other half of the sum total of diagnosed cancer patients die within five years after the diagnosis.

Because conventional cancer treatments are often a cause of adverse side effects and subsequent morbidity, growing numbers of diagnosed cancer patients are motivated to seek unconventional therapies. It is difficult to estimate the relative longevity and quality of life of the numbers of cancer patients who choose only alternative therapies or no therapy at all.

There are few studies that evaluate such a consideration. One, comparing the long-term outcome of 106 patients with slow growing brain tumors (oligodendroglioma and mixed glioma) given conventional therapies such as radiation and chemotherapy as opposed to patients who were given no treatment found that those patients who were given no treatment fared better and lived longer than those given radiation or chemotherapy.[1] What we do know from a huge and growing body of credible research is that complementary and alternative therapies are effective weapons against cancer and that they are, without a doubt, of benefit to cancer patients.

It doesn't seem that the tower of Babel that makes up the cancer industry is capable of bending to examine and compare the merits of its own vested procedures with the use of simpler, less invasive methods such as diet and herbs. The reason quite simply is that, if effective, these can undermine the ongoing opportunity for huge corporate profit. Sad to say that because of this, cancer patients are triply victimized. First by the growing concentration of environmental pollutants that are known to cause cancer, second by the disease itself and third by a medical establishment that continues to show itself blinded and incapable of prioritizing people over profits.

The unanswered question is not about conventional medicine's ability to cure cancer, for with few exceptions it is a fact that it is unable to do so, but whether the use of alternative therapies alone or in conjunction with conventional treatments are at least as effective or perhaps even superior to conventional aggressive cancer therapies. Certainly they are in terms of not causing adverse side effects such as chemotherapy induced neurotoxicities, radiation induced necrosis or increased susceptibility to cancer recurrence.

What is desperately needed is credible, unbiased scientific research separate from industry. Until then, encouraged by the undetermined numbers of people who have received significant benefit from alternative therapies, we must content ourselves with integrating these various methods as best as possible or in conjunction with conventional cancer treatment.

Mechanistic View

The secular worldview that has characterized the last 150 years has also informed our approach to healing the human body. Just as nature was reduced to a study of independent elements, the body was likened to a machine, a compilation of separately functioning parts. With such a focus, it is easy to lose perspective of the relationship of the body with itself and outer nature. The physician's role increasingly is towards specialization with an emphasis on mending or replacing the broken part(s). With the advent of genetic medicine, the focus continues towards greater physiological specificity as physicians receive little guidance or training on the interrelatedness of body, mind and spirit or our relationship with outer nature.

This mechanistic view has become the reigning theory of modern medical training, where medical students usually focus on the treatment of diseases based on the worst-case scenario, rather than the patient's immediate level of need. But most healing demands a more holistic view of the body. Where conventional practice falls short, traditional medicine, including dietary, herbal and other comparatively low-level invasive approaches can offer positive support or even a better alternative to what conventional medicine has to offer for a given condition.

When Louis Pasteur introduced his germ theory in the mid-1800s, he proposed that disease was located outside the body. Once the germs invaded, medicine's role was to eliminate the intruders, much like exterminating termites in a house, thereby curing the disease. Even if this were true, once the termites were gone, the weakened structural support might eventually lead to a crumbling home. If just one insect survived, its task could more easily be accomplished unless the foundation was strengthened anew. Remember, disease results from imbalance within the body and its interaction with external elements. Therefore, we must concern ourselves not only with the manifestation of the disease – the termites – but the environment from which the disease stems.

Similarly, the reigning conception and consequent approach to the treatment of cancer up until very recently, has been based on the theory of W.S. Halstead (1852-1922). This theory views solid cancers from the perspective of the development of a tumor rather than a more systemic model based on the underlying condition of the patient.

During the 1950's and 60's the late herbalist Dr. John R. Christopher described cancer as a condition of the blood rather than a mere local tumor manifestation. Because he used herbs such as red clover or burdock root, which are classified as blood purifiers or alteratives, he was at odds with the prevailing medical view. The western mechanistic view of cancer focused its attention only on removing or destroying the tumor.

In 1999, according to Dr. Zajicek,[2] as expounded in his book, *A New Cancer Hypothesis*, carcinogens deplete the body of a vital essence that eventually leads to wasting and cachexia. He further states that the actual tumor may be part of a self-protecting compromise for the body to generate what is missing. However, as the tumor grows, it poses a serious threat to its host by exhausting the body's resources in its effort.

Thus the approach of only focusing on the tumor is doomed to failure since it is based on the false premise that the cancer will be cured when the tumor is removed. The millions who have suffered the blow of cancer recurrence certainly can attest to this. Dr. Zajicek emphatically insists that merely removing the tumor will not cure the disease because it represents a chronic metabolic deficiency.

Again, despite this gradual shift away from viewing cancer as merely a local phenomenon, the mechanistic view of cancer persists with literally billions of dollars in research.

Today, increasing numbers of individual health practitioners, including medical researchers and oncologists, are embracing the concept of metabolic breakdown as the root cause of cancer. This is also beginning to reflect an integrative approach between conventional medicine and the use of therapeutic diet, nutritional supplements and herbs as adjunctive treatment of cancer.

Challenging the Norm

Humans are creatures of habit. Oftentimes, we follow standard practice because "it's the way we've always done it." In 1848, Austrian doctor Ignaz Semmelweis wondered if the high death rate of women in childbirth was related to the fact that physicians neglected to wash their hands between deliveries. His colleagues ridiculed these implications and he was expelled from his hospital position in Vienna, even though the death rate in Semmelweis's clinic dropped after adopting a new protocol of cleanliness. Thirty years later, cleanliness became standard practice, with Semmelweis remembered today as the "father of antiseptics."

This tendency toward habit often turns theory into fact, as seen in a surprising report from the Office of Technology Assessment, an extension of the U.S. Congress, which states that only 10 to 20 percent of conventional medical practices are based on scientifically validated evidence, leaving the remaining 80 to 90 percent based on anecdotal data.[3] This makes the practice of western medicine a contradiction in terms and opens the door to accepting proven alternative therapies that have become a 'habit' in alternative treatment protocols.

Ralph Moss, a former public affairs director at Memorial Sloan-Kettering Cancer Center, quotes a high official from that institute confiding behind closed doors in 1976, "So you want to know where we get all our new ideas?" The scientist picked up his copy of the American Cancer Society's *Unproven Methods in Cancer Management,* a blacklist of alternative therapies, and said to Moss, "This is our Bible." [4]

It is not merely an alternative to standard medical practice that is called for but an integration of that which is of value from the past with that of the present. In China, it is accepted that a combination of Traditional Chinese Medicine that is better able to deal with supporting the immune system and well being of the patient together with conventional medical approaches offers patients a better outcome.

Nor should any alternative cancer treatment that has established itself as popular 'habit' such as the use of Essiac tea or Hoxsey formula be blindly accepted as efficacious – these and many other herbs and supplements claimed to be efficacious for cancer need to be subjected to unbiased study and research to determine the extent of their value. Patients should be educated to question whether the currently accepted procedures of conventional medicine represent their best interests or the interests of a self-perpetuating medical bureaucracy.

Current Conventional Treatment of Cancer

Treatment can be divided into either local or systemic. Conventional local treatment may involve surgery or radiation. Systemic treatment with the intention of destroying cancer cells that may exist in areas beyond the primary site of a tumor usually means resorting to some form of chemotherapy. In alternative therapy, a local treatment might be the use of an escharotic salve, herbal poultice or the application of a strong negative facing magnet topically applied over a tumor site with the intention of destroying it in some way. Systemic treatment may involve the use of diet and herbs.

There are three primary characteristics of malignant cells: 1) they are malignant or deformed cells, 2) they exhibit the power of unlimited growth and proliferation, and 3) they tend to not die. They share similar characteristics with certain normally occurring cells such as those of the stomach lining, hair, and the bone marrow in their ability to subdivide and multiply at a rapid rate (unless it is a slow growing tumor). Because of this, chemotherapy in its ability to target quickly growing and subdividing cells often shows an acute adverse effect on the stomach mucosa with loss of appetite and nausea and hair loss. The recurrence of cancer and opportunistic infections is heightened as a result of the adverse reaction to the bone marrow, which is integral to the integrity of the immune system.

Of course, there is variable and sometimes considerable damage to healthy cells and this in turn has a devastating effect on the immune system, greatly increasing the risk of acute infectious diseases and the future recurrence of cancer. A medical oncology text states that patients receiving radiation therapy alone incur a threefold risk of recurring secondary cancers while a more extensive course of both radiation and chemotherapy is increased as much as 1000 times greater than normal.[5]

The advantage of the use of dietary and herbal therapy is clear. First, they do not compromise the immune system. In fact, with their immune enhancing properties they actually help to protect against cancer recurrence. The disadvantage is that alternative therapy is usually less aggressive in reducing the actual tumor in comparison to conventional Western treatments. However, whether one chooses alternative therapy alone or a combination of conventional and alternative therapies, there is clear benefit in the employment of herbs and diet for the treatment of cancer.

Chemotherapy

Chemotherapy, a term coined in 1907 by Nobel laureate Paul Erlich, means the treatment of disease with chemicals. A daughter of the chemical warfare of World Wars I and II, chemotherapy arose through government study of antidotes to mustard gas, which had been found to damage human bone marrow and deplete white blood cells. When a nitrogen compound derived from the gas was injected into laboratory mice with induced cancer of the lymphoid tissue, it produced remission. Scientists then experimented with this concept on a human patient using a substance they termed "compound X." At first, the patient experienced rapid tumor and lymph node reduction, but within four weeks his white blood cell count dove from 5,000 per cubic centimeter to almost 200, he developed severe clotting problems, the tumor regenerated and the man eventually died. [6]

Inspiration for the chemical approach to cancer treatment came from the antibiotic revolution of the 1930s. The idea of a "magic bullet" like penicillin was promising – a pharmaceutical that could destroy cancer as if it were an infection. While we have yet to find this "bullet," chemotherapy remains a thriving business. But its use can be attributed more to the economic structure of our drug-oriented society than its actual effectiveness, and to its acceptance as a standard procedure. As Ralph Moss states, "Drugs are central to the American economy, and it is perfectly logical from a business point of view to seek a cure for cancer in the form of a patentable and marketable drug." [7]

It is worth noting the close interconnection of drug companies, cancer research institutes and hospitals, and even petrochemical corporations – officials of one board often advise on another. Not that this makes their activities illegal or dishonest, but these advisors will naturally have greater personal interest in the success of all their related endeavors.

Chemotherapy has many limitations that require serious consideration. It seems to be most beneficial for childhood leukemias that only constitute about 2% of cancer deaths of patients under age 30, and reducing the mortality rate of adults with Hodgkin's disease, lymphoma, ovarian cancer, testicular cancer and a few other rare cancers. It can also be a beneficial adjunct in some instances for treating breast, colon and small cell lung cancer.

Side effects of chemotherapy range from self-limiting short term reactions to long-term conditions and even to death. Many are in themselves carcinogenic and can increase the risk of recurring secondary cancers. Since 1980 it was reported that over the previous 10 years of use for patients with breast cancer, chemotherapy did not improve the survival rate and may indeed have shortened it. [8] In an article published in Scientific American the author states "Apart from the success with Hodgkin's disease, childhood leukemia, and a few other cancers, it is not possible to detect any sudden change in death rates for any of the major cancers that could be credited to chemotherapy." [9] Bailar and Smith from the Harvard School of Public Health and the University of Iowa Medical Center further echoed this when they stated "The main conclusion we draw is that some 35 years of intense effort focused largely on improving treatment must be judged a qualified failure." [10] In general, the advent of chemotherapy has not greatly affected mortality rates from 1930 to 1990 for either males or females. In fact, between the years 1950 and 1989, with population adjustment, the incidence of cancer has actually increased about 10%.

Any claims in improved survival have to be considered in terms of earlier detection in relation to the highly controversial 5-year survival rate. With earlier detection, it may be found that many more people have cancer for a longer period of time than five years. Any survival statistics need to be evaluated in light of this important consideration. For patients and alternative therapists these considerations pose some real issues and conflicts regarding the choice of treatment.

Many claim that the use of alternative approaches might endanger a cancer patient's life because it causes them to delay conventional medical intervention, thus allowing the cancer to grow and proliferate. But what if the choices available to the patient neither prolong nor increase their quality of life? As New York cancer specialist, Albert Braverman, M.D. stated in the

British medical journal, *The Lancet*, "Chemotherapy should be prescribed only when there is a reasonable prospect of either cure or benefit in quantity and quality of life."[11]

According to Ralph Moss, "for solid tumors of adults, such benefit has rarely been proven and consequently chemotherapy should just as rarely be given." [12] He also names the relatively limited number of conditions for which chemotherapy can offer a positive and life saving possibility. These have been previously mentioned. It is also useful with surgery for the treatment of Wilm's tumor, Ewing's sarcoma, rhabdomyosarcoma, and retinoblastoma. It can extend the life of patients with small-cell lung cancer and in some cases of ovarian cancer. There is considerable controversy whether it is of significant value as adjunctive therapy for earlier stages of lung and colon cancer.

For breast cancer, the adjunctive use of chemotherapy provided no advantage in terms of survival rate. In fact, in June of 1990, the NIH issued a statement that "All patients with node-negative breast cancer should be made aware of the benefits and risks of adjuvant systemic therapy, a thorough discussion of which should include the likely risk of recurrence without adjuvant therapy, the expected reduction in risk with adjuvant therapy, the toxic effects of therapy, and the impact on quality of life. Some degrees of improvement may be so small that the disadvantages of therapy outweigh them." [13] They later found that adjuvant use of chemotherapy did reduce the rate of recurrence by about 1/3rd but there was nevertheless no improvement in longevity.

In general, 90% of women diagnosed with stage one breast cancer who undergo a lumpectomy will not experience a recurrence. Of the remaining 10% three may have some benefit from adjuvant chemotherapy. The question is whether all women who undergo surgery for early stage breast cancer should be subjected to the physical hardship and expense of chemotherapy. Obviously this is a difficult but individual decision. It might be that for those who choose not to undergo chemotherapy, given that the odds of survival are so much in their favor, the adjunctive use of an anticancer diet, lifestyle and herbs offers the added physical and emotional support that would further empower them in their decision.

There is similar controversy involved in the use of adjunctive chemotherapy, namely fluorouracil (5-FU) and levamisole for early stage colorectal cancer. The National Cancer Institute (NCI) maintains that there is "significant improvement in disease-free survival," but later states that "the overall survival benefits were of borderline statistical significance." [14]

About 35 chemotherapeutic drugs are currently approved for use in the United States. These are generally cytotoxic and, as stated, will attack any rapidly-dividing cells. Recently, a new class of drugs is being developed that are specific to certain tumor cells. For oncologists, these represent the most promising development in cancer treatment, as these drugs are antiangiogenic, meaning they inhibit and break down the formation of fragile capillaries formed to circulate blood within a tumor. Shark and bovine cartilage, soy products, and certain herbs such as red clover are also considered to have antiangiogenic properties. Western antiangiogenic drugs hold the promise of being far less damaging than the former broader acting cytotoxic drugs.

Perhaps one of the most difficult issues is in the recognized fact that chemotherapeutic drugs can actually cause an acceleration and metastasis of cancer following their use. One study quoted by Ralph Moss states that "cytotoxic drugs could promote the occurrence of metastases; suppress the immune system; damage the vascular system; and act directly and in a thoroughly unpredictable way on tumor cells." [15, 16]

Radiotherapy

In 1896, French physicist Marie Curie discovered a radioactive metal called radium. The recipient of two Nobel prizes, Madame Curie is considered one of the founders of radiation therapy, most notably the advent of x-rays, and of the nuclear age. Ironically and sadly, she died of leukemia at a young age related to unprotected exposure to radioactive materials.

Radiotherapy involves using x-rays, gamma rays and electrons to damage tumor cells. Radiation causes intercellular water molecules to ionize (break apart) which result in the formation of free radicals.

Radiotherapy is useful and can effect a cure for Stage 1 cancers including Hodgkin's disease, lymph node cancers of the neck and head, brain tumors, lung cancer, esophageal cancer, breast cancer and cancer of the uterus and cervix. In more advanced cancers it can offer palliative pain relief by temporarily shrinking tumors.

Direct side effects are generally local depending on where it is applied. These include rashes, burning, and loss of taste, lung fibrosis, pneumonitis, neurological problems, dysphagia, colitis, enteritis, malabsorption, diarrhea, hepatitis and sterility. More general effects may include digestive disturbance, weight loss, anorexia, nausea and vomiting. Because of the burning that occurs as a result of radiation, this approach is not usually suitable for recurring cancers. Long-term side effects involve the increased risk of contracting cancer again as a result of the radiation-damaged DNA cells.

The x-ray has unparalleled potential for diagnoses, but its value must be carefully weighed against its dangers. In 1902, a German doctor recorded the first case of human cancer caused by radiation; by 1922, over 100 radiologists had died from x-ray-induced cancer. Even with improved safety of contemporary methods of radiation and x-rays compared to the older methods, it remains a fact that radiation in any form is one of the most severe carcinogenic "hits" a patient endures. Again, whether these "hits" develop into cancer or cause its recurrence depends on the innate resistance of the body. Despite the risk involved it may be warranted in view of the possible immediate danger posed by a tumor.

Supportive dietary and herbal treatment should be undertaken to lessen the negative effects of radiation. This may include the internal use of aloe vera juice and the Indian herb, Ashwagandha (withania somnifera). Based on the considerable amount of respectable research that exists showing the benefit to patients who were given Ashwagandha[1] (also called "Indian ginseng") to lessen some of the negative effects on the nervous system, the healthy tissues of the body near the site where radiation is administered and the immune system generally, its use should be a routine procedure. Besides helping the patient weather the severe stress of radiation itself, Ashwagandha has been found to enhance the benefits of radiation treatment by inducing increased radio sensitization and helping to stimulate stem cell proliferation.[17,18,19,20,21,22] Holy Basil (ocimum sanctum) is another East Indian herb that has been found to be generally anti-carcinogenic as well as protective during radiation therapy. Other herbs that should be taken include mushrooms such as shiitake, maitake and reishi mushrooms as well as astragalus membranaceus root. Miso soup with seaweed and brown rice and soy are also known to counteract the effects of radiation as well as chemotherapy.

Surgery

Surgery as a cancer treatment dates back to the Egyptians, although it was not highly regarded in ancient times. The Greek physician Hippocrates (460 B.C. to 377 B.C.) believed, above all, in avoiding harm to the patient, stating: "It is better not to apply any treatment in cases of occult cancer; for, if treated, the patients die quickly; but if not treated, they hold out for a long time."

Surgery has not always been the illustrious profession it is now. From the twelfth century to the late 1800s, surgeons held the rank of mere craftsmen – they weren't allowed to perform surgeries in the absence of a physician or even to write prescriptions. Due to the advancement of x-ray technology, anesthesia and operating room antiseptics, the field of surgery rose rapidly at the turn of the twentieth century along with the status of surgeons in recognition of their fine-tuned levels of expertise. Regardless of the surgeon's skill, however, in at least temporarily removing tumors, it does not necessarily cure the patient of cancer.

---

[1] The Sanskrit name for the herb literally translates as "like a horse" based on its peculiar smell.

Surgery can often cure localized Stage 1 cancers. However, there are many areas where surgery cannot be used, such as brain tumors and non-solid cancers such as leukemias. It is also not useful for solid tumors that have already metastasized.

Surgery can be radical or conservative. Radical surgery involves removing much of the surrounding tissue along with the tumor. Conservative surgery, as in breast "lumpectomies," removes only the lump or tumor. If a tumor has metastasized prior to surgery, neither radical nor conservative surgery would make much difference. Surgery is a radical treatment modality that warrants the most conservative respect.

Summary of Risks Versus Benefits of Surgery, Radiation and Chemotherapy

Chemotherapy, radiation and surgery are most effective when combined with each other. This is because of the billions of cells that need to be destroyed; some may be more resistant to one form of therapy over another. Faced with a diagnosis of cancer, patients are understandably reluctant to subject themselves to the well-known debilitating effects of radiation and chemotherapy. On the one hand, even without research to support any significant claims, it seems more than reasonable to assume that alternative treatment approaches such as diet, herbs and health supplements have been and will be of considerable benefit. Furthermore, this benefit would be available whether or not the patient chose conventional treatment.

In early stage cancer such as breast or colorectal cancer, the collagen surrounding the tumor remains intact and under this circumstance, surgery offers odds of no recurrence that are definitely in the patient's favor. For certain forms of cancers of the chest, lymph and other specific areas radiation may be useful. Chemotherapy is useful in apoptosis or small-fractionated doses over a prolonged period or in arterial infusion in well-nourished patients. Either or both chemotherapy and radiation therapy may be recommended adjunctively with their usefulness evaluated on an individual basis. Whether the patient chooses to undergo these treatments should be their own prerogative. In advanced stages of cancer, conventional treatment is at best only palliative, offering no advantage in terms of survival or quality of life. Given the limited number of options alternative approaches, especially diet and herbs, offer significant benefit in both these areas as well as an all-important degree of hope.

From a Western medical perspective, chemotherapy, radiation and surgery are often considered more effective when combined together. This is because of the billions of cells that need to be affected; some may be more resistant than others to a single cytotoxic agent.

From this we see that unfortunately there are no easy answers and a treatment protocol may be best evaluated following a discussion between the patient, their primary oncologist and the alternative practitioner. It is to the patient's best interest that they work with therapists who are open to considering the best course of treatment.[2]

State of the Industry

As of February 4, 1990, a United Press International news wire declared cancer the leading killer of people between the ages of 35 to 64 and the leading cause of death among women in the United States. On Thursday, February 3, two thousand doctors, patients, scientists and advocacy groups gathered in Paris for an unprecedented World Summit Against Cancer conference. At this summit it was declared that based on more recent findings, cancer is expected to surpass heart disease as the number one cause of death in the United States and by the year 2020 the rise in cancer is estimated to reach 20 million worldwide. It is difficult to estimate the strain this rise in cancer will cause on financial, social and medical resources of the world.

Despite President Nixon's declared "war on cancer" in 1971 where he optimistically promised the nation a cure for the disease within five years, cancer is an end stage disease that remains difficult to treat. This is due to the wide array of variables from genetic, environment, dietary and psychosocial forces. For instance, a person may smoke tobacco despite the overwhelming proof that smoking tobacco "is the single largest risk factor for a variety of malignancies, including lung cancer. Worldwide, about 3 million people die each year of smoking-related disease, and this is expected to increase to 10 million deaths per year." [3]

As it stands, currently more than a half million Americans are expected to die from cancer in each year – more than twice the death rate of 1971. According to Richard Walters in The Alternative Cancer Therapy Book, "Death rates for the most common cancers – cancers of the lung, colon, breast, prostate, pancreas, and ovary – have either stayed the same or increased during the past fifty years." [4] Although the industry continues to pour money into the advancement of standard therapies, it seems to be having little effect on a cure. The good news is that death rates have dramatically fallen for less

---

[2] In the Moss Reports, cancer researcher Ralph Moss has prepared current and extensive reports on all aspects including alternative therapies for individual cancers. They are available for a fee from The Moss Reports, 144 St. John's Place, Brooklyn, NY 11217, USA. 718-636-4433, fax: 718-636-0186.

[3] Emmons, K.M., "Smoking cessation and tobacco control: an overview"; Dana-Farber Cancer Institute and Harvard School of Public Health, Boston, MA, USA. Karen_emmons@dfci.harvard.edu

[4] Business Week, September 22, 1986

common malignancies, such as childhood leukemia, Hodgkin's disease and testicular cancer – diseases often fatal just twenty-five years ago.[23]

Since the call to arms of the '70s, the National Cancer Institute (NCI) has invested $29 billion into the anti-cancer industry, although only 5 percent of their $1.8 billion annual budget is spent on prevention.[24] The astronomical costs of standard treatments such as chemotherapy, a $750 million a year business, is largely responsible for the $107 billion annual cost of cancer care in the United States. In 1995, in an issue of The New York Times (1/10/95) it was estimated that standard drug treatment for breast cancer, for example, cost between $5,000 and $25,000. If a bone marrow transplant is required, that price increases by $60,000 to $200,000. New drugs, such as alpha interferon, can cost anywhere from $6,500 to $75,000, not including supportive care, which can run into the tens of thousands.

It would seem that if there were a simpler, low-tech approach to the treatment of cancer, it would be welcomed or at least investigated. Instead, alternative methods that integrate herbs and therapeutic diets are engaged in ongoing battles for their legality. The problem lies in an economic system that pays huge profits for greed. At least at this time, cancer research – and alternative medicine, in general – must be supported by public funds through publicly funded organizations such as the National Institute of Health (NIH), independent of industrial sponsorship.

Control in the Hands of the Few

The anti-cancer industry is not controlled by doctors or scientists, but by committees within hospitals and medical societies, by insurance companies and by the U.S. government. Although the FDA and other regulatory institutions were established with good intention to monitor industry claims, this concentration of power heavily influences decision-making, weighing the scales in favor of conventional treatment rather than prevention.

As our technological society's progress is driven forward by carcinogenic fossil fuels that in turn are misted into the atmosphere from our engines or ploughed into the earth for fertilizer and used as a base for many of our drugs, we see an obvious increase in the proliferation of cancer.

While it is the leading cause of lung cancer, smoking tobacco is not the only cause. Furthermore, the carcinogenic effects of tobacco are greatly increased with the various chemical additives routinely used in the manufacture of tobacco for smoking. Nevertheless, it is clear that environmental causes play a major role in the proliferation of cancer. These range from the

---

[5] Ko, Y.C., Cheng, L.S., Lee, C.H., Huang, J.J., Huang, M.S., Kao, E.L., Wang, H.Z., Lin, H.J., "Chinese food cooking and lung cancer in women nonsmokers," Institute of Medicine, School of Medicine, Kaohsiung Medical University, Taiwan, Republic of China.

addition of carcinogenic food additives, air and water pollution, to inhaling the fumes of various gases, cooking oils.[5] The proliferation of the petroleum industry and various industrial pollutants that has adversely affected the air, water and food is a major cause of cancer worldwide. Despite all of the evidence on environmental and dietary influence on cancer the industry seems frustrated in its ability to deal with underlying causes. Instead, as of late it is increasingly focused on genetic causes and treatment as the ultimate goal. My question is even supposing through genetics we were able to successfully treat human cancer, this certainly will have no effect in eliminating the cancer in the environmental pollution in our natural world. Can the humans thrive in a world where air, soil and water are polluted? From this perspective, the majority of cancers are merely a reflection of a greater problem.

According to Ralph Moss, the cancer establishment "favor[s] cure over prevention. They emphasize the use of patentable and/or synthetic chemicals over readily available or natural methods. They set the trends in research, and are careful to stay within the bounds of what is acceptable and fashionable at the moment." [25]

The nation's most prominent cancer institutes, led by Memorial Sloan-Kettering Cancer Center, often owe their existence to the gifts of wealthy families, a natural result of the government's limited interest in health care in the 1800s. These families frequently have ties to other related industries, which greatly inform an institute's decisions. The Rockefellers, for example, were instrumental in creating the American Society for the Control of Cancer, predecessor to today's American Cancer Society (ACS), as well as the Sloan-Kettering Memorial Hospital. The family also dominated Standard Oil of New Jersey (ESSO), which was in business with I.G. Farben Company, a German trust that controlled a plethora of chemical and drug industries. The far-reaching efforts of the Rockefeller family remind us that control is not restricted to the United States, but is an issue of global proportions.

No Support for Botanical Research

Pharmaceutical companies are regular supporters of cancer centers, providing these centers use their brands of drugs in treatment. But new research remains confined to high-priced laboratory chemicals. Why study an herb that can easily be picked by anyone? If scientists can't synthesize its constituents into a chemical drug, there is no research incentive.

Alternative therapists often avoid seeking research grants. This is due not only to the high cost of developing a new drug (which has skyrocketed from $1.2 million in 1962 to $125 million in 1988 and today is estimated to be from $250,000 to $500,000 per drug) but also because of the illegality of botanical and related therapies. By publishing their findings on not yet approved techniques, they put themselves at risk of losing their license to practice. Consequently, much information is not shared or is lost.

In addition, the methods of research for conventional medicine are not always applicable to botanical treatments. There are so many components in any given herb, it is impossible to isolate enough factors to have objectively controlled studies. Furthermore, more than the presence of a particular bio-chemical agent, pharmacological action is based on the dynamic interaction of the various components with each other. Add to this the unique physi-ological reaction between an individual and a particular herbal treatment, and the control factors are even more obscured. Empiricism, based on 'what works' has always been the basis of herbal medicine. There are literally eons of empirical evidence of the effectiveness of herbs passed down in various cultures throughout the world. More than enough to keep science busy in evaluating, elucidating and refining this information to better adapt to the needs of our time.

Despite the difficulties surrounding the acceptance of alternative approaches to cancer treatment, it's estimated that at least half of all cancer patients use some form of alternative therapy. Where there is the 'smoke' in the rampant claims of herbal or other unconventional cancer treatments, there must also be the 'fire' of some truth. This implies that what is being offered by the medical establishment is insufficient to satisfy the desperate needs of patients diagnosed with cancer. Hearing that an herbal formula or health supplement can support the immune system during chemotherapy or radiation or cause a patient's cancer to go into remission is enough impetus for cancer patients to bypass the provider systems and pay for these out of their own pockets.

It is time that the healing benefits of herbs, acupuncture, moxibustion, food supplements, special diets, magnet therapy, psycho-spiritual counseling and other procedures that have been of benefit to at least 50 percent of the population be made more acceptable and available to the increasing numbers of people who will be forced to have to deal with a cancer diagnosis either for themselves or others among their friends and family.

Endnotes

[1] Olson, Jon D. M.D.; Riedel, Elyn; DeAngelis, Lisa M. M.D., "Long-term outcome of low-grade oligodendroglioma and mixed glioma," Neurology (April, 2000), p. 1442-1447.

[2] Zajicek, G. "A New Cancer Hypothesis." Medical Hypotheses 47 (1996). p. 111-115.

[3] Accessing the Efficacy and Safety of Medical Technologies, Sept, 1978, OTA report.

[4] Cancer Scandal: The Policies and Politics of Failure, one-hour video with Robert Houston, Patrick McGrady, Jr., and Ralph Moss, available from Patient Rights Legal Action Fund, 202 West 78th Street, Suite 3E, New York, NY 10024

[5] Calabresi, P.; Schein, P., Medical Oncology, Second Edition. New York: McGraw-Hill. Inc; 1993, pg. 362.

[6] Moss, Ralph W., Questioning Chemotherapy, 1995, Equinox, p. 18

[7] Moss, Ralph W., The Cancer Industry, revised ed. Brooklyn, New York; Equinox Press, 1996 [1989]

[8] Powles, T.J.; Coombes, R.C.; Smith, I.E., et al: "Failure of chemotherapy to prolong survival in a group of patients with metastic breast cancer." Lancet 1980: March 15:580-2

[9] Cairns, J., "The Treatment of Disease and the War Against Cancer," Scientific American, (1985;253(5):51-59)

[10] Bailar, J.C.; Smith, E.M.: "Progress against cancer?" The New England J of Med 1986; 314(19):1226-32.

[11] Braverman, A., Medical Oncology in the 1990's. Lancet 1991;337; 901-902

[12] Moss, Ralph W., Questioning Chemotherapy, p. 8. Equinox Press, 1995

[13] National Institutes of Health. NIH consensus conference: treatment of early stage breast cancer. Reported in JAMA 1991;265:391-395

[14] National Cancer Institute, PDQ. On colon cancer 4/14/94

[15] McMillan, T.J. and Hart, I.R., "Can cancer chemotherapy enhance the malignant behavior of tumors" – Cancer and Metas Rev 1987;6:503-520

[16] Moss, Ralph, PhD., Questioning Chemotherapy, 1005, Equinox

[17] Kuttan, G.: "Use of Withania somnifera Dunal As An Adjuvant During Radiation Therapy." Indian Journal of Experimental Biology, 1996; 34(9): 854-856.

[18] Ganasoundari, A.; Zare, S.M.; Devi, P.U., "Modification of bone marrow radiosensitivity by medicinal plant extracts," Department of Radiobiology, Kasturba Medical College, Manipal, India.

[19] Devi. P.U., "Withania somnifera Dunal (Ashwagandha): potential plant source of a promising drug for cancer chemotherapy and radiosensitization," Department of Radiobiology, Kasturba Medical College, Manipal, India.

[20] Devi, P.U.; Akagi, K.; Ostapenko, V.; Tanaka, Y.; Sugahara, T., "Withaferin A: a new radiosensitizer from the Indian medicinal plant Withania somnifera," Department of Radiobiology, Kasturba Medical College, Manipal, India.

[21] Sharad, A.C.; Solomon, F.E.; Devi, P.U.; Udupa, N.; Srinivasan, K.K., "Antitumor and radiosensitizing effects of withaferin A on mouse Ehrlich ascites carcinoma in vivo," Department of Radiobiology, Kasturba Medical College, Manipal, Karnataka, India.

[22] Devi, P.U.; Sharada, A.C.; Solomon, F.E., "In vivo growth inhibitory and radiosensitizing effects of withaferin A on mouse Ehrlich ascites carcinoma," Department of Radiobiology, Kasturba Medical College, Karnataka, India.

[23] Moss, Ralph W., Cancer Therapy, 1997, Equinox Press, p. 12

[24] See number 7.

[25] ibid

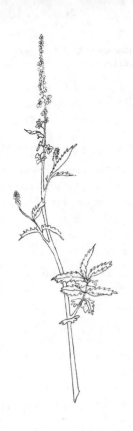

CHAPTER TWO

CANCER: WHAT IT IS

Cancer is the proliferation of aberrant mutated cells, which grow into tumors that eventually starve surrounding healthy cells of vital nutrients. Thus cachexia, or protein malabsorption, rather than the actual cancer itself, is considered by oncologists to be responsible for anywhere from 40% to 80% of all cancer deaths. As stated, malignant cell growth by definition is chaotic, erratic and undifferentiated in appearance and tends to not mature and die, as do normal cells. It may be ironic that cancer ultimately destroys itself by killing its host victim.

Cancer is described in terms of whether it is a solid palpable mass or present in a more fluid form in the blood and lymphatic system as with leukemia and lymphatic cancer. It is also described in terms of where it originates such as cancer of the lung, breast, prostate, brain, liver, etc. It is also described in terms of its general morphology, meaning its shape or form. It is finally described in terms of its stage or type.

The Types of Cancer

Treatment depends upon knowing the type of cancer one has. This is determined by its place of origin as well as the type and appearance of the cancer cell that is produced.

The initial tumor is called the "primary" tumor while its metastatic spread to other site and organs are secondary manifestations. If colon cancer spreads to the liver it is still called colon cancer. If breast cancer metastasizes to the bone it is still called breast cancer.

In some cases, several different types of cancers can start in the same organ. For example, when dealing with kidney cancer one can have the most common renal cell cancer as well as Wilm's tumor, which usually affects children and is a transitional cancer similar to bladder cancer. Treatment is complicated by the fact that these are all treated differently in conventional medicine.

Following is a brief overview of the different types of cancers:

- Carcinomas affect the epithelial cells of the skin, mouth, nose, throat, lung airways, genitourinary and gastrointestinal tract or that constitute the lining of the breast or thyroid. Lung, breast, prostate, skin, stomach and colon cancers are all called carcinomas and are solid tumors. Conventional treatment may include one or a combination of surgery, chemotherapy or radiation. Alternative medical treatment might include soy, red clover blossoms, seaweeds, andrographis, garlic, scutellaria or barberry as well as quercetin, essential fatty acids, laetrile (apricot or peach seeds) various antioxidants such as vitamins C, E, mixed carotenes, selenium, lipoic acid and N-acetyl cysteine.

- Adenocarcinomas specifically affect the glands and resemble the cells associated with each gland such as cervix, prostate, thyroid, breast, etc. Alternative treatment might include various anti-cancer herbs, scutellaria, coptis, barberry, poke root, red clover or burdock root together with essential fatty acids, apricot seeds and selected antioxidants including vitamins C, E, mixed carotenes, selenium, lipoic acid, N-acetyl cysteine and bromelain.

- Sarcomas affect the bones or soft connective and supportive tissues surrounding the organs and tissues including cartilage, muscles, tendons, fat and the outer linings of the lungs, abdomen, heart, central nervous system and blood vessels. Sarcomas are also solid tumors and are the most rare and malignant of all tumors. Alternative treatment might include reishi or maitake mushrooms, astragalus, tienchi ginseng, salvia milthiorhiza, barberry root, burdock root, red clover or Pau d'Arco together with various antioxidants including vitamins C, E, mixed carotenes, selenium, lipoic acid, N-acetyl cysteine, calcium orotate and vitamin D.

- Leukemias affect the blood and bone marrow and travel through the system effecting other organs such as the spleen. They are characterized by abnormal white blood cells and are non-solid tumors. Alternative herbs and supplements might include tienchi ginseng, astragalus, reishi, maitake, coriolus and cordyceps mushrooms, andrographis, indigo or isatis together with various antioxidants including vitamins C, E, mixed carotenes, selenium, lipoic acid and N-acetyl cysteine.

- Lymphomas are comprised of abnormal lymphocytes (white blood cells) that accumulate in the lymph glands and produce solid soft tumors. Hodgkin's and non-Hodgkin's lymphomas are the two that are most common. Less common in the U.S. is Burkitt's lymphoma. The lymph glands are concentrated mostly around the neck, groin, armpits, spleen, and the center of the chest and near the intestines. They serve partially as filters to remove impurities from the system. Lymphomas are usually treated with radiation or chemotherapy.[1] Alternative treatments involve the use of anti-cancer herbs such as herbs that detoxify, drain dampness (lymph) and move blood. These may include reishi mushroom, gallium (cleavers), poke root, Pau D' Arco and Tienchi ginseng. Nutritional supplements should include, among other substances, quercetin and hydrazine sulfate.

- Myelomas are rare tumors that occur in the antibody-producing cells of the bone marrow. Alternative treatments should include, among other substances, immune potentiating herbs such as reishi and maitake mushroom, astragalus root, scorpion, centipede and thymus extract.

Other types of cancers include:
- Melanoma represents a group of cancers primarily affecting the skin pigment. They are comprised of cancerous cells called melanocytes. Because of the depletion of the protective ozone layer, there has been a marked increase of melanomas. These occur most commonly in fair-skinned people having light-colored eyes. Previous sunburn increases a person's risk. Most melanomas form flat, dark skin patches that develop over several months or years. Any black or brown spot having an irregular border, a red, black and blue color seen on close examination or a node-like surface may mean there is a melanoma. It is usually removed by surgery for laboratory examination. Melanomas may spread throughout the body and are one of the most malignant of all skin cancers. Outcome depends on the kind of melanoma, its size and depth, its location, and the age and condition of the patient.

---

[1] Stage I lymphoma involves a single lymph node region while Stage II includes two or more lymph node regions on the same side of the diaphragm. In Stage III, lymph nodes on both sides of the diaphragm are affected with possible involvement of the spleen or of another organ or site. In Stage IV there is widespread involvement of one or more body organs or sites with or without lymph node involvement.

The different types of melanoma are amelanotic melanoma, benign juvenile melanoma, lentigo-maligna melanoma, nodular melanoma, primary cutaneous melanoma and superficial spreading melanoma. Treatment of melanomas involves surgery, and because they can be fast spreading if they are not immediately found in the associated lymph glands, a considerable margin of skin tissue is removed to help prevent further spread. Alternative treatment involves the use of anticancer herbs such as andrographis, lycii bark and lithospermum and immune tonic herbs such as reishi mushrooms taken internally. Externally, if it is inoperable for any reason, the lesion is debrided as much as possible either through surgery or radiation and then a topical application of sanguinaria ointment and/or escharotic pastes may be applied. Often small suspicious looking moles are easily removed with the topical application of a piece of cotton soaked in sanguinaria tincture or the more radical use of the escharotic paste.

Cancer Staging

Cancer staging describes the degree of proliferation from the primary site. Stage 1 cancers are small-localized tumors that are the most curable. Stage 2 and 3 cancers are usually locally advanced or metastasized to the lymph nodes. Stage 4 is considered inoperable cancer that has widely metastasized in different areas of the body.

Non-solid cancers such as leukemia that involve the blood cannot be staged in the same way and are classified according to the stage of advancement. Prostate and colon cancers are stages A through D rather than 1 through 4. Staging can be further subdivided into classifications such as 11a or 11b.

Another more complicated system of classification called "TNM" stands for Tumor, Nodes and Metastases. So that a cancer classified as T1 N1 M0 means that the tumor and lymph node involvement is at the first stage with no metastasis. T0 means that the cancer is "in situ" without invading any of the local tissues and T4 means a large, inoperable tumor. Similarly, N0 means no lymph node involvement; N4 refers to extensive involvement with metastases to other areas of the body.

A recurring cancer is generally more difficult to treat. If it recurs in a distant area it is called distant recurrent and is still classified based on its former primary site.

Tumors are also graded from 1 to 4 according to their increasing aggressive rate of growth. The grade of some cancers is of less consequence than it is for others. For instance, certain lymphomas and brain tumors may be very slow growing compared to others. Obviously this would have a strong influence on treatment and prognosis.

Another characteristic of cancer cells is that they have little or no cell-to-cell adhesion as opposed to normal cells that are able to form into well-defined tissues (except for circulating blood cells). The growth of a tumor that eventually causes it to break through its site of origin plus the lack of adhesion of cancer cells facilitates metastasis. This occurs when cancer cells circulate via the blood and lymphatic system and take root and grow into tumors at distant sites of the body. The type of cancer, however, is always based on its point of origin.

Causes of Cancer

Cancer affects the genetic core of our being. This is as a result of damage to the DNA (deoxyribonucleic acid) information in each cell, which if not repaired, will result in the formation of a neoplastic (i.e. newly formed) cell.

Oncogenes are a class of genes that initiate, cause and stimulate the growth of tumors. They are also able to transform healthy cells into cancer cells whose characteristic is their ability to bypass the normal growth-control mechanism of the organism. In fact, cancer-causing oncogenes are believed to evolve from Proto-oncogenes that at certain stages of fetal and early childhood growth are necessary for various tissue growth factors. They are normally inactivated by 'tumor suppressor genes' that are part of the immune system. This is at least part of the genetic predisposition that plays a significant role in the development of certain types of cancers.

Other than genetic causes, it is clear that by far the main causes of cancer are primarily based on the continued exposure to chemical-causing carcinogens. These can be either external or internal in origin.

Some external causes include:

1. Electromagnetic energy (x-rays, the ultra-violet rays of the sun, the geopathic stress rays, etc.)
2. Aflatoxins (mold on peanuts and other foods)
3. Nuclear radiation
4. Viruses
5. Carcinogenic food additives
6. Dietary and nutritional deficiencies
7. Irradiated and genetically altered food
8. Pesticides
9. Parasites
10. Mercury
11. Fluoride
12. Chlorinated drinking water
13. Tobacco and smoking
14. Hormones secondarily introduced from food sources such as the meat industry
15. Hormone supplementation
16. Dental factors
17. Industrial toxins
18. Polluted water
19. Immune suppressive drugs
20. Ionizing radiation
21. Sick building syndrome

Internal causes may include:

1. Physical and emotional stress
2. Impaired detoxification
3. Genetic predisposition (as is recognized with certain instances of colo-rectal cancers, ovarian and breast cancer)

These are probably only a few of the claimed causes and are not grouped in any order of preeminence. In most cases, each of these causes constitutes carcinogenic 'hits' that in one who is so predisposed may eventually develop into cancer.

The number of carcinogenic hits eventually causes the formation of free radicals that in turn directly mediates the development of cancer. Free radicals are molecules that contain an odd number of electrons. This in turn causes them to react with other cellular electrons leading to a proliferation of unstable molecules and cells throughout the body. Free radicals damage DNA, protein and lipids and are believed to be the cause of a variety of damaging diseases associated with aging, cancer, cardiovascular disease, immune dysfunction, brain dysfunction and cataracts.

The degree of chemical pollution in the world today is virtually incalculable. According to Patrick Quillin,[1] of the 5 million registered chemicals in the world, mankind comes in contact with 70,000 of them. At least 20,000 of these chemicals are known carcinogens, or cancer-causing agents. He goes on to describe how "each year, America alone sprays 1.2 billion pounds of pesticides on our food crops, feeds 90 billion pounds of antibiotics into our farm animals, as well as generally bombarding the environment with questionable amounts of electromagnetic radiation."

According to Bruce Ames, Ph.D. of the University of California at Berkeley, each of the 60 million cells in our bodies undergoes from 1,000 to 10,000 potentially cancer causing DNA "hits" daily. What saves us from developing full-blown cancer are DNA repairing mechanisms and our immune system. In order for such a hit to become cancer it must undergo a process of *initiation*, *promotion* and *progression*. Each of these describes a process over time that eventually results in cancer. Nevertheless, Dr. John Gant, a prominent authority on cancer at Duke University, estimates that at least 40% or more of cancer patients do not die of cancer but of malnutrition. Nutrients from food and herbs can intercept the progression of cancer at any of the three stages.

Inherent in the process of evolution is the generation of a certain number of mutated genes and cells that probably enhance the possibilities of adaptation and biodiversity. Generally these are controlled by the immune system, especially the Natural Killer (NK) cells that are able to recognize and destroy undesirable malignant cells before they develop into cancer. Therefore the immune system is intimately connected with the ability of the patient to thrive and survive cancer and is behind the various reported cases of "spontaneous remission" of cancer in many patients. Any nutritional supplement or herb that optimizes the cancer killing NK cells would be of significant benefit.

Overexposure to carcinogens constituting too many "hits" to the immune system will overwhelm even the healthiest individual and will eventually lead to cancer. Equally obvious is that factors such as developing positive lifestyle changes, positive dietary changes and developing a more positive emotional outlook are bound to influence the body's ability to prevent and survive cancer.

Cancer detection is difficult because by the time it is detected it has been growing for a long time. An aggressive cancer doubles in size in 60 days or less, a moderately aggressive cancer doubles in 61 to 150 days, a slow growing cancer doubles in size from 151-300 days and a very slow growing cancer may take 300 days or more. A million cancer cells are undetectable by the most sensitive medical instruments while a billion cells constitutes barely less than an undetectable lump. The average breast cancer detected through mammography is around 600 million cells, which measures approximately ¼ inch across. In contrast manual detection of breast cancer is only detectable when the mass measures 1¼ inches in diameter and has about 45 billion cells. One of the problems in detecting and treating cancer, therefore, is that even the most advanced modern diagnostic equipment is unable to detect a tumor until it has achieved a minimum weight of approximately one-gram. Successful chemotherapy or radiation therapy only occurs when the tumor is no longer detectable. While cell kill in a few cancers is able to cure some patients, tragically, with the majority of adult cancers, neither chemotherapy nor radiation is capable of killing all remaining cancer cells. What this means for the patient is that when the doctor says "I think we got it all" the battle must go on with the integration of an anti-cancer diet, herbs and positive lifestyle habits to prevent against further recurrence.

Again, lifestyle adjustment, maintaining a positive mental outlook, diet, herbs and acupuncture and other physio-therapies that tend to harmonize and balance the system can play a decisive role in the adjunctive treatment of patients undergoing conventional therapies as well as preventing the recurrence of cancer. Further, many cancers untreatable with conventional methods quite often may result in longer than predicted survival and in some cases spontaneous remission of cancer. No one can be sure of the large number of people who are not part of the "fatal" statistics who go on living their lives, often outliving their oncologists, refusing all medical intervention.

Precancerous cells with malignant tendencies are called *oncogenes*. In order to qualify as a legitimate cancer cell, however, the cell has to mutate in exactly the same way twice. Continuous and repetitive irritation from chemical substances such as aniline dye derivatives, asbestos and the tars, toxins and nicotine from cigarette smoke, pollution, bad air, food and water as well as the final insult of the use of chemotherapy and radiation treatments all encourage the production of mutated cells from various tissues of the body in the same way. This is cancer and if it were not for the normal biological controls of a healthy immune system even more would have it.

Most cell mutations are weaker than healthy cells and simply die. Of those that survive, their proliferation is limited by normal feedback controls that prevent their growth. Cells that may form cancer are able to produce abnormal protein that triggers the B-lymphocytes and natural killer cells to form an army of antibodies that in turn destroys the mutated cancer cells.[2]

Oncogenes or precancerous cells can be inherited. However, until the requisite number of mutations occurs in life, cancer will not develop. Viruses can also produce oncogenes. Because they proliferate by invading and taking over surrounding healthy cells, a coat of protein protects them. The science of virology substantiates that there are mechanisms in a healthy organism that can and does inhibit the invasion of viruses. Again this depends on a healthy immune system with the support of herbs such as scutellaria, coptis, barberry, burdock and dandelion that have anti-cancer properties and are effective in overcoming viruses and harmful bacteria.

A brief statistical analysis of selected cancers:

Melanoma in the white population has increased 321% since 1950 – more than any other cancer. This is believed to be due to a depletion of the ozone layer that allows for the increase in ultra-violet radiation. This is especially noticed in South latitude countries such as Australia where the ozone is particularly damaged.

Lung cancer has the second highest incidence (263%) with a close association with cigarette smoking. Though the rate of growth for melanoma is faster, the incidence of lung cancer is much greater.

Stomach cancer has decreased by 73% in the white population since 1950. The reasons are not certain but increased refrigeration, decreased use of salt and the addition of vitamin C to nitrite-containing products are suspected as being highly beneficial.

---

[2] In fact this is the basis of the ancient strategy of treating cancer with various toxic insects such as scorpions, centipedes and cantharides. One method used by the Chinese is to boil an egg with 6 grams of each of these and only one gram of cantharides. The insects are placed in a cloth bag so that they can be removed after cooking the egg. Both the egg and its fluid are consumed once daily. The theory is that cancer cells are attracted to the egg protein and in the process take in the strange insect protein and are killed.

Cervical cancer has decreased 76% since 1950 in the white population. This is believed to be due to improved living standards and the increase of hysterectomies. Early detection with PAP smears is also a significant factor. Mortality from cervical cancer has decreased 74% because of early detection and local treatment.

Colorectal cancer has increased 10% since 1950 in the white population but mortality has decreased 25%. Better diagnostic procedures and improvement in surgical treatments as well as adjuvant chemotherapy all demonstrate benefit in the treatment of colorectal cancer.

Prostate cancer has increased 108% in the white population since 1950 largely due to improved diagnostic procedures. Mortality, however, has increased about 23%.

Breast cancer is the leading cause of death in women between the ages of 40 and 55 and is the most common cancer among women, excluding skin cancer. There are approximately 180,000 new cases of diagnosed breast cancer each year in the U.S. Early detection has resulted in cancers being found earlier, smaller and in less advanced stages. This results in the misleading conclusion that while 72% of women diagnosed with cancer survived for 5 years in 1950, today the 5-year survival rate is up to 97%. One out of 8 women in the U.S. are at risk of developing breast cancer and 1 out of 28 are at risk of dying from breast cancer. Low income and African American women are approximately three times more likely to be diagnosed with breast cancer than white women are. This is probably attributed to reduced detection and monitoring that is lower among poorer minorities than among whites.

In general the rate of incidence of breast cancer has remained relatively stable over the last 50 years with a slight rise. Known and suspected risk factors for breast cancer include a possible inherited predisposition, ovarian or indometrial cancer, exposure to radiation, breast abnormalities, early puberty, late menopause, alcohol, oral contraceptives, postmenopausal estrogen therapy, diet and pesticide exposure. However, even when considering these risk factors, 70% of women diagnosed with breast cancer have none of the presumed risk factors.

Clinical Cancer Markers

A cancer or tumor marker is a laboratory blood test that measures the level of protein or other material produced by cancer cells. These markers become elevated in the presence of a cancer or tumor. Some of the different cancer markers for different kinds of cancer are as follows:

- CEA (carcinoembryonic antigen) test for colon cancer.
- AFP (alpha-fetoprotein) test for liver cancer (primary hepatocellular carcinoma.)
- PSA (prostate specific antigen) for prostate cancer.
- CA (carcinoma) 27.29 for breast cancer.
- CA 125 for ovarian cancer.

If the treatment numbers go down it indicates the cancer has been eliminated. If they become elevated then the cancer has recurred or has become active either locally or in some other site of the body.

AMAS (Anti-Malignin Antibody Screen) is a simple blood test that detects any type of cancer only in its earliest stages. It does not work for leukemia or non-malignant tumors and growth. There is much misunderstanding of the value of this test because in advanced stages of cancer or when the tumor is larger than two centimeters it will register a false negative. The reason for this becomes clear when we understand that an AMAS test measures levels of an antibody, not an antigen as indicated by the tests described above. AMAS is elevated only in early non-terminal stages of cancer before the advanced stages of tumor growth and metastasis causes antibody failure. This is precisely opposite of the antigen tests previously described, which will not indicate a positive reading until the cancer or tumor is in an advanced stage.

There have been numerous studies conducted between 1977 and 1988 confirming the value of the AMAS test. Generally one needs to obtain two readings since the first becomes a baseline reading with subsequent tests indicating an increase or decrease of the AMA marker. With repeats of the tests within 24 hours using freshly extracted serum, the false-positives and false-negatives are less than 1% (specificity and sensitivity greater than 99%). When the serum needs to be stored for periods greater than 24 hours, the false positives are 5% and the false negatives 7% (based on a controlled double blind study with 3,315 patients [2,3,4]). Because antibodies can be detected earlier than antigens, AMAS may provide useful early clinical detection for those who are known to be at risk. This would include individuals who work in toxic or high-risk environments, those who have a hereditary predisposition to a variety of cancers such as colorectal or breast cancer or individuals who have undergone conventional or alternative therapies such as surgery, chemotherapy or radiation where cancer is no longer apparent. The higher the AMAS values the longer the predicted survival.

As with all clinical laboratory tests, the AMAS test cannot be solely relied upon to determine the absence or presence of disease. It is a valuable aid to diagnosis, detection or monitoring of disease in relation to the history, medical signs and symptoms and the overall condition of the patient.

AMAS tests may be useful when patients that have undergone treatment want some reassurance that the cancer is not recurring. As such, it may offer another possibility to patients who, after a treatment such as surgery, do not wish to undergo debilitating adjunctive chemotherapy.

Endnotes

[1] Quillin, Patrick, Dr. Beating Cancer with Nutrition, Nutritional Times Press, Tulsa, 1994, p.4

[2] J. Medicine 13:49-69, 1982

[3] Protides Biol. Fluids 30:337-352, 1983

[4] Protides Biol. Fluids 31:739-747,1984

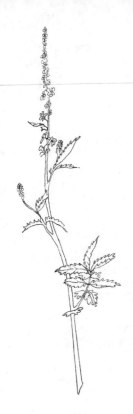

CHAPTER THREE

CONVENTIONAL CANCER THERAPIES

U nusual physiological indications such as a mark on the skin that seems to be changing, a palpable lump in the breast or other part of the body, unusual prolonged pain in the head or some other area of the body, unusual signs of bleeding from the lungs, rectum, etc. or a common symptom such as a persistent cough that is not relieved over time or through normal treatment all warrant seeking further medical evaluation.

In and of themselves, none of these may be a definitive indication of cancer. Superficial marks and lumps can be benign, meaning they are non-malignant. The next stage may be an x-ray, CAT scan or MRI of the area in question or it might involve a biopsy. Biopsies are the most definitive indicator of cancer and involve extracting a small amount of the tissue, which is then studied to determine the presence of malignancy.

In many cases, it is possible through a blood or urine test to generally assess the cancer risk before further, more expensive and invasive procedures are undergone. This is highly desirable since the use of other measures may be more traumatic and expensive. There is also a risk of further spreading the cancer through biopsies, which are regarded as controversial by some. An intermediate step is the use of tumor markers.

Tumor markers are substances created by a tumor and released into the body that are indicative of the presence of certain types of cancer. Usually these are in the form of unusual proteins, enzymes and hormones. Some of the more common tumor markers follow.

Tumor Markers and Their Common Indications

Carcinobryonic antigen (CEA)	This is the most common tumor marker and indicates various cancers including breast, thyroid and prostate cancer.
CA-125	Ovarian carcinomas and other solid cancers.
CA19-9	Gastrointestinal and colon cancers.
CA15-3	Metastatic breast and ovarian cancers.
CA27-29	Similar marker to CA15-3 antigen used to detect the recurrence of breast cancer.
Prostate-specific antigen (PSA)	Standard marker for prostate cancer.
Prostate acid ahosphatase (PAP)	Prostate cancer.
Plasminogen activators (PA)	Prostate cancer.
Human chorionic gonadotropin (HCG)	Trophoblastic tumors, breast, ovarian, liver and lung cancers.
Ovarian cancer antigen (OCA)	Ovarian carcinomas.
Ferritin	Used to detect liver cancer.
Alkaline phosphatase	Bone cancer and bone metastasis.
Antimalignin antibody (AMAS)	Used for early detection of cancer. It is not useful for fully developed cancers.
Fibroblastic Growth Factor (FGF)	A blood or urine test that detects the presence of cells secreting fibroblastic growth factor (FGF) created by tumors for the creation of new blood vessels to feed tumors. The degree of elevation of FGF in the urine may indicate the size and possible risk of metastasis of cancers.

Treatment

The four main approaches used by conventional medicine for the treatment of cancer are surgery, radiation, chemotherapy and immunotherapy. Which one or combination thereof utilized is based on the type of cancer. Specifically, its vulnerability to the mode of treatment, its size, aggressiveness, whether it is recurring, whether it has metastasized or spread to surrounding or distant areas, prognosis and the age and health of the patient based upon their ability to undergo the strain of treatment.

All of these approaches aim in some way to eradicate cancer directly. This would be a reasonable proposition if it were not for the fact that in most cases, cancer is the end result of a number of systemic flaws that have occurred over many years and that has caused it to opportunistically occur. Therefore, any direct treatment of cancer aimed at removing the tumor or offending agent must be accompanied, at least, by a more systemic approach involving the use of special diet, lifestyle modification, herbs and various supplements.

One of the problems with conventional medical approaches is that they are to varying degrees non-specific. As a result of this well recognized problem, there are increased attempts at pharmaceutical and medical refinements to make chemo and radiation treatments as specific as possible to particular types of cancers. The problem remains that cancer arises as a result of a number of imbalances created by environmental degradation, lifestyle, diet, stress, genetic predisposition, age and other factors. While it is desirable to limit such invasive therapies to a particular type of cancer, the condition is likely to reoccur if the causes preceding it have not been addressed.

The success of conventional therapies is usually determined by a reduction of the tumor size or other diagnostic indications that signal a favorable response to treatment. Because the presence of cancer cells is virtually undetectable until there are literally billions of cells (this is where the AMAS tumor marker test may be useful), most oncologists will then consider adjunctive therapies to prevent further recurrence of cancer. Generally, any recurrence of a secondary cancer following its primary treatment by such methods is bound to be far more aggressive. Further treatment with the same means with methods that are known to be carcinogenic and deplete the immune system would at that stage be, at best, only temporary and palliative.

Adjunctive therapies may include removal of a wider margin of tissue around the cancer, hormonal suppressing agents, the adjunctive use of radiation or chemotherapy or the removal of surrounding lymph nodes. All of these are accompanied by various debilities and side effects that range from minor to serious.

Because of this, patients should feel encouraged to get an independent second and perhaps even a third opinion. There are considerable differences as to how different physicians might approach the treatment of the same cancer. Cancer patients should become informed about their particular cancer as much as possible. Once a diagnosis is confirmed I recommend purchasing the corresponding report that outlines a description of the particular cancer and an outline of the conventional and alternative treatments for it. These are available online from Ralph Moss' website at www.ralphmoss.com. I also strongly encourage patients to read Ralph Moss' books, including Questioning Chemotherapy and The Cancer Industry, to gain a perspective of what they are about to become involved with. The nature of a difficult disease such as cancer is that there are often not clear-cut choices and alternatives so that one is frequently left with accepting the lesser of two evils.

Patients should assess their own personal state of vulnerability both from therapists as well as loved ones that may interfere with their making an independent judgment based upon what best suits their needs and intentions. In this, the greatest obstacle is fear. This should be lessened through various methods of prayer, meditation, journal writing or counseling, as one is so predisposed.

Surgery

Since pre-Egyptian times the customary method for dealing with solid tumors has been surgery. Obviously, it is only useful if the tumor is accessible and is still localized. Often, in order to assure that it is completely removed, the surgeon may opt to remove a wider margin around the tumor and some closely associated lymph glands at the same time. Surgery may be only palliative if the tumor has already progressed but, because of its size or location, may be interfering with normal physiological functions. Precancerous growth and early stage melanomas may also be surgically removed. Based upon equivalent long-term survival rates, in early stage breast cancer lumpectomy is considered more the standard than radical mastectomy.

Herbal and nutritional approaches can be very beneficial both before surgery to strengthen the body and afterward to promote healing. In general, one would use tonic and blood moving herbs such as tienchi ginseng, salvia milthiorhiza, dang gui angelica, astragalus and reishi mushrooms.

Radiation Therapy

Radiation therapy is a method of using radiation either from an external source or injected directly into an area or organ with the purpose of destroying adjacent cancer cells. This is often done adjunctively with either or both surgery and chemotherapy in the hope that the cancer will be completely destroyed. It is also performed to reduce tumors to a size more suitable for their removal through some other means such as surgery. Finally, radiation is administered to relieve pain on bone tumors or tumors that are placing pressure on a nerve center such as the spinal cord.

Radiation therapy has controversial side effects, not the least of which is the fact that radiation itself causes malignancies. Besides this there are a number of side effects that must be treated including a variety of skin reactions, hair loss, upper respiratory infections and other inflammations caused by a weakening of the immune system, peripheral nerve damage, organ damage, permanent hoarseness, dry mouth and other moist areas of the body, gastrointestinal problems, genito-reproductive problems and the list could extend out to include every area and function of the body.

If it appears that radiation therapy is the best choice given all the options and circumstances, there are a number of herbal and nutritional alternatives that can reduce the often considerable negative impact of radiation. I certainly recommend various supplements including vitamins, antioxidants, essential fatty acids, enzymes and amino acids. Ashwagandha (Withania somnifera)[1] should be taken immediately before, during and after radiation therapy. Aloe vera gel is also used to offset the adverse reactions to radiation therapy. An immune strengthening food, which is easily digested, consists of soft white rice and mung beans. Combine one part of the mixture to seven parts water. Cook slowly with 4 to 9 grams each astragalus root, shiitake mushrooms and pseudostellaria ginseng.

Chemotherapy

There are approximately 100 drugs used as chemotherapy for the treatment of cancer. The goal is to destroy cancer cells with the use of various poisonous drugs and compounds of either plant or chemical origin. Used for a wide variety of cancers, chemotherapeutic drugs are especially intended to attack and destroy fast growing cells typical of the behavior of cancer cells. Unfortunately other fast growing cells include hair, gastrointestinal cells and important immune potentiating cells of the bone marrow. This is why individuals commonly experience gastrointestinal upset together with acute hair loss. However, the effect on the immune system in most cases is even more devastating with patients often experiencing severe weakness and depression. While this approach may destroy cancer cells short term by adversely affecting the immune system, it leaves the body at risk for further cancer recurrence. Subsequently, with the body's defenses compromised, such a recurrence is accompanied with an even greater immunity to chemotherapeutic drugs.

---

[1] See Chapter Six, the materia medica

Because many cancers are immune in varying degrees to specific chemo-therapeutic drugs, it is not uncommon to make a chemo-cocktail combining a number of drugs together. These can be administered on a regular schedule by mouth, intravenously, topically on the skin, injected arterially, muscularly or into a specific area or organ of the body by catheter. The general protocol is to administer as high a dose as is tolerated.

For some cancers, however, a low dosage of select chemotherapeutic drugs in pill form is taken twice daily over a period of weeks or months. Rather than killing cancer cells directly this method, called apoptosis, creates an unfavorable environment for cancer cells to thrive so that they will self destruct and die off gradually. This latter method is probably the way anticancer herbs work. However, so far there have been no significant clinical trials to compare the effectiveness of anticancer herbs used to induce apoptosis as opposed to harsher chemotherapeutic drugs.

Like radiation, chime-therapeutic drugs tend to be indiscriminate in the cell it destroys. The immune system is overwhelmed and healthy cells are destroyed along with cancer cells. This is where herbs and various health supplements can be used in conjunction with wholesome nutrition to strengthen what the Chinese call the "righteous qi," or normal protective energy, while the strong chemotherapeutic drugs are used to destroy the cancer cells. Besides using such supportive therapy while undergoing conventional treatment, herbs and health supplements can be used long term to prevent recurrence. Further, as we will show, many studies corroborate how these natural agents actually increase the beneficial effects of radiation and chemotherapy against cancer.

There are continual efforts to discover specific chemotherapeutic drugs and methods of administration that refine and make chemotherapy more precise and less traumatic. However this effort still tends to focus only on the actual site of the cancer and not the broader systemic imbalances from which it arises.

Some of the latest approaches under investigation in the use of chemo-therapy drugs are as follows:

- Attaching a chemotherapeutic drug to various cells that will eventually seek out and destroy cancer cells, leaving normal cells alone.

- Isolating cancer cells extracted from patients in the laboratory to determine which chemotherapy drug is most specific for destroying it.

- Implanting refillable pumps into various parts of the body or organs to deliver the chemotherapy more directly to the cancer rather than allowing it to be introduced through the entire system.

- Making chemotherapy drugs from material derived from the body itself.

- Giving intense chemotherapy drugs as quickly as possible, in sequence, for shorter periods of time to ensure the patient gets a strong concentrated dose all at once accompanied by immune potentiating drugs to offset their side effects.

Major Types of Chemotherapeutic Drugs
(Modified from Boik[1] and Yance[2])

DNA Alkylating Agents

These were the original cytotoxic agents derived from mustard gas used during the First World War. These include bisulfan, cisplatin, carboplatin, cyclophosphamide, decarbazine, ifoside, etoposide IV, etoposide oral, lomustine, mechloretyamine, melphalan, mitomycin and thiotepa.

Used for lymphomas, Hodgkin's disease, leukemias, breast cancer, ovarian cancer, multiple myeloma, ovarian carcinoma, testicular cancers, brain tumors, endocrine cancers, bladder, and lung and head cancers.

Mitotic Modifiers

These include the plant derived agents vinblastine and vincristine from the rosy periwinkle (*catharanthus rosaceae*) and taxol from the yew tree (Taxus brevifolia). They are used for Hodgkin's disease, choriocarcinoma, neuroblastoma, acute lymphocytic leukemia, Kaposi's carcinoma, leukemia, Wilm's tumor, breast, lung, testicular cancers and other solid tumors.

Antibiotics

Antibiotics are derived from various funguses and have a variety of ways of working. They include doxorubicin (Adriamycin, ADR), bleomycin sulfate, dactinomycin (actinomycin D; ACT), mitomycin (Mitomysin-C; MTC) and fludarbine (Fludara). They are used for squamous cell carcinoma, lymphomas, testicular cancer, Wilm's tumor, choriocarcinoma, Ewing's sarcoma, acute leukemia, neuroblastoma, sarcomas, breast, ovarian, gastric, thyroid and bladder carcinomas, adenocarcinoma of the pancreas, stomach, colon, breast and lung cancers.

Cellular Modifiers

These modify and alter the growth, reproduction and proliferation of cancer cells. They include interferon and interleukin-2 and are used for leukemias, melanoma, Kaposi's sarcoma, and cancer of the ovaries, kidney, colon and bladder.

Combination Therapy

As previously stated, generally cytotoxic chemotherapeutic drugs are given in combination. The reason is to maximize the possibilities of destroying any cancer cells that may be resistant to a single chemotherapeutic agent.

Side Effects

Cytotoxic drugs by their very nature have a host of varying side effects ranging from short term, long term, and permanent to death. As with radiation, cytotoxic drugs are in themselves carcinogenic and may cause recurrence or different cancers to arise. Chemotherapy drugs are intended to destroy fast-dividing cells. Besides cancer cells, this unfortunately also includes healthy cells such as hair and cells lining the gastrointestinal tract and others. As with most drugs, they frequently cause liver damage but other organs such as the kidneys can also be injured. Adriamycin has a known risk of heart injury for which Vitamin E and CoQ10 have been found to be protective.

In so many cases, chemotherapy has caused more harm than good and may compromise both quality and longevity of life. This does not mean that it has no value. Cancer is a difficult disease with any modality. Sometimes choosing to live with cancer and manage its complications in as noninvasive a way as possible through diet, herbs, nutritional supplements, etc. is the best choice. However, it is a frightening disease and the plain fact is that no one has all the answers.

I try to make whatever opinions and information I have available to my cancer patients and work with them regardless of the course they choose to follow. There are times when less is more and despite what statistics may indicate, they do not reflect the considerable number of people I have encountered in lectures throughout the country who have, through one means or another, managed to exceed all statistical survival estimates without any medical intervention. When we read or are confronted with official survival statistics, these individuals are not included in the computation.

Nevertheless, I believe that there is rational and effective use of chemotherapeutic and other conventional cancer treatments and there is also irrational use. The same can certainly be said for alternative medical modalities. It is possible in many instances that a rational integration of conventional and alternative medical treatment is the best course for treating the majority of cancers.

Evaluation of Chemotherapy

Cancer mortality rates have been available since 1950. Before that it may be that many cancers went unnoticed or were misdiagnosed. Nevertheless, in the chemotherapy era from 1950 to 1989, mortality rates have risen some 10%, even with age and population adjustment.

We also know that from 1970 to 1980 the overall survival rate of patients diagnosed with breast cancer has not improved. In fact, inappropriately administered, chemotherapy has been shown to shorten the life expectancy of some patients.

Environmental factors, such as the depletion of the ozone layer, do play a major role in cancers as evidenced by an increase of melanoma in the white population of 321% since 1950. Lung cancer has had the second highest increase of 263% since 1950 as a result of tobacco smoking. The increases of both of these types of cancers may account for a significant part of the general 10% mortality increase of all cancers since 1950.

The standard for cancer survival rate calculated from the time of observation and diagnosis is 5 years. What this means is that any claims of increased survival by the proponents of conventional cancer treatments has more to do with earlier detection than any real survival. In the case of prostate cancer it was shown that 25% of all males who died over the age of 70 had small prostate cancers. It is estimated, however, that fewer than 10% of these would have grown to a size to produce symptoms. Improved diagnostic methods are diagnosing these slow growing prostate cancers, thus increasing the survival rate of prostate cancer patients between the years 1950 to 1985 from 43% to 77%.

Early detection also makes a big difference in the survival rate statistics of women with breast cancer. In general, early detection can make a big difference in cancer prognosis. However, despite earlier detection of breast cancer, mortality rates may have actually increased in the white population from 1950. The incidence rate has increased over 50%; however, due to earlier detection, survival rates have increased about 20%. Unfortunately, this does not mean that women with breast cancer are living longer but that they were diagnosed earlier.

Chemotherapy is big business but its value must be assessed on an individual basis depending on the physical health of the patient and their ability to withstand the assault on their immune system.

Herbal and nutritional support is of inestimable value for all patients undergoing conventional surgery, chemo and radiation therapies for cancer. Further, contrary to the misinformation currently circulating among some oncologists, nutritional supplements including herbs, antioxidants, vitamins and minerals will not only offer a margin of protection for cancer patients undergoing these therapies but have actually been shown to enhance their effect.

Following is a basic herbal and nutritional protocol for patients undergoing chemo or radiation therapies:

- Reishi Mushroom Supreme (Planetary Formula): 4 tablets, 3 times daily.
- Red Clover Cleanser (Planetary Formula): 4 tablets, 3 times daily.
- Triphala (Planetary Formula): 2 tablets, 3 times daily.
- Maitake Mushroom (Planetary Formula): 2 tablets, 3 times daily.
- Ashwagandha (Planetary Formula): take the indicated dose 3 times daily.
- Multi Vitamin: Advanced Nutritional System (Rainbow Light).
- Vitamin E (d-alpha-tocopherol): 400 to 1200 IU's daily.
- Selenium: 200 mcg.
- Vitamin C ascorbate: from 1000 to 2000 mg.
- Quercetin (Activated Quercetin with Bromelain by Source Naturals): 600 to 1500 mg.
- CoQ10 (Now Foods): 100 to 400 mg.
- Alpha Lipoic Acid (Metabolic Response Modifiers): 200 to 600 mg.
- N-Acetyl cysteine (NAC) (Jarrow): 1500 to 2000 mg.
- Grape Seed Extract (Olympian Labs Incorporated): 200 to 800 mg.
- L.Acidophilus (Ultradophilus by Metagenics): take freely a half-hour before meals or three times daily.

Be sure to <u>not</u> eat your favorite food on the days you receive chemotherapy since, in most cases, the negative effect on digestion that occurs as a result of the chemotherapy treatments will be transferred and associated with that particular food. For digestive upset I recommend Digestive Comfort taken with a combination of ginger and camomile tea. Use 3 slices of fresh ginger and 2 heaping tablespoons of camomile steeped in a cup of boiling water. Take freely as needed.

Hormone Therapy

Some cancers such as certain breast, ovarian, testicular and prostate cancers are hormone dependent. For these, hormone-suppressing drugs such as tamoxifen and raloxifene that block estrogen uptake in the breast and uterus are effective in stopping or limiting cancer growth. Progesteronic and testicular androgenic hormones are also used to block estrogenic hormones. Antiandrogenic hormones that block testosterone and other androgenic hormones include administering a female hormone called DES-flutamide (Eulexin).

One of the challenges of hormone therapy is that a particular cancer may actually thrive under the influence of its antagonist. It has been found that among women with a congenital predisposition to breast cancer, tamoxifen can increase their risk further by stimulating cancer growth. However, using hormone-blocking agents in men with hormonally sensitive prostate cancer may be a reasonable solution.

As with any other conventional treatment, hormone treatment is a drastic measure intended ultimately to prolong or save lives. In general it is less drastic than chemotherapy but it does have possible adverse side effects some of which include:

- In women there may be increased body hair, deepening of the voice, menopausal symptoms, increased libido and bleeding in postmenopausal women.
- In men there may be a decrease of libido, impotence, enlarged breasts and raising of the voice.
- Nausea and vomiting may also be an issue.

Some of these symptoms are only temporary but others may be permanent. Counseling may be appropriate for those who have difficulty reconciling themselves to the changes that are occurring.

There are newer therapies that are being developed including immunotherapy, vaccines and gene therapy. The problem remains, however, that if the causes, in the form of environmental pollution, food, air, water degradation, stress and poor life habits persist, treatment, whether conventional or alternative, can at best have only short-term temporary value.

Endnotes

[1] Boik, John, Cancer and Natural Medicine, pub. by Oregon Medical Press, 1995-6

[2] Yance, Donald, AHG, Herbal Medicine, Healing & Cancer, pub. by Keats, 1999

Part Two

COMPLEMENTARY & ALTERNATIVE CANCER TREATMENTS

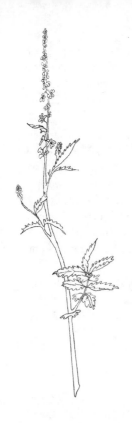

CHAPTER FOUR

TRADITIONAL CHINESE MEDICINE

PRINCIPLES & DIFFERENTIAL DIAGNOSIS

Traditional Chinese Medicine (TCM) offers an integrated holistic approach to the treatment of cancer. It is based on the principles of achieving homeostasis through balancing yin and yang, and addressing the outer manifestation of the disease as the branch while treating the inner cause as the root. Treatment integrates aspects of lifestyle, diet, herbs, acupuncture and other physiotherapies with the aggressive therapies of conventional medicine.

Fuzheng therapy means to "protect the normal." It is a branch of TCM that specifically supports the 'root' called *Zheng Qi* or "righteous qi," which represents the person's fundamental constitution or essence. This includes the immune system, digestion and overall organic vitality created through proper diet and herbs. Aggressive cancer treatments with conventional drugs are known to have an adverse effect on the righteous qi, or root. These adverse effects are greatly reduced when appropriate herbs are used.

Besides identifying and treating the root, 'branch' treatment involves methods of directly attacking the accompanying symptoms and manifestation of cancer such as reducing the tumor mass, gastrointestinal, respiratory, urinary and other problems including pain relief. Chemotherapy, radiation and surgery are considered aggressive branch treatments while herbs that clear heat, move blood, purge, clear dampness, resolve phlegm, soften and dissolve tumors are milder branch treatments.

Many herbs are capable of treating both the root and branch of cancers. This is important because if we only choose herbs that treat the root we may optimize the growth and survival of the cancer. If, on the other hand, we only choose herbs that treat the branch, the individual might be too weak to utilize the more active therapeutic detoxifying herbs, optimizing the growth or recurrence of the cancer. In fact this is what so often happens in conventional therapy where a strong 'branch' treatment using chemotherapy or radiation actually weakens the host so that the chances for metastasis and cancer recurrence is greatly increased.

In stronger patients we can use more aggressive detoxifying branch treatments while in patients with a weaker constitution, we must use more tonifying root treatments, emphasizing the use of those tonic herbs and foods that are also anti-carcinogenic.

Differential Diagnosis

From a traditional medical perspective one should focus on treating not only the disease but also the underlying imbalances. Often in the early stages of cancer it is difficult to determine what these may be. Fortunately, Chinese differential diagnosis can be used to evaluate a variety of signs and symptoms according to different diagnostic methods. A diagnosis is made when the majority of the signs tend to confirm each other.

Diagnosis according to the Eight Principles

The most basic level of discrimination in TCM is based on the Eight Principles. They are as follows:

1. External	Referring to the location of a cancer on the surface of the skin or to acute inflammatory and feverish conditions.
2. Internal	Referring to the effect of cancer on the internal parts of the body and the chronicity of the symptoms.
3. Excess	A condition that arises usually in a stronger, heavyset individual who would have a stronger voice, strong odors, more outgoing temperament and excessive symptoms.

4. Deficiency	A condition that arises in a weaker, thin individual who may have a more timid temperament, softer voice and symptoms that are more auto consumptive in nature.
5. Hot	Someone whose symptoms are aggravated by heat, who generally prefers a cooler climate, food and drink.
6. Cold	Someone whose symptoms are exacerbated by coldness, who generally prefers a warm climate, food and drink.
7. Yang	An individual who exhibits a majority of acute, excess and hot symptoms.
8. Yin	An individual who exhibits a majority of chronic, deficient and cold symptoms.

Following are a number of symptoms that correspond to the Eight Principles:

External: acute conditions, including colds, influenza, fevers, rashes, acute joint pains and injuries. The pulse would feel more superficial than normal. The tongue is not remarkable for either external or internal conditions.

Internal: chronic conditions including constipation, gastritis, ulcers, genitourinary infections, cholecystitis, low energy, weakness, diabetes, hypoglycemia, cancer, epilepsy, infertility, impotence. One might have to press deeper than normal to feel the pulse.

Excess: obesity, constipation, hypertension, high fever, severe infections, purulent discharges, and manic behavior. The pulse would feel strong, large and full and the tongue would have a thicker coat.

Deficiency: tiredness, weakness, weak digestion, low hydrochloric acid, hypothyroid, hypo-adrenal, anemia and wasting diseases such as TB and AIDS. The pulse would feel thin, thready or soft and the tongue would tend to lack a coat.

Hot: high fever, mild chills, thirst, flushed complexion, heat sensitivity, severe inflammations, infections, hepatitis and yellowish discharges. The pulse would be faster than 80 BPM and the tongue would have a red body and a yellowish coat.

Cold: severe chills, lack of thirst, pale complexion, sensitivity to coldness or cold weather, low hypothalamus function, weak digestion, hypoglycemia, lowered immunity, anemia, all hypo-conditions and clear or whitish discharges. The pulse would be lower than 60 BPM and the tongue would have a paler body and a whitish coat.

Yang: a majority of symptoms under the External, Excess and Hot categories. This refers to fundamental endocrine imbalances associated with hypertension, hyper-adrenalism, hyper-thyroidism and an overbearing aggressive behavior.

Yin: a majority of symptoms under the Internal, Deficient and Cold categories. This refers to overall endocrine imbalances associated with hypothyroidism, hypo-adrenalism, hypothyroid, hypoglycemia, pale complexion, fluid retention and timidity.

Yin and Yang, being the summation of the Eight Principles, is an expression of the hormonal or constitutional essence of the individual. Yang represents the condition of the immune system, which is so vital in our ability to inhibit the growth of cancer cells and prevent further metastasis. Yang energy is also required for our will to live and a healthy appetite and digestion. Yin represents our nutritional and fluidic essence. One who is yin deficient is in a state of autoconsumption as they manifest symptoms of heat caused by yin deficiency. Broadly speaking yin and yang are described as being rooted in the 'kidneys,' which more properly includes the adrenal glands attached to the kidneys and the entire endocrine system.

Both yin and yang qualities are often deficient in cancer patients and this deficiency is greatly exacerbated with the progress of the cancer as well as aggressive therapies such as chemotherapy, radiation and surgery. Once again, it is in this area that TCM anticancer herbal therapy plays a vital role in protecting against the depletion of yin and yang energy.

Cancer in the early stages may not be remarkable in terms of yin or yang deficiency. However, in the intermediate to advanced stages yin deficiency is present in 85 to 90 percent of all patients.

There are several studies indicating how Chinese herbs and traditional formulas exert significant benefit to patients undergoing conventional western treatment. One study administered the Kidney-Yin tonifying Liu wei di huang (Rehmannia Six Combination) or Jin gui shen qi wan (Rehmannia Eight combination) decoction to 83 patients diagnosed with small cell lung cancer and undergoing chemotherapy. There was a statistically significant positive response difference of 91.5% for those taking the herb formula as opposed to 46.9% for those in the control group. Immune studies of both groups were evaluated frequently through the course and it was noted that those in the Chinese herb group experienced ongoing immune enhancement as opposed to those in the control group. This same positive response to Chinese herbs was also found in animal experiments, which confirmed the value of kidney-tonifying herbs in enhancing non-specific immunology for solid cancer patients in adjuvant treatment.[1] Similar studies using the same formula conducted in Qidong county of Jiangsu Province involving liver cancer measured a 27.3% improved response compared to 1.1% of the control group undergoing chemotherapy only. Still, other studies employing the polysaccharides of coriolus versicoloris saw an 86.96% improvement rate as compared to the 11.11% of the control group not using Chinese herbal fungi.[2]

Diagnosis involving the Four Treasures

TCM utilizes several overlapping systems of analysis of a patient's condition and their cancer. This allows for somewhat different but still overlapping treatment strategies using herbs, diet and lifestyle. A practitioner must learn to evaluate a patient with cancer in terms of the Four Treasures. These are Qi, Blood, Yin and Yang and in turn represent the deepest levels of physiological processes involving hormones, metabolic processes, acetylcholine transformation, etc. The important consideration is that an analysis of symptoms manifesting deficiencies in any of these allows for the use of herbs similarly classified as Qi, Blood, Yin or Yang tonics.

Here is an outline of the Four Treasures, their meaning, diagnostic signs and herbs used for treatment:

Four Treasures	Meaning	Diagnosis Signs	Herbs for Treatment
Yin	The fluidic and cooling aspects of the body, bodily substance, internal or chronic conditions.	Symptoms of deficiency manifest with night sweats, a burning sensation of the feet and/or palms of the hands, flushed face, fever and inflammatory symptoms, a thin fast pulse (more than 80 BPM) and a dry, red tongue lacking a coat.	Processed Rehmannia Ophiopogon Ligustrum Asparagus root Lily bulb Black sesame seeds Cordyceps
Yang	The warming and motivating aspects of the body, more external or acute conditions.	Symptoms of deficiency manifest with coldness, lethargy, edema, back and joint pains, constipation, lack of libido, slow pulse (less than 60 BPM) and a pale tongue.	Deer antler Cinnamon Aconite Psoralea Eucommia Cordyceps

Four Treasures	Meaning	Diagnosis Signs	Herbs for Treatment
Qi	Vital energy or nerve force.	Low energy, weak digestion or edema.	Chinese ginseng Codonopsis
Blood	Both the blood itself and its circulatory power.	Paleness, anemia, low energy, scanty or irregular menstruation, numbness in the limbs, loss of hair, restless sleep, the pulse is thin and thready and the tongue is pale.	Angelica sinensis (Dang gui) Processed Rehmannia American Ginseng

Diagnosis according to the Chinese Three Humours

The Chinese three humours are Qi, Blood and Fluid. They are used to diagnose underlying imbalances of three vital bodily substances. In this way they are similar but significantly different from the Ayurvedic three humours, which are Water, Air and Fire. While the Chinese use their three humours to diagnose disease imbalances, the Ayurvedic three humours are significantly different in that besides defining states of disease, they also refer to predisposed constitutional types present in all people. The Ayurvedic model is close to the three constitutional types defined in the West, which are Ectomorphic, Endomorphic and Mesomorphic.

A brief outline of the Chinese Three Humours

Qi represents the circulation of vital energy in the body, which can be deficient or stagnant. It is treated with herbs that tonify or move (regulate) qi. These include Qi tonics such as ginseng, codonopsis and astragalus, or qi regulating carminatives such as saussurea and citrus peel.

Water refers to any problem associated with bodily fluids including urine, saliva, sweat, lymph, reproductive fluids and joint lubrication. A water imbalance, for instance, can manifest as dryness or edema. Water disease imbalances are treated with fluid and mucus eliminating herbs such as poria, pinellia, arisaematis and fritillary to clear mucus or ophiopogon, asparagus root and rehmannia for dryness.

Blood represents blood and its circulation throughout the body. It can manifest as anemia and problems with circulation. It is treated with blood tonics such as angelica sinica (dang gui) and rehmannia glutinosa and blood moving herbs such as tienchi ginseng, ligusticum and sparganis.

Diagnosis according to the Twelve Organs

Yin cancers primarily involve the internal yin organs while yang cancers are more external and involve the yang organs. In TCM the yin organs are primarily regarded because they involve the deeper processes of transformation of energy while the yang organs are regarded as vessels that hold or transport various substances including waste, food and fluids throughout the body.

The Chinese Organ System

Yin Organs	Yang Organs
Heart	Small Intestine
Pericardium	Triple Warmer (an organ function)
Spleen	Stomach
Lungs	Large intestines
Kidneys	Bladder
Liver	Gallbladder

The "organs" of TCM go beyond the conventional anatomical description to include complex functions and even distant relationships that might not normally be immediately apparent to one trained in Western medical anatomy. For example, there are specific emotional states associated with each of the yin organs that one would never find described in Western scientific anatomy. The following offers a brief description of the correspondence of various physiological and emotional conditions with each of the five yin organs. The description also forces one to define the "kidneys," for instance, to include the entire endocrine system represented by the adrenal glands and the spleen which involves the utilization and transformation of carbohydrates, implying that the TCM "spleen" includes the function of the pancreas.

The emotions and mental states associated with the "Five Yin Organs"[1] are as follows:

---

[1] They are described as "five" yin organs because the triple warmer and pericardium together are regarded as an extension of the heart and small intestine.

Five Yin Organs

Heart	Responsible for blood circulation and a calm mental state.
	Physical diagnostic symptoms include palpitations and irregular heartbeat, insomnia and restlessness.
	Mental symptoms include forgetfulness, mania, psychosis, hallucinations and dream-disturbed sleep.
Spleen-pancreas	Responsible for the assimilation and transformation of food and fluids and the transportation of blood.
	Physical diagnostic symptoms include digestive problems, problems with appetite, diarrhea, nausea and bloated abdomen, vomiting, tiredness and edema.
	Mental symptoms include symptoms associated with hypoglycemia and dwelling on the past and not in the moment.
Lungs	Needed to regulate the descending energy of the body and the immune and respiratory system.
	Physical diagnostic symptoms include any respiratory problems including cough, phlegm, and shortness of breath and skin problems.
	Mental symptoms include excessive grief or sadness and the inability to release past negative experiences.
Kidney-adrenals	Regarded as the root of yin and yang[2] throughout the body and is a reflection of the endocrine system.
	Physical diagnostic symptoms include urinary problems, lower back and joint problems, fatigue and infertility and impotence.
	Mental symptoms include inappropriate fear, paranoia and insecurity.
Liver	Needed for regulating the flow of qi and blood throughout the body.
	Physical diagnostic symptoms include a feeling of fullness in the chest, sub-costal pain, mood swings, dizziness or vertigo and problems with the eyes.
	Mental symptoms include aggressive temperament, anger, restlessness and depression.

As stated, the five yang organs (including the triple warmer and small intestine together as an extension of each other) are considered more superficially. Their indications are as follows:

---

[2] Yang generally corresponds to the sympathetic nervous system while yin is the parasympathetic.

Five Yang Organs

Large Intestine	Eliminates waste from digested food and fluids. Problems of constipation should be of primary concern in any natural treatment of cancer and the safest and mildest corrective is the Ayurvedic formula called triphala. Diarrhea and loose stool is also of concern. In cancer treatment, keeping the bowels open is very important because it is fundamental to the process of detoxification and eliminating 'lysing,' or the prevention of autointoxication from the elimination of dead cancer cells.
Small intestine	Continues the process of digestion begun in the stomach and separates waste from nutrients. Symptoms include abdominal pains, intestinal rumbling (borborygmus), diarrhea, constipation and urinary problems.
Stomach	Regarded as the "sea of food and fluid" and responsible for the initial processes of digestion. It also has a descending function (bringing food and fluids down). Symptoms include indigestion, nausea, stomachache, abdominal distention, belching and vomiting.
Bladder	Symptoms involve any dysfunction associated with urine excretion, including cystitis.
Gallbladder	Considered "the mysterious organ" because of all the yang organs, the gallbladder has associated mental indications such as timidity and indecisiveness. Physical symptoms are closely associated with those of the liver and may include pain over the region of the gallbladder or a bitter taste in the mouth.

Usually if there is an imbalance in one or a number of the internal organs there will be corroborating symptoms as outlined above that will serve as an indication. This becomes useful in prescribing herbs since they are classified as "affecting" or "entering" one or a number of the 12 organs.

TCM diagnostics is founded on first identifying the patient according to the Eight Principles, the three humours, the Four Treasures and finally Symptom-sign Organ diagnosis. One may concomitantly identify deficient qi, coldness and lack of appetite as "deficient qi and yang of the spleen," or depression and tightness in the chest as "stagnant liver qi," or lung problems with associated clear or whitish mucus as "cold dampness of the lung."

TCM diagnosis is a very complex and subtle study requiring many years to master. For a more thorough understanding of the system, I recommend my other books including *Chinese Traditional Herbal Medicine* (Lotus Press, 1998) or *The Way of Chinese Herbs* (Pocket Books, 1998). For the present limited purposes, this presentation should be sufficient to understand and utilize the approaches described throughout this book.

The Four Diagnoses

Various differential diagnostic principles are understood under the principles of the Four Methods of Diagnosis. These principles are *Interrogation*, *Observation*, *Palpation* and *Audition*.

I. Interrogation

Interrogation includes gathering all information possible through asking questions. This should include inquiring how the cancer was diagnosed and who the presiding oncologist is. If the patient does not have an oncologist they should be appropriately referred to one who will be sympathetic with the patient's desire to incorporate herbal and other non-conventional treatment as part of their care. The patient should be advised to obtain at least a second opinion independent of the first diagnosis.

Following are the basic ten questions to ask:

1. **Chills or fever:** This is part of understanding which stage of Qi, Yin, Blood or Yang deficiency is involved. Coldness points to Qi and/or Yang (low metabolism) deficiency and may be associated with, or be one of, the causes of qi stagnation, phlegm and dampness. Blood and Qi deficiency are particularly involved with leukemia as well as other types of cancers and blood and Qi stagnation. Heat can also be an indication of inflammation associated with the cancer and a reflection of excess yang stagnation or Yin deficiency, especially when there are signs of fever. Many anti-carcinogenic herbs are also heat clearing and these include lonicera, oldenlandia, andrographis, forsythia, coptis, phellodendron (good for yin deficiency) and isatis.

2. **Perspiration:** This may be an indication of exhaustion and/or yin deficiency, especially if it is involuntary, which includes night sweats. If it is yin deficiency, yin tonics need to be added to the formula such as raw rehmannia, asparagus root or ophiopogon. If it is caused by exhaustion, use herbs such as ginseng, codonopsis and astragalus to tonify energy.

3. **Pain:** This can be caused by the cancer or its metastases to different areas of the body. Sharp pains signify blood stagnation; dull pains signify phlegm or damp stagnation and pains that move or alternate can be caused by Qi stagnation. For Blood stagnation pain we use blood-moving herbs such as sparganii, dang gui, tienchi ginseng, ligusticum or salvia milthiorrhiza. For Qi stagnation pains, often associated with eating or emotional issues, we use bupleurum, ligusticum or citrus peel. For Phlegm and damp stagnation we use arisaematis, pinellia and citrus peel. Often a lack of pain with the known presence of cancer means that the condition is more chronic.

The external application of herbs can relieve pains. These may include a combination of the following: Semen strychnii, arsenicum, olibanum (frankincense), myrrh, ligusticum and dang gui. The herbs are finely powdered and mixed with enough flour and water to form a paste. This is then topically applied. Other pain-relieving medicated herbal plasters are available from Chinese herb pharmacies.

4. **Defecation:** One should have regular daily bowel movements. Bowel sluggishness is a repeated lack of daily bowel movement while full-blown constipation is a lack of bowel movement over several successive days. However, incomplete bowel elimination, even if one seems to have a daily bowel movement, can over time create toxicity. Constipation can indicate obstruction and even tumors in the large intestine, especially if there are signs of blood in the stool. Since the large intestine is the receptacle of waste from food and the liver, it is important to maintain regular elimination. Additionally, having more than one bowel movement daily will optimize chances of recovery from cancer. Herbs such as rhubarb (da huang), which is a highly effective anti-carcinogenic herb, and the Ayurvedic formula called triphala are extremely important to maintain bowel regularity and help limit the growth and proliferation of cancer.

   The dose of a purgative depends on the reserves of righteous Qi (innate reserves). If one is thinner and weak, we use a smaller dose of purgatives. If stronger, then more may be added. Many herbs that are heat clearing are also classified as cholagogues (stimulate production of bile.) For instance, the berberis species including Oregon grape, coptis (huang lian) and philodendron bark (huang bai) also have purgative action because of the increased discharge of bile into the large intestine. It is at least to be expected that taking these herbs may cause a looser stool than normal. In any case, any degree of constipation will negatively affect the outcome of any healing.

   Finally, the accelerated destruction of cancer and other cells in the body is called 'lysing.' The accumulation of these dead cells can overload the eliminatory systems and cause mild to severe autointoxication. This is one of the reasons for the daily coffee enema.

5. **Urination:** This is important because as with the stool and sputum, signs of blood in the urine may indicate possible cancer. Patients who have any suspicious or abnormal signs of blood or reddish-colored urine should be referred to a physician for further evaluation. Frequent urination is also indicative of high blood sugar with corresponding spleen and/or kidney deficiency. This is often associated with cancer. Light urination indicates coldness while dark urine signifies heat.

6. **Appetite:** This indicates the condition of the digestive system and the process of food metabolism and assimilation. Appetite is closely associated with the state of the immune system as well as general Qi and vitality. Digestion is of primary importance in the treatment of cancer. Chemotherapy, radiation and the use of certain supplements and cold natured herbs can adversely effect digestion and appetite. This is why Six Gentlemen Combination (Liu junza tang) with ginger is so important to counteract the negative effects of these substances and to increase digestive power.

7. **Hearing:** This is not of great consequence in cancer diagnosis.

8. **Thirst:** This indicates a condition of heat, dryness or yin deficiency and is treated by using heat clearing herbs, yin tonics or demulcent herbs that lubricate dryness.

9. **Mental condition:** This is important because not only will negative mental states contribute to most cancers that are completely or partially caused by qi stagnation, they will also affect one's ability to consistently follow treatment. Bupleurum and Peony Combination (xiao yao wan) are used for qi stagnation; however, one can also consider adding spirit calming herbs, which are mild sedatives, such as zizyphus (suan zao ren), ganoderma (ling zhi) and scutellaria (huang chien) to a cancer formula to counteract anxiety and nervousness. These last two are also important anticancer herbs.

10. **Menstruation:** This is indicative of the state of blood in women. If it is scanty, irregular and clotted, it may indicate blood stagnation. If it is scanty and light colored it can signify blood deficiency. Angelica sinensis (dang gui) and ligusticum (chuan xiong) are both important to tonify and move blood. Polygonum multiflorum (hou shou wou) and yellow dock root (rumex crispus) are very valuable for reversing blood deficiency and the latter has potent anticancer properties as well.

II. Observation

Tongue Diagnosis

Tongue diagnosis is one of the easiest and most graphic representations of the state of the body. It is generally divided between the tongue body, the coat and the areas that designate the specific state of the internal organs. The tongue body describes the more constitutional aspects of the patient while the coat is an indication of metabolism and digestion. It is a simple yet valuable diagnostic system to learn and should be reinstated as part of western medical diagnosis.

Tongue Body

- If the tongue exhibits uneven patches and ruts it can be a sign of either weak digestion or possible yin deficiency. If the tongue has had these traits since birth it could be what is known as a 'geographic' or mapped looking tongue, which is normal.
- A swollen tongue, scalloped on the sides and lacking color, indicates qi deficiency. If it is wet and shiny it indicates edema.

Tongue Coat

- If the coat is white it is an indication of coldness. It can be a sign of low thyroid, high cholesterol or overeating of rich fatty foods and baked goods.
- If the coat is yellowish it indicates damp heat. It is usually an indication of problems associated with the spleen-pancreas and/or the liver.
- If the coat is thick, either white or yellow it indicates poor digestion and food stagnation. This is a sign of stagnation caused by overeating.
- Dark or black color of the tongue coat is an indication of a serious condition and discharge from the kidney-adrenals.
- If there is mucus on the tongue it indicates dampness.
- If the coat appears only on the front of the tongue it indicates an acute, superficial illness while a thick coat at the back or root of the tongue indicates a chronic condition.
- Purplish or black spots on either side of the tongue indicate blood stagnation affecting corresponding organs on the right or left side of the body.

Organ Correspondences on the Tongue

- A normal tongue should appear not too large or small, clean and clear with a thin whitish coat.
- A red tipped tongue indicates nervous tension affecting the heart. It can be a sign of stress and possible insomnia.
- A deep rut down the middle of the tongue indicates weak digestion.
- A coat or other unusual signs on the front area of the tongue indicates the condition of the lungs and gastric organs.
- A coat or absence of coat on the sides of the tongue may be an indication of an imbalance in the liver.
- A coat or unusual signs towards the back of the tongue is an indication of the state of the Large intestine and Kidney-adrenals.

Fingernail Diagnosis (Compiled by Lesley Tierra)

Various people, including the Chinese and Greeks, have used fingernail diagnosis over millennia. Because the nails are always growing, they have the potential for being an accurate record of a person's physical condition. However, these markers of organ function are slow to appear and disappear as they can take between six and eight months to grow out in an adult. Thus, any nail indicators seen mean the dysfunction has been occurring for several months, and as the body condition improves, it may take a few months before the change is reflected in the nails. If there are any horizontal dips in the nail, the actual time of the problem starting can be determined by measuring the distance of the dip from the matrix, or bottom of the nail.

Healthy nails are shiny, pink colored and transparent, with an even, smooth arch and a hard epithelial cornea layer. They are between .5 and .75 mm in thickness, slightly curved, horizontally arched, elastic and strong, with a smooth even face. There should be eight moons, located on every nail but those of the pinkies. The face of the nail should be proportional in size to the hands and the rest of the body.

Nails are comprised of a tough protein called Keratin. The various nail parts include the nail bed (the area under the nail), the nail matrix (the area under the nail at its root where nails grow), the nail plate (the nail itself), the lunula (moon at the base of the nail), the cuticle (skin attached to the nail at its root), and the nail fold (the skin area at the sides of the nail). (See diagram) The nail matrix, where the matrix cells collect and make keratin, contains the nerves, lymph vessels and blood vessels vital for nourishing the nails.

Each fingernail reflects a certain part of the body. If only that fingernail has a problem, it may indicate only a localized or associated system malady.

Thumbnail: brain, excretory system, and reproductive system.

Index fingernail: liver, gallbladder, and nervous system, especially if this nail is brittle, grayish yellow or dark green.

Middle fingernail: circulatory system, presence of heat in the body.

Ring fingernail: reproductive organ function, hormonal balance.

Pinkie fingernail: digestive system, gastrointestinal tract, including the stomach and small and large intestines.

In using the nails to diagnosis bodily conditions it is important to keep a few things in mind. First of all, it is possible to have nail conditions but not have any of the associated physical problems. Sometimes just an external trauma to the nail bed or nail matrix is enough to cause nail deformities. If the nails chronically display particular characteristics, however, it is worth checking other signs in the body to see if any of the associated conditions could be developing. Other times, the nail signs may simply indicate a propensity for the associated conditions to develop if you don't take care of your health.

Traditionally, nail diagnosis was done on the fingernails. However, many of these indications hold for the toenails as well.

A well-known way to test for anemia is to press down on the nail, release and then immediately count one-thousand-one. The pink color should return within the second. If it returns slower, then there is anemia.

If when pressing down on the tip of the fingernail the blood still carries over, this indicates the artery valve isn't closing well and the veins aren't functioning properly. It can also indicate hyperthyroidism.

Nails that have fine horizontal stripes or are brittle and crack easily are one indication of low thyroid.

Fingernail Moons

The first and most important diagnostic factor is the moons at the base of the nails. These represent a person's cellular oxygen levels and lung function as well as their energy and strength. There should be eight moons on the fingernails, on all but the pinkies, and they should decrease in size from the largest on the thumb to the smallest on the ring finger. They should take up no more than ¼ the size of the nail. The smaller the moon, the lower the hormone function. Moon size can be hereditary; therefore, compare the size of your moons with your family's first. If they are the same, then overly large or small moons may be normal for your family.

Large moons on every fingernail, including the pinkie: (especially if there is also a noticeable reddish strawberry-like area or narrow, pointy tip at the front of the tongue) indicates a high chance of heart disease and other heart conditions. The individual will normally be hyper-excitable and generally have a ruddy complexion. Stroke is possible and hyperthyroidism.

Moons markedly smaller on one hand than the other: chance of a stroke (if the person doesn't use the hand with larger moons a great deal more often than the other hand. i.e., pitchers, writers, etc.) and circulation blockage.

Over large moons: overactive thyroid.

Over large moons, seeming to reach to the tip of the nail with just a little bit of red left: liver cirrhosis.

Fewer than 8 moons: poor circulation.

No moons on 3 to 7 fingernails: fatigue, low energy, weak-spirited, poor circulation, cold hands and feet, numbness, memory loss and coldness.

Two large moons on the pinkies: over-worked heart and prone to high blood pressure and heart disease.

No moons at all: coldness, anemia, depression, low blood pressure, weak immune system and under-active thyroid.

Shoot-like growth sprouting from the border of the moon: thyroid problem.

Ear Diagnosis

The Chinese associate the ears with the kidney-adrenals. Since these encompass the entire endocrine system they are also considered the root of yin and yang for the entire body. Therefore, the ears are an indication of one's constitution potential.

Buddhist art depicts the Buddha with long, well-formed ears, which indicate a strong constitution and great understanding. The ideal ears are ears that are large, well shaped, rounded at the top, with the middle fairly wide and tapering down to a large lobe.

If the outer rim is thick and wide it is associated with good circulation and good body temperature. Such a person will have a strong, well-grounded personality.

Individuals with thin or no ear rim indicates a weak circulatory system. An expectant mother who over-eats rich fatty foods during pregnancy can pass on a tendency towards poor circulation to her offspring. Such individuals innately feel more vulnerable and defensive and are therefore prone to argue and fight.

At the top area just below the rim there is an indented line that moves down and forward. This ridge is an indication of the condition of the nervous system.

The ridge on the inner part of the ear that circles from above to below the ear hole indicates the state of digestion. If this is strong and well formed it indicates strong digestion and a greater ability to assimilate the experiences of life. If it is thin and shallow it indicates weak digestion and less tolerance for shocking or new experiences.

Large earlobes indicate long life, endurance, tolerance and understanding. Small earlobes indicate less tolerance, a narrower life view and less tolerance and understanding of others.

A horizontal ridgeline on the ear lobe indicates a tendency towards diabetes while a vertical line in front of the nub near the ear hole indicates a tendency towards high blood pressure and heart problems.

III. Auditory and Olfactory

A weak, soft-spoken voice indicates coldness and deficiency. The opposite of a strong, loud voice indicates excess. If the voice is low pitched it signifies coldness while a heavy, unclear sounding voice indicates heat stagnation. A faint thin voice indicates a serious illness.

A strong smell of the breath, urine or feces indicates heat. Patients with advanced stages of serious disease such as cancer will emit a foul, fetid odor indicating further deterioration.

IV. Palpation

Pulse Diagnosis

Pulse diagnosis is one of the subtlest and most difficult diagnostic systems to master. For most, it requires years of daily practice. Yet it remains as one of the defining hallmarks of an experienced practitioner. Today, its use for the less experienced is based on discerning the six basic pulses, which anyone with a fair amount of sensitivity and patience can master relatively quickly. Equipped with this basic skill, the pulse is, for all practical purposes, primarily used to confirm previously learned diagnostic signs.

All traditional diagnostic methods begin with what is most apparent down to increasingly more subtle signs. It is from this progression that one eventually employs intuitive awareness as part of diagnosis. To claim to discern the condition of a specific organ associated with a specific area no larger than a finger's breadth on the small radial artery of the wrist, when one is unable to accurately tell the difference between the six pulses represents the height of foolish ignorance.

Begin by lightly grasping the patient's left hand with your right as in the act of a friendly handshake. With your left hand place your middle finger lightly over the patient's styloid process (the bump on the wrist) located on the right radial artery. This is located on the thumb side of the wrist. Press with just enough pressure so that the pulse beat is clearly felt.

The Six Basic Pulses

Rate of Speed: To arrive at the number of beats per minute, count the pulse beats on the radial artery for 15 seconds and multiply this times four. A pulse that has less than 60 BPM is regarded as a slow pulse, which is an indication of low metabolism, coldness and hypo function. A pulse that is faster than 82 is regarded as a fast pulse. This indicates hyper metabolism, heat or hyper function. The exceptions are athletes who tend to have slower pulses without signs of coldness. For these, the rate of speed may not be a reliable indication of heat or coldness.

Superficial or Deep: With relatively lighter pressure one is aware of the pulse that is close to the surface. With relatively deeper or firmer pressure, one perceives the deeper pulse quality. This reflects strength of the internal organs based on the resistance of the circulating blood as it encounters the deeper finger pressure.

During a cold, flu or fever, the pulse is always beating strongly at the surface because this is the area where the body is engaged in defending itself from invading pathogens. For chronic disease, the pulse is located deeper, reflecting problems with the internal organs. If there is speed plus a deep pulse then it is internal heat or inflammation. If it is slow at the deeper position then it reflects internal coldness or organic hypofunction. If it is full at the deep position then it reflects excess, congestion or fullness at the deep level. We then evaluate if it is excess, deep and either fast or slow indicating internal excess heat or coldness. If it is deep, thin, hollow (like a soft straw) or thready and fast or slow it indicates internal deficient heat or coldness. If it is deep, weak and fast then it indicates yin deficiency or consumptive internal wasting and heat.

A pulse that is surface, full and fast means external excess heat; if it is surface, thin and fast then it indicates surface, deficient heat, which is again a sign of yin deficiency. If it is surface full and fast then it indicates excess heat. If is surface and slow it indicates external coldness.

Full or Empty: This equates with an excess or deficient condition, which, depending on the rate of speed and depth may be associated with heat or coldness, acute or chronic conditions.

The reader can readily see how these basic six pulses relate to Eight Principle Diagnosis as previously described.

In addition to these basic pulses one can then learn to discern a few other qualities:

Slippery pulse: This has a gliding, more globulous feeling and indicates dampness. To learn this pulse feel the pulse of a woman who is at least one to two months pregnant since, with the additional fluid, they will always exhibit a slippery quality. Next, check someone who is struggling with an obvious mucus problem.

Bowstring pulse: This has a taught and tense quality like the string of a musical instrument that is overly tight. This pulse indicates nervous tension and usually is an indication of liver qi stagnation. Again, to learn to discern this pulse, make it a point to check someone's pulse when they are fired up, angry or tense.

Irregular or Intermittent pulses: There are two basic types. Regularly irregular, which can either be normal for that individual or a sign of stagnation, or irregularly irregular which can indicate, if it is weak, a sign of impending death. If it is normal strength but irregular or intermittent, it can be a sign of stagnation and congestion.

The pulse, along with symptom-sign and tongue diagnosis, can serve as important adjunctive diagnosis tools for evaluating patients with cancer. It can inform us of the areas of the body that are affected, the constitutional strength, the degree of stagnation, acute or chronic symptoms as well as the state of qi, blood, yin or yang.

For cancer, one may find a pulse that is both floating and deep but difficult to feel in the middle. This represents a lack of spleen or nutritive qi. Cancer is indeed a metabolic imbalance that ultimately leads to severe malnutrition (cachexia) of the host while the cancer uses up the first quality protein for unregulated proliferation. This is why it seems at first that cancer is cured by a protein deficient macrobiotic, or raw food, diet.

Audition and Smelling

Voice: A loud and clear voice indicates the presence of strong qi and abundant yang. If it is soft and low it indicates a yin condition.

Coughing: If the cough is productive it represents phlegm and damp-ness. If it is dry, it indicates dryness, heat and lung deficiency. If there is blood, with or without shortness of breath, one should consider lung cancer. Refer the patient to a medical doctor for further diagnosis.

Vomiting: This can be an indication of excess if it is strong and forceful, or deficiency if it is weak. It is, of course, also a side effect of chemotherapy and radiation treatment and should be treated with ginger. Vomiting is also an indication of obstruction in the stomach and esophagus and could be a symptom of cancer in those areas. Again, any abnormal blood stained excretion; sputum, phlegm, stool or urine should be referred to a medical doctor for further evaluation.

Abdominal rumbling sounds: These represent coldness and fluid in the gastrointestinal tract. In cancer patients, it is an indication of weak digestion.

Body odor: In advanced cancer this is usually putrid and/or rancid, indicating deficiency of Kidneys and Liver.

The Five Stagnations

Traditional Chinese Medicine views stagnation as a fundamental aspect of all imbalance and disease. Diet, herbs, acupuncture and various other physiotherapies can be used to move and clear stagnation. The concept of stagnation is equivalent but of deeper significance to the concept of toxicity in western herbal medicine since anything that accumulates and does not move in the body will have a potentially toxic effect. The difference is that while western healing approaches identify specific toxic substances as 'good or bad,' Chinese medicine only sees them as bad when a substance causes stagnation in the body.

This allows us to better understand how two individuals exposed to the same carcinogen may result in one individual developing cancer but not another. Radiation is toxic because it damages Qi and Blood and impairs circulation. The same is true of other suspected carcinogenic substances and phenomena introduced in the food and water supply. Individuals also have constitutional predispositions that will allow one to be more adversely affected by a particular carcinogen or cancer causing experience than another does.

The Five Stagnations that one should consider are Qi, Blood, Damp, Phlegm and Cold. Heat, rather than stagnation in and of itself, can result from any of these five.

A basic treatment strategy is to first clear toxicity and then, if necessary, give tonics. It may appear that toxins are all physical, but in fact they are also mental, or at least can be aggravated by emotional stress.

Abstinence or light fasting from food to clear many types of Stagnations, as well as appropriate exercise, must always be considered an option. On the other hand, abstinence from emotional stress and meditation is, for some, another important stagnation clearing strategy. As for exercise, Qi Gong and yoga exercise combining conscious movement, breath and internal visualization is probably the best physical exercise for relieving stagnation.

Indications for the Upper Warmer Stagnations

Qi Stagnation	Emotional and mental signs, depression, hysteria, headaches, dizziness, etc.
Blood Stagnation	Discoloration, varicosities, blueness, heaviness of the head and arms.
Fluid Stagnation	Edema, dampness of the head and chest, damp, swollen and scalloped tongue, slippery pulse.
Cold Stagnation	Cold extremities.

Indications for the Middle Warmer Stagnations

Qi Stagnation	Burping, gas, bloating, tight abdomen.
Blood Stagnation	Blood stagnation felt as a lump in the abdomen.
Fluid Stagnation	Borborygmus or gurgling abdominal sounds.
Cold Stagnation	Cold digestion (essentially poor digestion), anorexia, diarrhea.
Food Stagnation	Greasy tongue coat, epigastric spasms.

Indications for the Lower Warmer Stagnations

Qi Stagnation	Stiffness, heaviness, tightness in the lower abdomen and extremities.
Blood Stagnation	Palpable lumps (oketsu) in the lower abdomen, menstrual irregularities, and varicosities.
Fluid Stagnation	Edema, dampness.
Cold Stagnation	Cold abdomen, back, legs and feet.
Food Stagnation	Constipation.

As in western herbal medicine, cancer is not seen as a local condition but a condition that involves the whole person. Even if we consider cancer to have a genetic predisposition, there will always be, from the perspective of TCM, predisposing bodily and life factors that will contribute to or cause the development of, cancer. Traditional Chinese Medicine diagnosis requires years of study and practice to gain any consummate proficiency. However, even in a short time, anyone can learn some of the above principles and methods and use them for evaluating the different underlying imbalance of cancer patients. Based on that, it is possible to formulate a treatment strategy appropriate for each individual.

Endnotes

[1] Liu, X.Y.; Ang, N.Q., [Effect of liu wei di huang or jin gui shen qi decoction as on adjuvant treatment to a randomized group of 83 patients diagnosed with small cell lung cancer.], Beijing Institute for Cancer Research, Chung Hsi I Chieh Ho Tsa Chih, 10(12): 720-2, 708 1990 Dec

[2] Pan Mingji, MD, *Cancer Treatment with Fu Zheng Pei Ben Principle*, pg. 30, (Fugian Science and Technology Publishing house, 1992.)

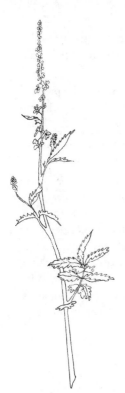

CHAPTER FIVE

TREATMENT SED ON THE SIX METHODS OF TRADITIONAL CHINESE MEDICINE

I n the *Yellow Emperor's Classic of Internal Medicine (Huangdi Nei Jing)*, compiled over 2000 years ago, cancer was described as an attack of cold evil that causes Qi and Blood to stagnate and form cancerous tumors. With no distinction between cancerous and non-cancerous tumors, no definite treatment protocols were offered. Later in 1264 in the *Wei Ji Bao Shu* and the *Ren Zhai Zhi Zhi Fu Yi Fang Lun* the term 'cancer' appeared. It was described as a mass that projected above and sank below. It had a poisonous root that deeply penetrated the interior. Through this the nature and shape of tumors, as well as the process of their metastasis and etiology, was described.

To date, five causes of tumor foundation have been differentially described. What is interesting about these is how many seem to concur with contemporary understanding of the cause of disease.

1. **Deficiency of Zheng Qi** based on inherited constitution potential and innate health reserves. This corresponds today with our understanding of the genetic and immunological basis for the cause of cancer.

2. **Deeply rooted fire toxins (toxicity).** This corresponds with our understanding of the role of environmental and dietary carcinogenic pollutants as a cause of cancer.

3. **Qi and Blood stagnation.** This has to do with the effects of the previous two causes including genetics, pollutants, diet, etc and their impairment of normal physiological processes as a cause of cancer.

4. **Phlegm and fluid stagnation.** This reflects the role of a diet high in fats as causes of different types of cancers.

5. **Emotional disharmony.** This reflects the role of stress and the concurrent hormonal imbalance that occurs as a contributing cause of cancer.

What is interesting about these is that while today various authorities might expound on any one of the above causes of cancer, hardly anyone except the ancient Chinese are able to comprehensively take into account the multiple causes of cancer. This clearly points out the difficulties in treatment. With multiple causes there must be multiple approaches to treatment and, as we have learned, there is no single treatment for all cancers. These in turn gave rise to the Six Therapeutic Methods as follows:

The Six Therapeutic Methods

1. **Supplement Zheng Qi** by restoring normal health and supporting the immune system.

2. **Remove toxic heat.**

3. **Stimulate blood circulation.**

4. **Clear phlegm.**

5. **Relieve liver qi stagnation.**

6. **Soften and dissolve the mass.**

Treating cancer based on the theory of Five Causes and Six Methods is based on historical and recent approaches as advanced by Professor Yu Wenjun, director of the medical department of Chengdu College of TCM in 1978. It represents an integration of traditional Chinese medicine with conventional western medicine, presently including surgery, chemotherapy and radiation. Herbal formulas created according to the Six Methods are compounded based on the presenting indications and needs of each individual patient. Treatment according to the Six Methods involves selecting one or a number of herbs from each of the six categories based on the symptomology and the type of cancer intended for treatment.

By definition, herbs are seldom specific to a disease but they are specific to a symptomatic pattern. TCM is based on the evaluation of patterns rather than simply named diseases. Unless one is absolutely certain that an herb is indicated for a particular condition, it is usually better to synergistically use a combination of 2 to 4 herbs from a single category. By so doing, one is able to affect a broader sphere of influence while lessening the possibility of an adverse reaction to a single herb or substance. This does not mean that in one category one may never use only a single herb. When selecting an herb based on the type of cancer read the more detailed description of the uses of the herb in the materia medica and especially use it if it seems to conform to the secondary symptom pattern. The more we understand the sphere of influence of a single herb we may choose to use, the more effective our results will be.

Take burdock root as an example. It is a well-known desmutagenic, meaning that it inhibits the formation and growth of cancer cells. It is therapeutically classified as a cooling or antiinflammatory alterative, diuretic and antirheumatic. As an alterative it has great value for the prevention and treatment of cancer and for a wide range of chronic degenerative diseases. Alteratives clear heat and correct chemical imbalances in the blood. However, the diuretic properties of burdock root make it particularly apt for swelling, urinary, lymphatic and mucoid symptoms especially when these tend to exhibit a more inflammatory tendency. Because it is a nutrient herb it is not necessarily limited to the treatment of hot conditions and diseases; however, that is its special range of influence. From its indications we can assume that burdock root is particularly useful for individuals with a more phlegmatic constitution with symptoms of swelling, edema, mucus and urinary impairment. This does not mean that one needs to have all of these symptoms to receive benefit from burdock, but it will be beneficial for any one or a number of them.

The three most important effects of herbs used for the treatment of cancer are 1) to restore normal function and strengthen bodily resistance, 2) to remove toxic heat, and 3) to relieve pain by promoting the circulation of blood. These three methods are employed in the treatment of all types of cancer while the remaining three methods are used depending on the condition and symptomology of the patient. In general, one should choose 2-4 substances in each category.

In general, cancer formulas tend to include a large number of herbs in larger amounts than usual. Treating according to the Six Methods may mean that a single formula may contain anywhere from six or more herbs; however, it is not necessary to use an herb from each category on every patient. The Six Methods tells us what to look for and treat in most cancer patients and in some cases we may omit using an herb from a particular category. This may occur because that category is treated in some other way, such as a particular nutritional supplement or it may also occur because the cancer is being treated by conventional western medical treatment, as in the case of chemotherapy or radiation, which represents the category of strong anti-cancer treatment.

Some examples of the Six Methods formulas follow:

1. A woman with small cell lung cancer and a history of long-time tobacco use developed cancer a couple of years after finally quitting. She had good energy but a loud liver sounding voice and had high blood pressure.

Qi tonic(s)	Reishi mushroom Cordyceps Milk thistle seeds—also good for the liver
Anticancer herb(s)	Lonicera Houttuynia Solanum nigrum and agrimony (these should always be used together because they potentiate each other.) Trichosanthes root Apricot seed
Stimulating Blood Circulation	Tienchi ginseng, good for heart and lungs. Salvia, good for heart and lungs.
Regulating Qi	Strychnos Nux-vomica—good for lungs and strengthens the nervous system. Citrus aurantium—helps digestion and assimilation and dries phlegm.
Clearing Phlegm	Pinellia Fritillaria
Soften and Dissolve Lumps and Nodules	Sargassum Laminaria

2. A woman with diagnosed liver cancer. She exhibited a characteristic loud voice, dark, sallow complexion, severe mood swings and low energy.

Qi Tonic(s)	Reishi mushroom Maitake Astragalus Codonopsis

Anticancer	Andrographis
	Silybum marianum
	Sophora flavescentis
	Verbena
Stimulating Blood Circulation	Sparganium
	Paeoniae
	Trogopterorum faeces
Regulating Qi	Bupleurum
	Curcuma
Clearing Phlegm	There was no sign of phlegm.
Soften and Dissolve Lumps and Nodules	Prunella
	Bombyx

3. A man with colorectal cancer, some abdominal pain and a tendency to bloat with digestive weakness.

Qi Tonic(s)	Reishi mushroom
	Maitake mushroom
	Poria
	Milk thistle seeds
	Astragalus
Anticancer	Andrographis
	Celandine, coptis
	Patriniae
	Pau d' Arco
	Cat's Claw
Stimulating Blood Circulation	Tienchi ginseng
	Corydalis
	Persica
Regulating Qi	Citrus aurantium
	Corium Stomachichum
	Curcuma longa
Clearing Phlegm	Phlegm was not an issue.
Soften and Dissolve Lumps and Nodules	Prunella, Sargassum
	Laminaria

4. A man with blood vessel cancer, low energy, metastasis to the lungs, liver and bone, pale complexion and an anxious temperament. He also complained of a cough with phlegm and heart palpitations.

Qi Tonic(s)	Reishi mushroom Astragalus Ginseng
Anticancer	Silybum seeds Rumex crispus Garlic Andrographis
Stimulating Blood Circulation	Tienchi ginseng
Regulating Qi	Aurantium citrus peel with fresh ginger for phlegm.
Clearing Phlegm	Pinellia Fritillaria
Soften and Dissolve Lumps and Nodules	Ostrea gigas – also calms the spirit.

5. A young man in his 20's with leukemia, pale, blood deficient, frail constitution and cough with phlegm.

Qi tonic(s)	Reishi mushroom Maitake American ginseng Asparagus root Cordyceps Schizandra
Anticancer	Indigo Lonicera Rumex Scrophularia Milk thistle seeds
Stimulating Blood Circulation	Tienchi ginseng Ginkgo biloba (taken as a separate supplement)

Regulating Qi	Aurantium citrus
	Corium stomachichum – to aid digestion and assimilation.
	Strychnos Nux-vomica (taken separately as a homeopathic remedy)
Clearing Phlegm	Pinellia
Soften and Dissolve Lumps and Nodules	Not applicable

6. A young woman in her early 20's with thyroid cancer, surgically treated and involving lymph nodes, slight cough and some phlegm.

Qi Tonic(s)	Reishi mushroom
	Maitake
	Cordyceps
	Astragalus
	Schizandra
	Ashwagandha (given as a separate supplement)
Anticancer	Poke root
	Duchesnea
	Burdock root (given separately as a tea and also as food)
	Scrophularia
	Milk thistle seeds
Stimulating Blood Circulation	Tienchi ginseng
	Salvia Milthiorrhiza
Regulating Qi	Aurantium citrus
	Lindera
Clearing Phlegm	Pinellia
Dissipate and Soften Lumps and Nodules	Laminaria
	Sargassum
	Bombyx

7. A woman, age 48, breast tumor, surgically removed, metastasis to axillary region, signs of dampness (edemic constitution). She is pre-menopause.

Qi Tonic(s)	Reishi mushroom Cordyceps Poria Astragalus Codonopsis
Anticancer	Andrographis Burdock (given separately with red clover as a tea) Coptis Gleditsia Lobelia chinensis Lonicera
Stimulating Blood Circulation	Tienchi Ginseng Salvia Milthiorrhiza Leonurus Persica
Regulating Qi	Bupleurum Aurantium citrus peel Cyperus
Clearing Phlegm	Fritillaria – Because phlegm caused by fat malabsorption is usually an issue with breast cancer.
Dissipate and Soften Lumps and Nodules	Prunella Violet leaf Nine Times salt Ostrea

Treatment may take months and necessitate periodic adjustment of constituents based on the changing symptomology and needs of the patient. Because of this, the best form I have found for long-term compliance is granulated five to one herbal extracts available from sources offered in the appendix of this book. You can purchase these ingredients individually or have them custom-made to specifications. On the average a daily dose consists of 3 grams taken three times daily. Alternatively, one may calculate a minimum dose of one gram per 20 pounds of body weight divided in two or three doses throughout the day. Of course this dose must be adjusted based on individual tolerance; however, if the dose seems well-tolerated one can increase dosage up to 12 to 15 or more grams per day. Patients can, if they choose, take these as a tea or put the granules in capsules.

Description of the Five Causes

I. Deficiency of Zheng Qi, Strengthening the Immune System, Maintaining and Restoring Normal Health and Well Being

The concept of deficiency of Zheng Qi refers to genetically predisposing factors, which may lead to cancer. Zheng Qi represents what in TCM is described as "righteous" or "normal" qi. When Zheng Qi is deficient either through genetics, lifestyle, bad diet or stress of all kinds the body is unable to maintain normal physical homeostasis. This may involve one or a number of physiological processes including what is most immediately relevant to this category, the immune system. From the following we should develop an appreciation for the role of the immune system as one expression of Zheng Qi in the prevention and treatment of cancer.

A brief overview of the immune system:

As it is characterized, the multi-layered task of the immune system is to identify 'self' from 'not self.' How the potential invasion of pathogens in the form of bacteria and viruses in a normal functioning immune system are identified as 'not self' is accomplished in various ways. One is simply a method of blocking the intrusion of a chemical or pathogen into the system through physical means such as the skin, stomach and intestinal lining. Two others would be classified as chemical and microbial barriers. The secretion of stomach acids that are able to destroy many pathogens, for instance, would be a chemical barrier. A microbial barrier is most apparent in the production of beneficial intestinal micro flora that assists in the normal breakdown of waste. Their presence in the intestines also serves to displace and limit the proliferation of unfavorable bacteria and parasites; therefore it plays a vital role in immunology.

While all of these undoubtedly play a part in inhibiting the development of cancer, the method of greatest relevance is even more internal. It involves the way cells replicate, the production of blood cells, antibodies and other blood-borne entities called cytokines whose job it is to regulate cellular growth and function. Since the body generates many cells that could develop into cancer, the fact that they do in some and not in others is completely dependent on the strength and integrity of the deep immune system.

Cytokines are secreted by lymphocytes (white blood cells) and serve to regulate the growth of other lymphocytes that are in turn called lymphokines. When stimulated by specific antigens, lymphokines that are stimulated by the sensitized lymphocytes respond by forming antibodies whose job it is to specifically react against antigens. Fundamentally this antibody-antigen response is the basis of immunity. Antigens themselves are either introduced or are secreted by the body in reaction to the presence of bacteria, toxins, foreign blood cells and cancer cells.

The process of cellular immunity occurs as a result of the generation of various macrophages and monocytes including interleukins-1, initiated during the acute stage of fevers, and interleukins-2, which is a lymphokine that stimulates the growth of T-lymphocytes that can destroy renegade tumor cells. Interleukin-2 also stimulates interferon that is also able to destroy both cancer cells and viruses.

Unlike other types, T-lymphocytes only react to antigens called *histocompatibility* antigens found in cells that are incompatible with the host. They are so called because after being formed from stem cells in the bone marrow they migrate to the thymus gland, which in turn programs them to perform their various functions. It is through this mechanism that the body recognizes and tends to reject altered cells and cells from transplanted organs. An autoimmune disease occurs specifically when histocompatibility antigens created by the self are not recognized. From this we see the importance of both the bone marrow and the thymus gland to the immune system.

Still another level of immune reaction involved with the destruction and inhibition of pathogens and cancer cells are the natural killer cells (NK). Constituting up to 15% of the total lymphocytes in the body, according to John Boik they represent "the first line of defense against metastatic spread of tumors."[1] He further goes on to describe how "depressed NK cell activity and depressed NK cell populations may be associated with the development and progression of cancer, AIDS, chronic fatigue syndrome, psychiatric depression, various immunodeficiency syndromes, and certain autoimmune diseases."

Monocyte-macrophages are the last group of lymphocytes responsible for cellular immunity. They can be activated by bacterial pathogenic by-products, but also by direct contact with tumor cells. They are able, among other things, to inhibit the growth and metastasis of tumors.

Again this gets back to an inherent deficiency of 'Zheng Qi,' or the inability of the body to maintain homeostatic normalcy in cancer patients. Further, one of the reasons that the risk of metastasis or recurrence is increased up to 1000-fold in patients who have been treated with both radiation and chemotherapy is because the debilitating and destructive effect of these therapies has specifically further injured and depressed the immune system. Specifically, these herbs are of vital importance as a component in the treatment of all chronic degenerative diseases such as cancer. They are especially important for patients undergoing more aggressive western therapies such as chemotherapy, radiation and surgery to prevent further recurrence.

The category of tonic herbs benefiting the immune system, while one of the most important, is too often misunderstood from a Western medical point of view. While it would be contraindicated to use immuno-stimulating or immune-modulating herbs for someone with an organ transplant, it has been clearly demonstrated by Chinese practice that it is not only appropriate, but also vital to use herbs in this category for the treatment of cancer or to accompany conventional western medical treatment.

Surgery, radiation and chemotherapy all represent a serious immuno-suppressive threat to the body overall. Of these, chemotherapy is the most debilitating. This is because it is intended as a selective poison targeting any rapidly reproducing cells in the body. These include blood cells, stomach lining cells and hair follicles which, when damaged through chemotherapy result in a correspondent lowering of white cell count (called leukopenia), nausea and hair loss.

Chemotherapeutic agents are usually given in high doses for a relatively short period of time or in low doses over a long period of time. Administering a low dose of chemotherapeutic drugs over a prolonged period (ranging from a few months to a year or more) attempts to lessen adverse reaction on the host while slowly killing vulnerable cancer cells by creating an adverse environment for their proliferation. This method, called "apoptosis," is the subject of much research interest and may offer an explanation for the way certain anticancer heat-clearing herbs may work against cancer. The advantage with the use of herbs is that they have a milder adverse reaction on the body than chemotherapeutic drugs.

Since both radiation and chemotherapy have been found to greatly increase one's risk of recurrence (according to Ralph Moss, up to a thousand-fold), tonic herbs that restore the 'righteous qi' are used both to offset the negative effects of chemotherapy as well as to prevent the recurrence of cancer. By 'promoting the normal,' however, they do not interfere with the tumor killing effects of radiation or chemotherapy. In fact, through various means such as enhanced circulation, many of them have been shown to enhance the effect of radiation and the ability of chemotherapeutic drugs to destroy cancer cells, thus making the blood less 'sticky' and reducing the possibility of metastasis.

Herbs for Strengthening the Constitution and Restoring Normal Function

This category of herbs are important to offset the immune debilitating effects of cancer, the damaging side effects of aggressive western therapies (surgery, radiation and chemotherapy) and to prevent the recurrence of cancer.

The body naturally produces cancer antibodies that help to destroy cancer cells in their early stage. It is when these antibodies are overwhelmed that cancer develops. The production of cancer antibodies would therefore be considered part of the 'righteous qi' of the body so that tonic herbs support the vital process of promoting the production of cancer antibodies.

A major indication of the adverse effects of chemotherapy and radiation is the diminishing of defender white blood cells (leukocytes). If they diminish excessively, aggressive cancer therapy is stopped until the cells restore themselves to offer defense against possible life-threatening infections. With a compromised immune system, stopping chemotherapy or radiation may allow the cancer to rejuvenate with a vengeance. Therefore any supportive therapy, such as the integration of tonic Chinese herbs such as astragalus (huang qi) that are known to support the immune system by helping to maintain blood cell count, is of great value. Since the immune system is a complex interdependent process, those herbs that are known to stimulate the production of blood cells are of value in maintaining anti-malignin antibodies as well.

Astragalus is particularly rich in immune-potentiating polysaccharides (long chain sugar molecules) while its yellow color is indicative of its flavonoid content. The yellow to red pigments of flavonoids represents the most common pigments next to the green color of chlorophyll. They are responsible for protecting the plant from damaging UV radiation, acting as antioxidants, enzyme inhibitors, pigments and light screens. They are also involved in the process of photosensitization and energy transfer of plant growth hormones and growth regulators[2] (Middleton, 1988).

In the body, they are often regarded as "biological stress modifiers" because they offer protection from environmental stress.[3] They have anti-oxidant effects, protecting against the oxidative degeneration of polyunsaturated fatty acids that are implicated in all degenerative diseases including cancer. Plant flavonoids such as those found in astragalus and other tonic herbs also serve to strengthen against the permeability of capillaries and other membranes that are part of a variety of diseases ranging from diabetes, blood deficiency, hemorrhoids and varicose ulcers to easy bruising. They are also potent enzyme inhibitors and anti-inflammatories that can inhibit various metabolites such as prostaglandins, leukotrienes and histamines that are responsible for various types of swelling inflammatory conditions including chronic arthritis. (Prostaglandins are locally acting hormones that mediate inflammation and smooth muscle activity, which is an immune response, and regulate the size of blood vessels.)

In contrast to anti-inflammatory drugs that have immune suppressing effects, flavonoids naturally found in various plants represent a wide margin of safety. Some well-known plant flavonoids include sylamarin that protects liver mitochondria and microsomes from lipid peroxidation, and quercetin that is an effective inhibitor of histamines associated with upper respiratory allergic reactions.

Certain flavonoids characteristically found in the Fabaceae (legume) family, to which astragalus, red clover, soy and sophora are all members, contain isoflavones. These are flavonoids that rarely appear in their long chain glycosidal form. In fact they are similar to estrogens and serve to occupy and bind with the body's estrogen receptor sites regulating against possible uptake of estrogen that is implicated in the growth of many types of cancers including cancer of the breast, female reproductive organs and the male prostate. Astragalus, being in the Leguminosae family, also possesses these types of compounds as does licorice and red clover. Genistein, characteristically found in various beans, legumes and especially soy products, is known to be effective in the prevention of breast and other estrogen sensitive tumors.

The immune potentiating effects of the astragalus polysaccharide was validated through research at the M.D. Anderson hospital in Houston, Texas during the 1980's. No patentable drug resulted from this research because of the difficulty of patenting plant polysaccharides. However, both in China and Japan a wide range of anticancer herbs rich in immune potentiating polysaccharides are used including a variety of medicinal mushrooms such as ganoderma (reishi), lentinus (shiitake), grifola (maitake) and coriolus versicolor (turkey tails) and cordyceps (dong chong xia cao).

Herbs in this category are used to augment healing potential or to protect and optimize the immune system either from the effect of the cancer, its treatment or by the negative effects of anticancer herbs. One may either add herbs such as ganoderma and astragalus root, for instance, that have known anticancer properties, or give these or other tonic herbs as a supplemental formula. See the list of possible supplemental tonic formulas that may be used at the end of the list of individual herbs. These formulas are given in detail in another section of the book.

One may ask how or why two herbs with opposing energies can be used in the same formula? The answer is that they both work differently or have a different sphere of influence. For example, we can combine astragalus root, which is warm to the spleen with bupleurum, which is cool to the liver. Astragalus, a warm natured herb that enters the lungs also stimulates digestive metabolism. Despite its warm nature, it can be used with lonicera (honeysuckle flowers) and other cooling and detoxifying herbs that also enter the lungs. One may not want to combine these two herbs together in the same formula if the intention is to treat an acute upper respiratory infection. However, for a chronic condition such as cancer, the intention is to employ the cancer inhibiting properties of lonicera with the immune stimulating effects of astragalus.

Tonic Herbs

ALOE VERA	Liver, heart, spleen – Used for gastrointestinal and adjunctively for other cancers, it has vulnerary, laxative and cholagogue properties. It is especially indicated for radiation. Indications: externally for burns, abrasions, ulcers, hepatitis, constipation.
AMERICAN GINSENG **Xi yang shen**	Lung, heart, kidney, stomach – Nourishes yin essence, counteracts dryness and wasting. Glehnia has similar properties. Dose: 3-9g
ASPARAGUS COCHINENSIS **Tian men dong** (Asparagus root)	It is used for cancer of the breast, lungs and leukemia and enters the lungs and kidneys. It nourishes yin fluids especially of the lungs and expectorates phlegm and dampness. It is also indicated for yin deficiency, night sweats, muscular degeneration, dry throat, blood in the sputum and constipation. It is contraindicated for symptoms of diarrhea or symptoms of cold and dampness Dose: 6-24g
ASTRAGALUS MEMBRANICUS **Huang Qi**	It is used for all types of cancers when there is qi and blood deficiency, threatened immune system, especially for lung, breast and gastric cancer, to offset the adverse effects of chemotherapy and radiation. Dose: 9-30g
ATRACTYLODES MACROCEPHELA **Bai zhu**	Spleen and stomach – tonifies qi, promotes appetite, clears dampness, increases white blood cell count, inhibits cancer, stimulates phagocytosis, increases white blood cells. Dose: 3-9g
CHAGA (Inonotus sciurinus, I. Tabacinus, I. Orientalis, Poria obligua, Polyporus obliquus)	It is used for various types of cancers, especially breast cancer, lip cancer, gastric, parotid gland, pulmonary, stomach, skin, rectal cancers and Hodgkin's disease. It has both tonic and anticancer properties. Dose: Boil about 3 centimeters of the grated fungus for about 20 minutes and take as a tea. It must be taken long term for many months.

CODONOPSIS PILOSULA **Dang shen**	Spleen, lungs and all cancers, especially when there is qi deficiency. It is similar but more mild than ginseng. Dose: 9-30g
COIX (Coicis lachryma-jobi) **Yi yi ren**	Spleen, Stomach, Kidney, Lung and Large Intestine – used for most types of cancers but especially the lungs, breast, stomach and large intestine. It assists digestion, regulates fluid metabolism, clears heat. Dose: 9-30g
CORDYCEPS SINENSIS **Dong chong xia cao**	Lung, kidneys, breast – tonifies both yang and lung yin, inhibits cancer, strengthens the immune system. For lung cancer take 6 grams powdered twice daily. Dose: 6-15g
CORIOLUS VERSICOLOR (Trametes versicolor) (Turkey tails) **Yin zhi**	For all types of cancers but especially liver cancer. It is a major source for pharmaceutical polysaccharide krestin (PSK), recognized for its anticancer properties as well as improving blood vessel strength, supporting normal hepatic function, protecting the liver and general immune enhancement. Coriolus is useful. Dose: 5-20g 3x/day as tea.
EMBLICA OFFICINALIS (Phyllanthus emblica) (Amla or Amlaki)	Useful for liver, lung and other cancers. It has detoxifying, nutritive tonic, astringent, cholagogue, mild laxative properties. Dose: 6-30g
GINSENG, PANAX **Ren Shen**	All types of cancers when there is accompanying qi deficiency, especially gastric cancer, also to offset the adverse effects of chemotherapy and radiation. Dose: 3-9g
LICORICE (Glycyrrhiza species) **Gan cao**	For various types especially gastrointestinal and lungs. It tonifies and nourishes the Spleen Qi, clears Heat and dispels toxicity, lubricates the Lungs and relieves spasms and pain. Avoid or use with care concurrently with chemotherapy or when there are symptoms of edema, nausea or vomiting. Dose: 2-9g

LIGUSTRUM LUCIDUM **Nu zhen zi**	Liver, kidney and all types of cancer including non-solid cancers. It nourishes liver and kidney yin, clears deficient heat, counteracts wasting, strengthens and supports the immune system. Dose: 9-15g
LILIUM BROWNII **Bai he**	Heart, lungs, breast – Nourishes yin fluids, lubricates and expels dried mucus, calms spirit. Dose: 9-30g
LYCII BERRIES **Gou gi zi**	Liver and kidneys – Blood and yin tonic, high beta-carotene. Include as part of diet. Dose: 6-18g
MAITAKE MUSHROOM (Grifola frondosa)	Generally inhibits tumor growth for all cancers. It also has a protective effect on the liver and is an important immune tonic. Dose: 9-15g daily.
MILK THISTLE SEEDS, **SILYMARIN** (Silybum marianum or Carduus marianus)	For liver, kidneys, reproductive organs, skin and other cancers. It is hepatoprotective, bitter tonic, demulcent, antidepressant. Used for various acute and chronic liver conditions including hepatitis A, B and C as well as liver cirrhosis. It also helps the cardiovascular system by lowering blood lipids. Contraindications: None noted. Dose: At least 420 milligrams daily.
OPHIOPOGON **Mai men dong**	Lung, stomach and breast. It nourishes yin fluids and essence and is useful for cachexia associated with cancer. Dose: 6-12g
POLYGONATUM **ODORATUM** **Yu zhu**	Lung, heart, stomach and breast. It nourishes fluids of lung and stomach, for yin deficiency and wasting. Dose: 6-12g

PORIA COCOS **Fu ling**	For various types of solid tumors. It has tonic, diuretic and sedative properties. Contraindications: Not for someone with symptoms of frequent urination, spermatorrhea or prolapse of the uro-genital organs. Dose: 6-18g
PORIA UMBELLATA **Zhu Ling** (Grifola)	For various types of solid tumors. Contraindications: It is not indicated if there are no signs of dampness. Dose: 6-15g
PSORALEA CORYLIFOLIA **Bu gu zhi**	For Various types of cancers. It tonifies kidney and spleen yang (improves metabolism), for symptoms of coldness, lung qi weakness, and a tendency towards frequent urination. It should not be used if there are acute inflammatory symptoms and should be combined with digestive and carminative herbs, as it may be difficult to digest. Dose 3-9g
REHMANNIA GLUTINOSA (prepared) **Shou di huang**	Heart, liver and kidneys. It tonifies blood and kidneys, nourishes essence. Dose: 9-30g
REHMANNIA GLUTINOSA (unprepared) **Sheng Di huang**	It is used for various types of cancers associated with dryness, inflammation and yin deficiency. It is Antiinflammatory, tonifies Yin and promotes fluid production. Dose: 9-30g
REISHI MUSHROOM (Ganoderma lucidum) **Ling zhi**	All types of cancers when there is qi weakness, blood deficiency, low and/or threatened immune system, dampness, nervousness and anxiety. It is also used to offset the adverse effects of chemotherapy and radiation. Dose: 9-30g
SAW PALMETTO (Serenoa Serrulata)	It is useful for prostate and lung cancer. It is a nutritive yin tonic, diuretic, expectorant, roborant, sedative, endocrine and anabolic agent, aphrodisiac and is indicated for wasting diseases, underweight and cachexia associated with cancer. Dose: 3-12g three times daily.

SCHISANDRA CHINENSIS **Wu wei zi**	For all cancers. It enters the lung, heart, liver and kidney. Preserves essence, calms the mind and maintains liver function. Contraindicated for individuals with external symptoms of colds and flus. Dose: 2-9g
SHIITAKE MUSHROOM (Lentinus edodes) **Sean goo**	Particularly effective for the liver but generally effective against all cancers. It tonifies the immune system and is antiinflammatory against viruses and bacteria. It also helps regulate cholesterol. Dose: to treat cancer use 9-12g, fresh 90g.
WITHANIA SOMNIFERA (Ashwagandha) (Available in Planetary Herbal Extract)	It is useful for all types of cancers associated with immune deficiency, inflammation, anxiety and nervousness. It lessens the adverse effects of radiation therapy and optimizes its intended effects. It is tonic, antirheumatic, aphrodisiac, sedative, astringent, anodyne, anti-fungal, anti-hypertensive, anti-inflammatory and immuno-stimulant. Contraindications: Do not use during pregnancy. Dose: 3-12g or 3g of the powder boiled in warm milk for a tonic. The powder can be taken mixed with ghee (clarified butter) and honey.

Tonic Formulas

In general a tonic formula should be continuously taken for only 3 to 6 months, then either stopped altogether or another formula selected in its place. Depending on how much the tonic effect is required, one would avoid taking tonics at the same time as anticancer, detoxifying formulas as they may compromise the effects of each to some degree. Despite the fact that for convenience we may sometimes combine tonic herbs according to the Six Methods approach as stated previously, it is generally better to take detoxifying and tonic formulas at separate times rather than immediately together. Tonic herbs and formulas are best taken 20 minutes or so before eating while the more detoxifying and eliminative formulas are taken 10 to 20 minutes after meals. The reason for this is to gain full benefit from the tonic formula when the body is prepared to accept food. If it is a warming formula, it may even assist better digestion and food metabolism.

Tonic Formulas

BU ZHONG YI QI TANG (Ginseng & Astragalus combination also known as Ginseng Elixir) (Planetary Herb Formula)	A good formula to combat chemotherapy toxicity and radiation burn.
GINSENG COMPLEX (Planetary Herb Formula)	Panax ginseng, Panax ginseng extract, American ginseng, Siberian ginseng, Siberian ginseng extract, Codonopsis, Tienchi ginseng, Atractylodes alba, Polygonum multiflorum, Astragalus mongolicus, Dang quai, Poria, Ginger and Licorice.
LIU JUNZA TANG (Six Major Herbs)	Loss of appetite with dampness, to counteract the adverse effects of chemotherapy.
LI ZHONG WAN (Ginseng & Ginger Combination)	Great for diarrhea after chemotherapy.
MAITAKE EXTRACT (Planetary Herb Formula)	Single herb, full spectrum formulation.
REHMANNIA SIX **Liu Wei Di Huang**	Tonifies kidney and liver yin essence, strengthens the immune system. Use after radiation and surgery.
REISHI EXTRACT (Planetary Herb Formula)	Single herb, full spectrum formulation.
REISHI MUSHROOM SUPREME (Planetary Formula)	Immune tonic, fu zheng (support righteous qi) formula. Use ongoing to prevent recurrence and to counteract the adverse effects of radiation and chemotherapy. Contains: Reishi Mycelial Biomass, Shiitake Mycelial Biomass, Siberian Ginseng Extract, Schizandra, Astragalus, Atractylodes, Grifola, Ligustrum, Poria Cocos, Reishi Mushroom Extract, Polygala, Ginger Root and Green Citrus Peel.

SHIITAKE MUSHROOM SUPREME (Planetary Herb Formula)	Immune tonic, fu zheng formula. Especially for the liver and also for hepatitis B and C. Reishi Mycelial Biomass, Shiitake Mycelial Biomass, Siberian Ginseng Extract, Schizandra, Astragalus, Atractylodes, Grifola, Ligustrum, Poria Cocos, Reishi Mushroom Extract, Polygala, Ginger Root and Green Citrus Peel.
SHI CHUAN DA BU WAN (Ginseng and Dang Gui Combination)	For detoxifying from chemotherapy and stimulating the immune system. Also use as a tea for non-solid tumors including leukemia and non-Hodgkin's lymphoma.
SI JUNZA TANG (Four Major Herbs or Four Nobles) (Planetary Herb Formula)	For loss of appetite (anorexia) caused by stomach Qi deficiency of cancer patients.
SI WU TANG **Dang Gui Four**	Blood deficiency caused by chemotherapy, radiation and surgery. Can combine with with Si junza tang if there is qi deficiency as well.
WU ZI WAN (Schizandra Adrenal Tonic) (Planetary Herb Formula)	Tonifies and regulates the adrenals and hormone system generally. Used for "kidney-essence" deficiency, promoting health and increasing longevity.
XIAO CHAI HU TANG (Minor Bupleurum Combination)	Very good for nausea and anorexia due to chemotherapy.

II. Herbs for Removing Toxic Heat (Anticancer Herbs)

Herbs in this category possess heat-clearing properties, or what in western herbal medicine are called alteratives or anti-inflammatories. Research based on a few human studies, but considerable animal studies from countries throughout the world, abounds to substantiate the considerable anticancer properties of many of these herbs. Perhaps this research would be of much less interest if these herbs did not have a long standing empirical background of efficacy for various pathological conditions such as inflammations and even cancer. Choosing the herb or synergistic herbs from this category is based on the specific actions and effects they have on certain areas of the body. This is ultimately what makes them optimally effective for a particular type of cancer. An example is the use of seaweed for thyroid carcinoma or dandelion for breast cancer. The presence of iodine in kelp and other seaweeds indicates that particular herb has a particular affinity for the thyroid gland. The fact dandelion root is well known to stimulate the production of mother's milk demonstrates its affinity for the breasts. Such affinities increase specificity for a particular area but may not necessarily be exclusive to it.

Nevertheless, in treating a specific type of cancer, we should include as many specific or 'near-specific' herbs for the type of cancer as we can. There are also a number of herbs, such as many of the anti-cancer mushrooms like grifola frondosa (maitake) and herbs such as andrographis, red clover and berberine-containing herbs such as coptis and barberry, that while having a more or less specific action for certain types of cancers, have broad anti-cancer properties that are of value for a wide range of cancers.

Herbal Alteratives

Anticarcinogenic herbs are broadly derived from a category described by western herbalists as 'alteratives.' Western herbal alteratives are defined as substances that act through the lymphatic, serous, glandular and mucous membrane systems, and to a lesser degree through the skin. Their primary action is to facilitate and enhance the breakdown and elimination of metabolic wastes. Secondarily they are used to enhance the absorption and assimilation of nutrients. Alteratives, therefore, are broadly used as detoxifiers and purifiers intended to neutralize and/or eliminate toxins from environmental, nutritional or stress-related influences that generate the production of metabolites that the body may be unable to either utilize or eliminate. The function of herbs in this category is to optimize the body's normal eliminative channels via the liver, kidneys, intestines and lungs, or directly by chemically neutralizing the toxic wastes found in the blood, lymph and other bodily tissues.

Herbs in this category serve as primary substances for the treatment of cancer. They may also be variously classified as anti-inflammatories, chola-gogues and mild to stronger purgatives. These would include the well known western herbs such as chaparral, red clover, burdock root, dandelion root, stillingia, poke root, oregon grape root and pau d' arco to name a few. Traditional Chinese Medicine classifies most of the anticancer herbs in the category of 'heat-clearing,' with each herb subclassified in five separate sub-categories and according to different organ systems they influence. This is the basis for choosing which herb or herbs are best suited for particular cancers.

The 'official' TCM materia medica of Chinese medicine constitutes three to four hundred herbs at most. Nevertheless, it is roughly estimated that over 5,000 herbs are used either in folk or local practice and many of these may have more efficacious benefit against cancer and include many so-called western herbs such as red clover, burdock root and yellow dock, etc. As a result, many of these herbs have been researched in Chinese universities and found to have potent anticancer properties.

So what does it mean to "clear heat" or use an alterative for inflammatory or toxic diseases? Just as all herbs have multiple properties, herbs classified as heat clearing or alterative also possess multiple properties and functions.

For instance, besides having anti-inflammatory flavonoids including the isoflavone and genistein, a number of herbs such as red clover also contain blood-thinning coumarins. Herbs with these constituents, therefore, also break up blood stagnation and promote blood circulation, decidedly important for treating the stagnation aspect of cancer. Baicalein, a constituent of Scutellaria barbatae has antiinflammatory properties.

Alkaloids are another class of constituents in herbs that are associated with heat clearing, alterative and anticancer properties. Alkaloids tend to have a very strong therapeutic reaction and act upon the system in many diverse ways. They alter or counteract acid conditions. Other alkaloids, such as the pyrrolizidine class (implicated in comfrey toxicity and senecio) and aconitine found in aconite, are mild to strongly toxic. Alkaloids include a wide variety of compounds including caffeine, morphine, pilocarpine, reserpine, quinine, atropine, piperidine, colchicine and aparteine. Berberine, found in coptis, golden seal, Oregon grape root, and phellodendron inhibit cellular respiration of cancer cells. Matrine and oxymatrine, found in sophora is partially responsible for that herb's anti-carcinogenic properties. Essentially, the heat-clearing and anticancer properties of herbs are mostly found in their flavonoid and alkaloid content.

Certain animals and insects are also used for their anticancer properties. These include scorpions, centipedes, earthworms, silk worms, and hornet's nest to name a few. These also each have a slightly different action but essentially are considered according to the Chinese as "strange proteins." These are in the form of various amino acids, hemolytic proteins and other substances. As such, they are absorbed as part of the food chain but introduce a foreign element that has the potential, like chemotherapy, of compromising and disrupting those fast replicating cells such as cancer and yet have little or no effect on normal cells. This is why these substances are so widely used in China and, for that matter, historically in early western herbal medicine.

The herbs in this category affect the growth and proliferation of tumors both directly and indirectly. Some may have mild toxicity and for this and other reasons, it is a good idea to vary the formulation approximately every 3 months. Combining them with other herbs in compound formulas also greatly reduces their potential toxicity.

Anticancer Herbs

AGRIMONY (Agrimonia eupatoria) **Xian He Cao**	For various types of cancer including cancer of the liver, lungs, breast, abdomen, esophagus and bone. Contraindications: Not for an individual with acute inflammatory symptoms. Dose: 10-15g
AKEBIA TRIFOLIATA FRUIT **Ba Yue Zha**	For breast and digestive tract tumors. It has diuretic, cholagogue and tumor dissolving properties. It is contraindicated for pregnant women or individuals with a tendency to frequent urination or lack of energy. Aristolochic acid found in akebia has been found to cause pulmonary-cardiac arrest. It should be used starting with a small dose and gradually increased to the full-indicated dose according to the patient's tolerance. Dose: 6-12g
ANDROGRAPHIS PANICULATA **Chuan Xin Lian**	For all types of cancers, especially breast, lung, gastrointestinal, liver and pancreas. It clears heat and reduces inflammation and swelling. Contraindication: Use with caution for weak digestion or with digestive herbs. Do not use on pregnant women. Dose: 9-15g or 1 to 2g in powder form.
ARCTIUM LAPPA (Burdock) **Niu Bang Zi**	For various types of cancers including breast, lungs and gastrointestinal. It is detoxifying, diuretic, nutritive and desmutagenic (prevents cellular mutation). Contraindications: Limit use if there is diarrhea or loose stool unless other herbs are added to counterbalance it. Dose: 3-9g
BELAMCANDA CHINENSIS **She Gan**	For cancer of the pharynx and lungs. Actions: It clears heat, treats acute sore throat, clears phlegm. Contraindications: Not for pregnant women or individuals with weak digestion. Dose: 6-9g

BOS TAURUS DOMESTICUS (Cow gallstone) **Niu Huang**	*Mainly for use by experienced practitioners.* Especially for cancer of the liver, lung, brain and leukemia. It enters the heart and liver. It is anti-inflammatory, antispasmodic and detoxifying. It treats delirium, apoplexy, epilepsy, tetany, mouth inflammations and purulent skin inflammations. Contraindications: Not for pregnant woman. Dose: 0.15-0.3g
BUPLEURUM CHINENSIS **Chai Hu**	Liver, spleen, lungs, reproductive organs and abdomen. It is cholagogue and antiinflammatory. Contraindications: Should not be used by those with Yin deficiency or with extreme headaches or eye diseases such as conjunctivitis when caused by Liver Fire. Dose: 3-12g
CELANDINE (Chelidonium majus) Greater delandine	*Mainly for use by experienced practitioners.* For liver and gastrointestinal type cancers. It is alterative, cholagogue, diuretic, purgative, antispasmodic, diaphoretic, anodyne, antitussive, narcotic and mildly toxic. Contraindications: Not for an individual with a cold condition and diarrhea. Dose: Of the dried herb take 1 or 2g three times daily. Of the 20% tincture take 5 to 15 drops three times daily. **An overdose can be toxic.**
CHAPARRAL (Larrea tridentata)	For various types of cancers. Contraindications: Lactation, liver conditions (cirrhosis, hepatitis), MAOI drugs, pre-existing kidney disease and pregnancy. Dose: 3-6g in decoction, of the 1:5 in 75% alcohol, Dose: 20-60 drops up to 3x/day

COPTIS CHINENSIS **Huang lien**	Most types of cancers, especially liver, pancreas, esophagus, breast, and large intestine. It clears dampness and heat, and quiets the mind. Contraindications: It is contraindicated for weak digestion unless other herbs are added to protect digestion. It should also not be used by those with Yin deficiency when there is vomiting or nausea and Cold. Dose: 1-9g
DIONAE MUSCIPULA (Venus Flytrap) (Carnivora®)	For various types of cancers. Avoid during pregnancy. Dose: 30 drops of the extract in water, taken four times daily.
DUCHESNEA INDICA **She Mei**	*Mainly for use by experienced practitioners.* Cancer of the vocal cords, thyroid, lungs, stomach, nasopharynx, cervix, liver and chest. It is antiinflammatory and blood moving. Contraindications: Not for pregnant women, or individuals with a cold and deficient tendency. Dose: 30g in decoction.
ECHINACEA SPECIES (E. angustifolia, E. purpurea, E. pallida)	For various types of Cancers. It is useful for painful inflammatory conditions. Dose: 15 to 30 drops of the 5:1 tincture, four times daily.
CLEAVERS (Galium aparine)	For lymphomas, liver, leukemia and colon cancers. Contraindications: Not for cold, deficient conditions. Dose: 45g
GARLIC (Allium sativum)	For cancer of the lungs and gastrointestinal system. Contraindications: This herb should not be used by those with Yin deficiency and Heat signs. It should not be applied topically for long periods of time as it destroys tissue. Dose: 6-15g

GLEDITSIA SINENSIS **Xao Jiao Ci**	For breast cancer, nasopharyngeal carcinoma, lung cancer and cancer of the large intestine. It clears inflammation and purulence. Contraindications: Not for use during pregnancy. Dose: 3-9g
HOUTTUYNIAE CORDATA **Yu Xing Cao**	For lungs, breast and colon cancers. It is antiinflammatory and diuretic. Contraindications: Not for use with Cold deficiency unless there are herbs to counterbalance it. Dose: 15-40g only lightly decocted. It can also be taken freshly juiced or combined with other herbs in decoction. The leaves are sometimes eaten steamed or fresh as a potherb.
HYDRASTIS CANADENSIS (Goldenseal)	For breast, liver and gastrointestinal cancers. Contraindications: Do not use during pregnancy, for cases of hypertension or for yin deficient with symptoms of wasting. Dose: 1:5 tincture 20-40 drops, powder 1-2g
INDIGO NATURALIS **Qing Dai**	Used for leukemia and fevers associated with cancer. It is antiinflammatory, antiviral, detoxifying and inhibits leukemic cells. Contraindications: Not for use during pregnancy nor for an individual with weak, cold digestion. Dose: 1.5 to 3g
ISATIS TINCTORIA **Ban Lang Gen**	For all types of cancers including non-solid types and leukemia. It is antiviral and antiinflammatory. Contraindications: Not for those who are deficient or with signs of true Fire toxicity unless combined with other herbs to counterbalance it. Dose: 10-30g

LACCA SINICA EXSICCATA (Rhus vernicifera) **Gan Qi**	For cancer of the stomach, intestines and liver. Contraindications: Do not use during pregnancy. Use with caution for those who are very weak. Dose: 2.4 to 4.5g for each dose.
LOBELIAE CHINENSIS **Ban Bian Lian**	For cancer of the lungs, breast, kidneys, nose, liver and ascites cancer. Contraindications: Use with caution for individuals with all types of deficiencies. Dose: 15-30g
LONICERA JAPONICA **Jin Yin Hua**	For breast, lungs and various other cancers. Contraindications: Those with deficiency in the Spleen/Stomach should not use this herb especially when there is Coldness or diarrhea unless counterbalanced with other herbs in the formula. It should be used carefully when there is Qi or Yin deficiency. Dose: 6-15g; large doses (up to 60g) can be used effectively and safely in severe cases.
MOMORDICA CHARANTIA (Bitter melon)	For all types of cancers. Contraindications: Should not be taken by pregnant women. Dose: 9-30g
NYMPHAEA ODORATA (White Pond Lily)	For uterine and cervical cancer. It is astringent and antiinflammatory. Contraindications: Do not use if there is dryness and constipation. Dose: 4-8g
OLDENLANDIAE **CHRYSOTRICHAE** **Bai Hua She Shi Cao** (Oldenlandia)	For various cancers especially gastrointestinal, cervix, breast, rectum and fibrosarcoma. Contraindications: Not to be used by pregnant women. Dose: 15-30g (up to 60 for treating cancer).
PARIS POLYPHYLLA **Zao Xiu**	For many types of cancers. It is detoxifying, antiinflammatory and analgesic. Contraindications: For a weak or pregnant woman. Dose: 5-10g

PATRINIAE SCABIOSAEFOLIAE **Bai Jiang Cao** (Thlaspi) (Patrinia)	For colorectal cancer. It clears heat and toxicity. Contraindications: It should not be used alone in individuals with weak, cold digestion, lack of appetite or diarrhea. Dose: 6-15g
PAU D' ARCO (Tabebuia heptaphylla, Tabebuia impetiginosa) (Ipe Roxa, Ipe Roxo, Ipes, Lapacho, Lapacho Colorado, Lapacho Morado, Red Lapacho, Taheebo, Amapa, Tecoma, Trumpet Bush)	For various types of cancers including leukemia and lymphoma. Contraindications: It is a cool-natured herb and it should be used with caution in those with severe gastric weakness. Do not take during pregnancy. Normal dosage is well tolerated and has no side effects. However, high doses have been known to cause nausea, vomiting and slow blood clotting. Dose: Dried bark; 3-6g in decoction using three cups of water. One cup is taken three times daily. Liquid Extract: 1:1 in 50% alcohol, 15-60 drops up to 5x/day Tincture: 1:5 in 50% alcohol, 1 teaspoon to one tablespoon should be taken up to 4x/day
POKE ROOT (Phytolacca decandra or P. americana) **Shang Lu**	*Mainly for use by experienced practitioners.* For breast, glands, lungs and lymphatic cancers. It is antiinflammatory and diuretic. It detoxifies the glands and lymph system. Contraindications: Not for edema caused by qi deficiency. Dose: 4-9g. No more than five drops of the extract should be taken at a time. In higher doses, poke root is toxic.
PRUNELLA VULGARIS (Selfheal Spike) **Xia Ku Cao**	For all cancers. It is anticancer and helps soften and dissolve tumors. It also lowers blood pressure. Contraindications: Not for someone with weak digestion unless combined in a formula with herbs to counterbalance it. Dose: 6-18g

PRUNUS ARMENIACA (Apricot Seed) **Xing Ren**	Especially for lung and colorectal cancers but also for most other types as well. Contraindications: This herb should be used with caution when there is Yin deficiency and with infants. It should not be used when there is diarrhea. Dose: 3-9g
RABDOSIA RUBESCENS **Dong Ling Cao**	Especially for esophageal, breast and prostate cancers. It is probably useful for a wide variety of other solid type cancers as well. The standard dose is about 12 to 20g three times daily with a full course of treatment lasting 1 to 1.5 months. Contraindications: In higher doses it may cause nausea, vomiting, abdominal distension and diarrhea. The standard dosage should be first stopped until all symptoms subside and later resumed at a lower, more tolerated dosage.
RED CLOVER (Trifolium pratense)	For all types of cancers, especially lungs and breast cancer. Contraindications: Not for those who are taking other blood thinning agents. Dose: 9-15g
RHEUM PALMATUM (Rhubarb, Chinese rhubarb, Turkey rhubarb) **Da Huang**	For colorectal cancer, uterine and ovarian cancer, granulocytic leukemia. Contraindications: Because of its purging properties, rhubarb is contraindicated for patients with digestive weakness and low energy. Dose: 3-12g
RUMEX ACETOSELLA (Acetosella vulgaris) (Sheep Sorrel)	For different types of cancers. Contraindications: Generally very safe and mild but its cooling nature may need to be considered for individuals with symptoms of cold deficiency. The leaf is high in oxalic acid and over consumption has been known to cause toxicity. Dose: 6-9g daily. It is used in Essiac tea.

RUMEX CRISPUS (Yellow Dock, Broad leafed dock, Curly dock)	For leukemia, liver and colorectal cancers. Contraindications: Not for pregnant women. Use with caution for people with internal coldness. Dose: 3-6g of the tincture, 10 to 30 drops for each dose.
SANGUINAREA CANADENSIS (Bloodroot)	*Mainly for use by experienced practitioners.* For cancer of the lungs and liver. Contraindications: It is toxic in high doses and should not be taken by pregnant or lactating women. It should not be taken internally for more than three or four days at a time. Do not take with heparin and other anticoagulants that are opposed by berberine. Dose: 10 to 30 drops of the tincture. Externally it is combined with zinc chloride to make a famous escharotic paste.
SCROPHULARIA NODOSA ET SPECIES (Figwort, HealAll, Carpenter's square)	For cancer of the breast, lungs, glands and lymphomas as well as other cancers. It clears heat and dampness and detoxifies. Contraindications: It should not be used during pregnancy, lactation, diabetes, or with ventricular tachycardia. Large doses are poisonous. The use of any cardioactives can potentiate herbs with cardiac glycosides. It can also interfere with antidiabetic drugs. Dose: Of the tincture take from 5 to 30 drops three or four times daily. Of the whole herb use 6-9g daily.
SCUTELLARIAE BARBATAE (Barbat skullcap) **Ban Zhi Lian**	For cancer of the lungs, breast and various types of cancers. It is antiinflammatory and detoxifying. Contraindications: Not for use during pregnancy Dose: 15-30g
SILYBUM MARIANUM (Carduus marianus) (Milk thistle, Silymarin)	For liver, kidneys, reproductive organs, skin and other cancers. Contraindications: None noted. Dose: At least 420 milligrams daily

SOLANUM NIGRUM (Black Nightshade) (also Solani lyrati) **Long Kui**	*Mainly for use by experienced practitioners.* For cancer of the lungs, breast and liver. Contraindications: Do not use during pregnancy or if there are signs of deficiency and coldness. Dose: 30-60g
SOPHORA FLAVESCENTIS **Ku Shen**	For cancer of the cervix, stomach, pancreas and liver. Contraindications: Those with weakness and cold in the Spleen and Stomach should not use this herb. Dose: 3-12g
SOPHORA SUBPROSTRATA **Shan Dou Gen**	For cancer of the lungs, breast, gastrointestinal, large intestine, cervix, pancreas and urinary bladder. Contraindications: Those with weakness and cold in the Spleen and Stomach should not use this herb. Dose: 6-9g
STILLINGIA ROOT (Stillingia sylvatica, Stillingia ligustina, Stillingia treculeana) (Queen's Delight, Queen's Root, Queensroot, Silver Leaf, Stillingia, Yaw Root)	For various types of cancers. It is alterative, anti-inflammatory, diuretic and mildly laxative. Lactation and during pregnancy. Overdose can cause vertigo, burning sensation of the mouth, throat and gastrointestinal tract, diarrhea, nausea, vomiting, dysuria, pruritus, skin eruptions, cough, depression, fatigue and perspiration. Dose: (3x/day) Dried Root: 1-6g or by decoction Liquid Extract: 1:1 in 25% alcohol, dose 0.5-2 ml Tincture: 1:5 in 45 % alcohol, dose 1-4 ml Tincture, Dried Root: 1:5 in 50% alcohol, dose; 10-30 drops Tincture, Fresh Root: 1:2 in 50% alcohol, dose; 10-30 drops
TARAXACUM OFFICINALIS (Dandelion) **Pu Gong Yin**	For cancer of the breast, liver, lungs, pancreas. Contraindications: Overdose can cause mild diarrhea. Dose: 10-30g

THEA SINENSIS (Green tea)	For all types of cancers; however, used mostly for prevention and adjunctive treatment. Contraindications: Not for individuals with a tendency towards frequent or nighttime urination. Dose: 1 to 6 cups daily.
THUJA OCCIDENTALIS (Thuja, White cedar, Arbor vitae)	For various types of cancers. It is a lymphatic cleanser. Contraindications: Avoid high dosage and use during pregnancy. Dose: From one to ten drops every two or three hours for malignancy. For non-malignant growths such as warts, take a drop two or three times daily for four days. The excrescences will fall off, especially if it is also applied externally. One can use either the 1:1 fluid extract or the 1:5 tincture. Good results can also be obtained with homeopathic 30X dosage.
TINOSPORA CORDIFOLIA (T. Sinensis) **Kuan Jin Teng** (Guduchi)	Especially for liver cancer. It is antiinflammatory and detoxifying. Contraindications: Not to be used during pregnancy or immediately after childbirth. Dose: Of the root 6-9g, of the vine, 15-30g
TRAPAE BISPINOSAE, FRUCTUS **Chi Shih**	Mostly for gastrointestinal cancers. Contraindications: Not for individuals with weak digestion unless combined with digestive, carminative herbs. Dose: 9-30g
TRICHOSANTHES KIRILOWII (Trichosanthes root) **Tian Hua Fen**	For cancer of the lungs, breast and gastrointestinal system. It is antiinflammatory and detoxifying. Contraindications: Avoid during pregnancy. In high dosage it can be toxic and even fatal because of its ability to impair hepatic and renal function. It is also contraindicated for weak digestion. This means that its use for cancer patients should probably include digestives as part of the formula. Dose: 9-15g

TULIPA EDULIS, PSEUDOBULBUS (Tulip bulb) **Shan Ci Gu** (Cremastra variabilis) (Iphigenia indica, a toxic plant, is mistaken for this herb.)	*Mainly for use by experienced practitioners.* It is mostly used externally for a wide variety of cancers, especially breast and esophageal cancers. It is antiinflammatory and detoxifying to the blood and lymph. The major use of this herb is externally in the form of a plaster for skin cancers and other types of cancers that are closer to the surface of the body. In this way, it is similar to the use of bloodroot and zinc chloride salves used as escharotic salves in the west. Contraindications: Use with caution internally on weak patients. In general one should avoid internal use of this herb as it contains the toxic alkaloid colchicine, which is accumulative and can cause symptoms ranging from nausea to respiratory failure. It can also cause blood disorders such as granulocytopenia. Dose: 3-9g in decoctions.
UNCARIA TOMENTOSA (Cat's claw, Una de Gato)	For various types of cancers. Contraindications: No serious side effects have been reported. In Europe, health care providers avoid combining this herb with hormonal drugs, insulin, or vaccines. Avoid during pregnancy. It should be avoided or used with caution with other platelet blocking drugs such as aspirin. Dose: This product can be taken as a tincture (1-2 ml) up to 2 times per day, as a capsule (350-500mg) once or twice per day, or as a tea (1g of root bark per cup of boiling water). Drink 1-3 times each day. It can be combined with other herbs or therapies for cancer.

VERBENA HASTATA (Blue vervaine)	For cancer of the cervix, liver and ascites cancer. It is bitter and cold and enters the liver and stomach organ meridians. It has antiinflammatory, blood moving, cholagogue, diuretic and anthelmintic (parasites) properties.
	Contraindications: Not for pregnant women or those with a cold deficient constitution unless it is combined with other herbs to counterbalance it.
	Dose: 15–30g
VISCUM ALBUM (European mistletoe, birdlime, Iscador)	For all types of cancers. Widely used by Anthroposophical practitioners for the treatment of cancer based on the recommendation of the early 20th century visionary, Rudolf Steiner.
	Contraindications: Avoid during pregnancy. Large doses in animals have been known to cause vomiting and death.
	Dose: 2.5g infused in cold water for 10 to 12 hours taken up to two times daily. Blood pressure should be regularly monitored.

Anticancer Herbal Formulas

Hoxsey Formula:

Herb	Hoxsey Dosage	Antiseptic Compounds	Antitumor Compounds
Barberry root bark	10 mg	9	3
Buckthorne bark	20 mg	7	3
Burdock root	10 mg	2	2
Cascara sagrada root	5 mg	7	2
Red Clover blossoms	20 mg	18	5
Licorice root	20 mg	18	5
Poke root	10 mg	3	2
Prickly ash bark	5 mg	3	2
Stillingia root	10 mg	3	3
Blood root (used in an external salve or powder only)		5	5

Essiac Formula:

Sheep sorrel (Rumex acetosella)
Burdock root (Arctium lappa)
Slippery elm bark (Ulmus fulva)
Rhubarb root (Rheum palmatum)

Developed by Rene' Caisse,[1] this is perhaps the most popular herbal anticancer formula on the market. Both sheep sorrel and rhubarb contain anthraquinones known to be effective against cancer. Burdock root contains arctigenin, a weak inhibitor of experimental tumor growth;[2] a desmutagenic factor of high molecular weight that reduces the effect of a number of mutagens including those which do not require metabolic activity;[3] and antimicrobial properties possibly as a result of the polyacetylenes.[4] Part of the history surrounding Essiac is that it was first bequeathed to a Catholic nurse, Rene Caisse, in 1922 by a woman who 20 years earlier received it from an Ojibway Indian medicine man for the successful treatment of her breast cancer. Rene Caisse eventually set up practice, administering the formula to thousands of cancer sufferers with acclaimed success. However, of the four herbs, three are of European origin and only Slippery elm is an American native botanical.[5]

Eli Jones Compound Syrup of Scrophularia (Cancer Syrup):

Scrophularia leaves and roots	32 scruples or 1-1/4 oz.
Phytolacca root	8 scruples or 1/4 oz.
Rumex crispus (Yellow dock)	8 scruples or 1/4 oz.
Celastrus scandens bark and root (False Bittersweet, an introduced weedy vine found growing in New England)	4 scruples or 1/8 oz.
Podophyllum root (Mandrake)	4 scruples or 1/8 oz.
Juniper berries	3 scruples or a bit less than 1/8 oz. (approximate)
Prickly ash berries	1 scruple or 1/24 oz. (very little)
Guiacum wood	2 scruples or 1/16 oz.

---

[1] The name is derived from spelling "Caisse" in reverse.

[2] Dombradi, G. (1970) Chemotherapy 15, 582

[3] Morita, K. et al. (1984) Mutat. Res. 129 (1), 25

[4] Schulte, K. et al. (1967) Arzneim. Forsch. 17 829

[5] Richard Thomas (1993) The Essiac Report, publ. by The Alternative Treatment Information Network, 1244 Ozeta Terrace, L.A., CA. 90069, 1-310-278-6611

Use fresh herbs. Mix together and coarsely grind. Moisten with alcohol and let them stand for two or three days. Steam distill and pass through the vapor of three pints of alcohol; continue this displacement with the steam of water until the strength is exhausted. Set aside the three pints of tincture which passed first and evaporate the remainder to two pints. Mix these together and add syrum Ovi. (**Note:** serum Ovi is the oil expressed from hard boiled eggs that have been broken up and fried.) Add oil sassafras q.s. to flavor it. Dose: one tablespoonful three times a day or sufficient to keep the bowels regular every day.

To my knowledge, this formula is available from Herb Pharm and Herbalists and Alchemists.

III. Herbs for Stimulating Blood Circulation and Eliminating Blood Stagnation

The categories of qi and/or blood moving are extremely important for many diseases, including cancer. The concept of movement by normalizing the circulation of qi and blood is pivotal to the entire system of TCM. These herbs are important both for helping to remove the tumor as well as treating the associated pain of cancer. Many herbs that move blood seem to enhance the effects of conventional therapies, such as chemotherapy and radiation, by making a greater volume of blood exposed and available to radiation and the chemotherapeutic agents. Further, blood activating herbs are also able to lessen the tendency to form adhesions and scar tissue, which is a common complication following surgery as well as both radiation and chemotherapy. Finally, blood-activating herbs, contrary to the expectation that it would tend to transport metastatic cancer cells to distant areas of the body, actually diminish and slow metastasis. The reason is that by lessening the fibrinogen level of the blood, it becomes less viscous and sticky so that cancer cells are less able to adhere to other tissues.

The high concentration of fibrinogen, a clotting factor in the blood, is associated with the formation of tumors. Fibrin tends to surround a tumor and prevent the cancer fighting factors from entering it. Thus herbs that diminish fibrin help to break down a tumor mass, prevent its formation, and thereby greatly increases all other cancer fighting elements both from the body as well as from herbs and conventional cancer therapies such a chemotherapy and radiation. Therefore, by making blood more viscous, herbs that move blood also help to prevent metastasis.

One other extremely important benefit of blood moving herbs is their ability to relieve pain. Pain caused by blood stagnation is usually severe, fixed and stabbing. Herbs in this category relieve these kinds of pains by enhancing circulation.

Classical symptoms of blood stagnation are:

- Fixed, stabbing pain
- Lumps and swellings
- Hard, immobile masses
- Recurring, frequent hemorrhages
- Clots of dark, purple tinge
- Dark colored blood
- Dark complexion
- Purple lips, nails
- Tremors
- Swelling of the organs (such as enlarged liver or spleen)
- Pulse: choppy, irregular, wiry, tight
- Tongue: dark purplish tongue and/or with red spots.

There are many TCM herbs that are widely used and respected in this category. Two of the most important are tienchi ginseng (panax pseudoginseng) and red sage root (salvia milthiorrhiza). Tienchi, or Sanqi, ginseng because of its ability to tonify blood and qi, relieve pain and support the immune system, paradoxically is a primary antihemorrhagic herb as well. Both on its own and in the form of the famous first aid patent formula called "Yunnan Baiyao" whose principle ingredient is panax pseudoginseng, tienchi ginseng is the most popular herb throughout China.

Unlike Tienchi ginseng, which has a warm tonifying energy, red sage (salvia milthiorrhiza) or 'dan shen' has a cool energy, calms the mind, lowers cholesterol and triglycerides, relieves pain and is highly effective in the category of moving blood for the treatment of cancer.

The most experienced Chinese herbalists regard blood moving as one of the most effective therapies. Western herbal medicine has been very limited in this category because of its rather confining categorization describing these herbs as 'emmenagogues' that in theory at least confines them to regulating female menses. They are also regarded with great caution because of their abortifacient properties.

The herbs in this category, primarily used to relieve pain, paradoxically also have an angiogenic function in inhibiting blood supply to the tumor and counteracting the tendency towards metastasis. Still another important use is to enhance the effect of chemotherapy and radiation. This is the third most essential category to use for the treatment of all types of cancers.

Blood Moving Herbs

BUTHUS MARTENSI (Scorpion) **Quan Xie**	*Mainly for use by experienced practitioners.* For various types of cancers including brain tumors. It is pungent, neutral and toxic in high doses. It enters the liver organ meridian. It is anticonvulsant, detoxifying, reduces lumps and restores the flow of Qi and blood to relieve pain. It is contraindicated for individuals with spasmodic conditions caused by anemia. Dose: 2-5g or 0.6-1g in powder form in capsule. For cancer it is commonly combined with Scolopendra.
CORYDALIS YANHUSUO **Yan Hu Suo**	For various types of cancer. Used to relieve pain by invigorating the circulation of qi and blood. Contraindicated during pregnancy. Dose: 3-9g
EUPOLYPHAGIA SEU OPISTHOPLATIAE (Cockroach) **Tu Bie Chong**	*Mainly for use by experienced practitioners.* For various types of cancers including the cervix, liver and multiple myeloma. It also inhibits leukemic cells. It is salty, cold and mildly toxic. It enters the liver and spleen organ meridians. It promotes blood circulation, relieves pain and detoxifies. Contraindications: Not for use during pregnancy. Dose: 3-6g Or 0.6 to 1g of the powder in capsule. It can be combined with scorpion and centipede for the treatment of most cancers.
GINKGO BILOBA (Ginkgo, Maidenhair tree)	For all types of cancers. Contraindications: Care should be exerted on patients who are on other blood thinning medications, including aspirin. Other possible but rare adverse reactions include dermatitis, irritability, restlessness, diarrhea and vomiting. Dose: This should only be taken in its standard extract form of 50:1 concentration.

LEONURUS HETEROPHYLLUS (L.Cardiaca) (Motherwort, Chinese Motherwort) **Yi Mu Cao**	For cancer of the breast and uterus. Contraindications: Motherwort should not be used during pregnancy or by those with Blood deficiency or Yin deficiency. Dose: 9-30g
LIGUSTICUM WALLICHII **Chuan Xiong**	It is useful for relieving pain associated with various cancers. It is pungent and warm and enters the liver, pericardium and gallbladder organ meridians. It moves blood and qi, regulates menstruation, and is useful for vascular headaches. It is contraindicated for pregnant women, pains caused by yin deficiency or hypertension and for any abnormal bleeding. Dose: 3-9g
MANIS PENTADACTYA-DACTYLA (Pangolin) (anteater scales) **Chuan Shan Jia**	*Mainly for use by experienced practitioners.* For cancer of the breast, cervix and liver. Contraindications: Use with caution for the treatment of sores caused by Deficiency. Preparation: Presoak in warm water for 2 hours, then simmer 1 to 3 hours. Dose: 3-9g
NIDUS VESPAE (Hornet nest--It is from the honeycomb of Polistes mandarinus) **Lu Feng Fang**	*Mainly for use by experienced practitioners.* Cancer of the lungs, liver and gastrointestinal region. It clears heat, damp stagnation, moves blood and relieves pain. Contraindications: This herb should not be used by those with Qi or Blood deficiency. This herb should not be used when there are open sores. Dose: 6-12g decocted; 1-3g as a powder internally.

PAEONIAE ALBA **Bai Shao Yao**	It is useful for various types of cancer including ascites, stomach, intestinal, liver and bone cancers. It is bitter, sour and has a cool energy. It enters the liver, spleen and lung organ meridians. It balances the vital energy of the liver, relieves pain, nourishes blood and consolidates yin (vital essence and fluids). It is contraindicated for someone with diarrhea and cold abdomen. Dose: 9-18g
PERSICA SEED (Peach Seed) **Tao Ren**	It treats various types of cancers including lung, liver and large intestine cancers. It enters these organ meridians. It is sweet, bitter and neutral. It promotes blood circulation, relieves stagnation, cough and asthma. It also has mild laxative properties. Contraindicated during pregnancy. Dose: 6-10g
SALVIA MILTHIORRHIZA (Chinese red sage root) **Dan Shen**	Used for a wide variety of cancers including cancer of the thyroid, thymus, abdomen, breast, esophagus, liver and reproductive organs. It is both antiinflammatory and moves blood. It reduces blood lipids and has a general sedating and tranquilizing effect. Dose: 3-15g
SCOLOPENDRA (S. subspinipes) **Wu Gong**	*Mainly for use by experienced practitioners.* For cerebral tumors, malignant soft tissue tumors, bone tumors and pain caused by cancer. It is anticonvulsant, analgesic, detoxifying and it reduces lumps and swelling. It clears the channels and relieves pain. It is salty, warm and toxic in higher doses. It enters the liver organ meridian. Dose: 2-3g Or 0.6 to 1g in powder form in capsule. For cancer it is commonly combined with Buthus.

SPARGANIUM STOLONIFERIUM (Scirpus martimus) (Bur reed tuber, sparganium, scirpus) **San Leng**	For various cancers, especially liver cancer and cancer of the gastrointestinal and genitourinary organs. Contraindications: Not for a women who is pregnant or with symptoms of excess menstruation. Dose: 3-9g
TIENCHI GINSENG (Panax pseudoginseng) (Notoginseng) **(San Qi or Tien Qi ginseng)**	It is indicated for both solid cancers of all types and non-solid types such as lymphomas and leukemia. It stops bleeding and resolves Blood stasis, reduces inflammation and associated pain. Dose: 1-9g; 1-3g when taken as a powder, can be used topically
TROGOPTERORUM, FAECES (Trogopterus dung, Pteropus excrement) **Wu Ling Zhi**	*Mainly for use by experienced practitioners.* For cancer of the liver, spleen, reproductive organs, pancreas and abdomen. It moves blood and relieves pain. Contraindications: Not for someone with symptoms of anemia with blood stagnation. Traditionally it is said to be counteracted by ginseng, though this may not be true according to contemporary research. Dose: 3-9g
ZEDOARIA (Curcuma Zedoaria) **E Zhu**	For cancer of the abdomen, cervix, uterus, breast, testicles, liver and pancreas. Contraindications: Not for someone with deficiency of Qi and Blood, Spleen and Stomach. Dose and Directions: 4-9g

Blood Moving Formulas

Guggul is a traditional Ayurvedic compound made principally of the resinous exudate of a sub-species of myrrh that has been specially processed to make the guggul phospholipids more bio-available. It is traditionally used for relieving all types of pain, promoting blood circulation and reducing blood lipids.

Dang Quai Four (Si Wu Tang) with added ingredients consists of angelica sinensis, ligusticum wallichii, rehmannia glutinosa and white peony root. This is a basic formula for tonifying and moving blood. The blood moving properties are enhanced when ligusticum is increased and the prepared rehmannia is decreased. Blood moving and pain relieving properties are also enhanced by the addition of corydalis and sparganium.

Cinnamon and Poria Combination (Gui Zhi Fuling Wan) consists of cinnamon twigs, poria mushroom, moutan peony root, persica seed and red peony. It is specifically used to remove blood stagnation, relieve pain and soften hard lumps especially in the lower abdomen.

Patent Medicines

Compound Tablets of Salvia Miltiorrhiza
(Dan Shen Tablets)

Pills of Rheum and Eupolyphaga Sinensis
(Da Huang Zhe Chong Wan)

Yunnan Bai Yao: Used for leukemia or lymphatic cancers. The primary herb is Radix Notoginseng, commonly known as Tienchi.

IV. Regulating Qi

The process of metabolism has to do with using drying carminatives such as citrus peel, saussurea and magnolia bark to promote the movement of digestive qi. Other herbs such as ginger-fried pinellia and ginger-fried arisaema eliminate phlegm. Fritillaria bulbs act as phlegm clearing and expectorants. An herb such as apricot seed, apart from their well-known high content of cancer inhibiting B17, clears toxic phlegm from the lungs and at the same time supplies good quality lubrication for dry lungs.

The process of qi regulation through the use of carminatives causes a neurological response that stimulates gastric secretions and enzymes that support the movement of food through the intestines.

Some of the herbs in this category possess resins that are ultimately secreted by the mucus membranes and in the process promote the dissolution and flow of mucus. The process is aided by triterpenoid saponins found in many of these herbs. These include a large group of saponins found in plants that consist of naturally occurring glycosides whose active portions are water-soluble and produce lather. Many of these also have a detergent effect and were used by native people for soap such as "soap root" (Chlorogalum pomeridianum) used by the Native Americans. These water-soluble sugars combine with lipophilic aglycones (or sapogenins) that lower surface tension and produce the characteristic detergent or soap-like effect on the membranes of the skin. It is the combination of resins that act as a non-digestible surface stimulant to digestive and mucus membranes and mucus-dissolving saponins that is responsible for the action of most herbs that move or regulate qi and transform and dissolve phlegm.

The classical symptoms of qi stagnation are:

- Distention in the ribs and abdomen
- Fluctuating emotions, moodiness, depression
- Soreness and pains that change in severity and location
- Soft, palpable lumps
- Frequent sighing
- A sensation of constriction around the ribs or chest
- Feeling a lump or something stuck in the throat
- Irregular menses
- Swelling of the breasts during menses
- Pulse: wiry or tight
- Tongue: dark, purplish tinged

Qi stagnation is commonly associated with various types of cancer. Qi stagnation assumes many different forms including depression, the formation of nodules and lumps, weak and erratic digestion. Herbs in this category are chosen according to the patient's symptomology.

Regulating Qi

BUPLEURUM CHINENSIS Common name: Bupleurum, Hare's Ear **Chai Hu**	For cancer of the liver, spleen, lungs, reproductive organs, and abdomen. Contraindications: This herb should not be used by those with Yin deficiency or by those with extreme headaches or eye diseases such as conjunctivitis when caused by Liver Fire. Dose: 3-12g
CITRUS AURANTIUM (Orange peel, Citrus peel) **Chen Pi**	For most types of cancers. Contraindications: Not for a person who is spitting blood or has symptoms of extreme dryness. Dose: 3-9g

CORIUM STOMACHICHUM GALLI (Chicken gizzard skin) **Ji Nei Jin**	For esophagus, stomach, and cardiac cancer. It is sweet and neutral. Enters the spleen, stomach and urinary bladder organ meridians. It relieves indigestions, stimulates appetite, treats frequent urination, gall and urinary stones. It is very useful for supporting digestion and appetite in cancer patients. Dose: 3-9g
CURCUMA LONGA (Turmeric) (Radix Curcumae) (Turmeric root) **Jiang Huang**	For cancer of the Liver and reproductive organs. Contraindications: Do not use during pregnancy, or if there is blood deficiency with no symptoms of blood and qi stagnation. Dose: Each decoction consists of 4.5 to 15g
CYPERUS ROTUNDUS (Nutgrass) **Xiang Fu**	For cancer of the digestive tract, uterus, ovary and for the relief of pain. Contraindications: This herb should not be used when there is Yin or Qi deficiency especially when there is heat associated with the condition. Dose: 4-12g
FOENICULUM VULGARE (Fennel seeds) **Xiao Hui Xiang**	For cervical and stomach cancer. They also increase white blood cell count. Contraindications: Not for someone with yin deficiency with symptoms of acute inflammation. Dose: 3-8g
LINDERA STRYCHNIFOLIA (Lindera Root) **Wu Yao**	For cancers of the thyroid gland, breast and liver. Contraindications: This herb should not be used by those with Qi deficiency or interior Heat. Dose: 3-9g
MAGNOLIA OFFICINALIS (Magnolia Bark) **Hou Pou**	For cancer of the stomach and esophagus. Contraindications: This herb should not be used by pregnant women or by those with Stomach or Spleen deficiency. Dose: 3-9g

STRYCHNOS NUX-VOMICA (Nux vomica, Nux-vomica seeds) Ma Qian Zi	*Mainly for use by experienced practitioners.* For a wide variety of cancers including lungs, breast, nasopharyngeal, uterine, colorectal and leukemia. Contraindications: Strychnine, the primary constituent, is very toxic with 5-10mg causing poisoning and 30mg death so that it should be used with great caution internally and certainly not during pregnancy or for very weak individuals. Processing will greatly reduce its toxicity. The procedure to detoxify it is to boil it first, strip off the shell, cut into slices and stir fry or roast with sesame oil. Dose: 0.3 to 0.9g per day. An appropriate amount is powdered and applied topically for external application. It is also very safe and effective to use in homeopathic dilution up to 30X.

V. Clearing Phlegm

Herbs in this category treat internal phlegm stagnation, which according to Chinese medical theory is regarded as a component in the formation of tumors and nodules. Certainly this may be more obvious for lung cancer but the concept of phlegm in TCM represents a further congelation that can occur in a lymphatic-type constitution. Phlegm is also a by-product of imperfect digestion and assimilation. In this way, in TCM the spleen and stomach, representing the pervasive assimilative function not only in the GI tract but even down to the mitochondria of individual cells, is functioning imperfectly and leaving a toxic residue of dampness and phlegm as a result. A certain amount of lubricating fluid is necessary but in excess it becomes pathological.

Besides edema and phlegm, fat is also a form of dampness. In Ayurvedic medicine this moist waste accumulated in the various tissues of the body is called "ama" and also comes from imperfect metabolism. Western medicine sees a co-relationship between the accumulation of fatty deposits in the blood, arteries and other circulatory vessels as an underlying cause in cardiovascular disease. Other studies have substantiated a relationship between fat and its production with a number of different types of cancer including prostate, colon, cervical and breast cancers. [1,2,3]

From the TCM perspective, dampness, fat and phlegm are all a reflection of weakened spleen function. The TCM spleen represents the deepest levels of assimilation. When we eat too much or the wrong type of foods, such as the overconsumption of dairy products, cold, iced, frozen or raw foods over a period of time, these cause 'dampness' and can weaken our metabolism as they transform and manifest as phlegm.

Phlegm-Clearing Herbs

ARISAEMATIS (Arisaema Consanguineum) Jack In The Pulpit **Tian Nan Xing**	Mainly for cancer of the liver and breast. It dries and expels Phlegm in the lung and resolves coughs; it clears Wind and Phlegm in the channels and stops convulsions and spasms; it can be used topically to reduce inflammation and pain. Contraindications: Those with Yin deficient cough with dry Phlegm should not use this herb during pregnancy. Dose: 4-9 grams internally of the prepared rhizome. In this dose it should only be used when it is prepared with alum and ginger to detoxify it. Otherwise in raw form only take 0.3 to 1.0g daily.
FRITILLARIA CIRRHOSAE (Fritillaria) **Chuan Bei Mu**	For cervical, breast and lung cancer. Contraindications: This herb should not be used by those with Cold-Damp Phlegm conditions. Dose: 3-9g
INULA JAPONICA (Elecampane Flower) **Xuan Fu Hua**	For cancer of the lungs and breast. Contraindications: those with tuberculosis or cough due to Wind-Heat or deficiency should avoid this herb. Dose: 3-9g
PINELLIA TERNATAE (Pinellia) **Ban Xia**	It is useful for most cancers associated with the presence of phlegm, especially for stomach and lung cancer. It drains dampness and reduces phlegm; reverses the flow of rebellious Qi and reduces hard lumps and relieves distention. Contraindications: Pregnant women or those with any blood disorders associated with abnormal bleeding should not use this herb. Use *with caution* if there are symptoms of heat. Also generally contraindicated with Aconite (Fu Zi). Dose: 3-12g

V.   Softening and Dissolving Lumps and Nodules

Herbs and substances in this category are used to soften and dissolve masses, lumps and nodules. The mechanism affected is different with each herb or substance. Seaweeds regulate the thyroid function by supplying easily assimilable organic iodine. Even a subclinically low thyroid can contribute to an imbalance of many other hormones such as estrogen, progesterone and androgenic hormones. Considering that an imbalance of any of these can cause both benign and cancerous tumors, as well as certain types of goiters, fibrocystic breasts and uterine fibroids, it is quite remarkable that the ancient Chinese were able to see this relationship when they classified a group of sea herbs, minerals and other herbs under the category of substances that soften and dissolve lumps, and nodules. Of course this would also include various types of tumors.

However, besides their iodine content, seaweeds also have potent anti-coagulant properties that would also account for their ability to soften and dissolve lumps and nodules of various other kinds besides a swollen thyroid.[4] This same study, however, finds that the unique anticoagulant properties of seaweed have little effect in an elevated hemorrhagic risk.

While all of the seaweed type herbs exert this function, the antitumor properties of the brown sargassum seaweed used by both the Chinese and Japanese has been studied in Japan and its primary therapeutic effects seem to be largely due to a polysaccharide group known as L-fucon.[5]

Many cultures, such as the Japanese, wisely incorporate seaweeds as part of their diet. Besides iodine and most of the minerals (Mg, Ca, P, K and I) as well as valuable trace minerals, they are also a valuable source of vitamins including beta carotene, vitamin C and all of the B vitamins including the rare vegetable sources for B12. Their important dietary fiber content ranges from 33% to 75% of dry weight, and mainly consists of soluble polysaccharides (range from 17% to 59%), which have known immuno-tonic properties. Referenced data indicate that algal dietary fiber may show important functional activities, such as antioxidant, antimutagenic and anticoagulant effects, antitumor activity, and an important role in the modification of lipid metabolism in the human body.[6]

Seaweeds are traditionally consumed in Asia as sea vegetables, but in Western countries they have been used as gelling or thickening agents.

The iodine found in sea herbs is potent as an anti-inflammatory and detoxifier. The alginate binds with radioactive elements in the body, promoting their elimination from the system. Practically speaking, for the treatment of cancer seaweeds have powerful antioxidant and free radical scavenging properties.[7]

Perhaps partially because of their powerful anti-aging, antioxidant and free radical scavenging properties it was noted that of the survivors from exposure to radiation from the atomic bomb blast in Japan during the Second World War, those who were in a hospital close to the blast and who regularly consumed miso soup and seaweed had less adverse reaction to radiation exposure. This certainly would suggest that any cancer patients undergoing radiation or chemotherapy should be regularly consuming miso soup cooked with added seaweed (such as wakame). From the above, it is clear that sea vegetables play an important role in both the prevention and botanical treatment of cancer. Patients should be encouraged to include them daily as part of their diet or take them as a supplement.

Other substances and plants that seem to have similar softening and dissolving properties include oyster shell, ground tortoise shells (these are naturally shed from the animal and involve no cruelty) and prunella vulgaris spike (selfheal). The latter is one of the few herbs whose therapeutic properties are developed only in the dried and withered flower spikes as opposed to the fresh herb. Prunella is also very effective in lowering hypertension.

Herbs in this category soften and disperse swollen glands, hard lumps, nodules and certain types of tumors. Each have somewhat different ways of working and should be chosen according to the patient.

Herbs for Dissipating and Softening Lumps and Nodules

BOMBYX BATRYTICATUS (Silkworm) **Jiang Can**	For cancer of the throat, lungs and liver. Contraindications: Traditionally is contraindicated with Platycodon (Jie Geng), Poria (Fu Ling), Dioscorea Hypoglaucae (Bei Xie), and Ooetheca Mantidis (Sang Piao Xiao). Biochemical Constituents: Fat, protein, destruxin, organic acids, chitinase, bassianins, fibronolysin, and beauverician Dose: 3-10g; as a powder only 0.9 to 1.5g is taken.
LAMINARIA JAPONICA (Ecklonia kurome) (Kombu seaweed, kelp, Ecklonia) **Kombu**	For thyroid tumors, cancer of the neck, digestive tract and lungs. Contraindications: Use with caution for those with symptoms of coldness and dampness. It is also hard on the digestion so that it should also be used with symptoms of weakness and coldness of the digestive system. Dose: 9-15g

LEVISTONIA CHINENSIS (Palm root and/or leaf)	For various cancers including esophageal, nasopharyngeal cancers and leukemia. Contraindications: none known. Dose: of the seeds, 30 to 60g Of the seeds for various types of cancers, 30g can also be cooked with equal amount of lean pork for 1-2 hours.
NINE TIMES SALT (Prepared Sodium chloride) (Rock salt) **Zi Nao Sha**	Used for various types of cancers including esophageal cancer, thyroid and other glandular types of cancers and gastrointestinal tract cancers. Contraindications: None known. Dose: 1g (1/8th teaspoon) 3 times daily with food.
OSTREA GIGAS (Oyster Shell) **Mu Li**	For various cancers including lung, liver, stomach, breast, lymphomas and especially thyroid cancer. It is sedative, tranquilizing, astringent and softens and disperses hard lumps. Contraindications: Avoid using singly if there are symptoms of coldness and weakness or fevers without sweating. Dose: 15-30g; it should be cooked for 30-45 minutes before the other herbs are added.
PRUNELLA VULGARIS (Selfheal Spike) **Xia Ku Cao**	For all types of cancers. Contraindications: Not for someone with weak digestion. Dose: 6-18g
SARGASSUM PALLIDUM **Hai Zao**	It generally inhibits tumor cells but is especially useful for thyroid, stomach, liver and lung cancers and malignant lymphoma. It is salty and cold and enters the stomach and kidney organ meridians. It is expectorant, transforming phlegm, diuretic and softens and dissolves nodules. Useful for swollen glands and edema. Dose: 9-15g Commonly used with Konbu seaweed.
VIOLET (Viola odorata)	Especially for cancers of the breast, lungs and gastrointestinal organs. Contraindications: None noted. Dose: One ounce of the aerial portion of the plant steeped in three cups of boiling water. Consume a cupful three times daily.

Calming Spirit and Sedative Herbs and Therapies

While wishing to maintain the integrity of the Six Methods as developed in China, there is an obvious reason for the use of herbs to calm the spirit or act as a mild sedative. First, a patient who cannot sleep and maintain a certain level of inner centeredness and calm will not be able to heal properly. Sleep and relaxation is the recuperative essence or 'yin energy' of the body and must be supported through various means.

Counseling, meditation and Chinese yoga known as Qi-Gong practices must be encouraged. These have been shown to be profoundly healing and seem in many instances to cause spontaneous remission of cancer in more than a few patients. Following includes a number of sedative and calm spirit herbs that have already been described in the above categories but are listed again with a few that have not been mentioned thus far.

Calming Spirit and Sedative Herbs and Therapies

CANNABIS SATIVA (Marijuana) and **Huo Ma Ren** (Cannabis seed)	For all cancers. The leaf is spicy, sweet and neutral energy. While smoking will produce the most immediate response, in this form it is warm and toxic to the lungs. It is best, especially for lung cancer patients, to use internally in the form of capsules, tablets, tincture or some other internal preparation. It affects the liver, heart, spleen and stomach. It can be used to reduce nervousness, relieve hypertension, stimulate appetite and relieve nausea. The seeds are especially valuable as a lubricating yin tonic rich in valuable essential fatty oils (oleic, linoleic, linolenic acid), protein, choline, essential oil, vitamin B as well as non-intoxicating small amounts of cannabinol. Seeds are specifically effective as a lubricating laxative and increases peristalsis for promoting normal bowel evacuation. They are routinely included as an article of diet with rice porridge in China. Simply grind the seeds and add to food or eat directly. Contraindication and counteraction: Do not use if there are symptoms of diarrhea. Traditionally they are not used with oyster shell, poria and Cynanchum atrati.

LILIUM BROWNII (Tiger lily) **Bai He**	Heart, lungs, and breast, it nourishes yin fluids, lubricates and expels dried mucus, and calms the spirit, for lung and breast cancer. Dose: 9-30g
OSTREA GIGAS (Oyster Shell) **Mu Li**	For various cancers including lung, liver, stomach, breast, lymphomas and especially thyroid cancer. It is sedative, tranquilizing, astringent and softens and disperses hard lumps. Contraindications: Avoid using singly if there are symptoms of coldness and weakness or with fevers without sweating. Dose: 15-30g; it should be cooked for 30-45 minutes before the other herbs are added.
PORIA COCOS **Fu Ling and Fu Shen** (the part of the mushroom attached to the stem or root of the tree.)	For various types of solid tumors. It has tonic, diuretic and sedative properties. Fu shen has more calming spirit and sedative properties. Contraindication: For someone with frequent urination, spermatorrhea or prolapse of the uro-genital organs. Dose: 6-18g
REISHI MUSHROOM (Ganoderma lucidum) **Ling Zhi**	All types of cancers when there is qi, blood deficiency, low and/or threatened immune system, dampness, nervousness and anxiety. Also to offset the adverse effects of chemotherapy and radiation. Dose: 9-30g
SCHISANDRA CHINENSIS **Wu Wei Zi**	For various types of cancers. It enters the Lung, heart, liver and kidney. Preserves Essence, calms the mind, and maintains liver function. Contraindications: Not for those with signs of colds and flu or with excessive heat. Dose: 2-9g

ZIZYPHUS SPINOSA SEEDS Suan Zao Ren	For all cancers. It affects the heart-mind and liver. It treats insomnia, nervousness, palpitations, night sweats and spontaneous perspiration. It is a non-addictive mind tranquilizer and sedative but will not cause daytime drowsiness.
	Contraindicated only in the most severe acute inflammatory conditions.
	Dose: 9-18g. It can be taken throughout the day or put into capsules to be taken for insomnia.

The above list represents only a partial selection of some of the herbs I have used in my practice that have been found to have anticarcinogenic properties. Too often we are confronted with a simplistic one herb or herbal formula for all individuals sold at a high price, with unsubstantiated and exaggerated claims of success. In most cases the herbs or formulas that are sold are seldom as powerful as many of the less commercialized herbs described above. The reason should be obvious. Many of these herbs are simply too powerful and don't lend themselves to widespread profiteering and commercialization. This is not to say that some of the simpler herbs such as red clover, sheep sorrel, burdock root and dandelion are not as effective as others such as black nightshade, andrographis or isatis. Only that the most effective use of herbs is not based on a shotgun approach but tailoring and creating a combination based on the presenting symptoms and signs of each patient.

This is where the Six Methods from a TCM perspective offers a guide for creating the most effective herbal formula. The average cancer patient is bombarded with a plethora of possible therapies, supplements and herbs that may be useful in the treatment of cancer. In most cases there is scant research available and claims made are mostly unconfirmed. This does not mean that there is no validity to these therapies and supplements, only that one simply can't do them all. Further, I have found that an attempt to do as many as possible can be counterproductive.

For the most part pills, herbs and supplements when taken to excess can be hard on the stomach and digestion. TCM theory states that above all, one should attempt to maintain digestive strength in treating any chronic disease such as cancer. Therefore the objective is to take as much of anticancer supplementation directly from food and use other nutritional supplements and herbs judiciously, i.e. taking enough but not too much.

The Six Methods offers a valuable guideline whereby one can evaluate the totality of one's anticancer program including herbs, supplements and conventional drugs and therapies. For instance, chemotherapy and radiation would be in the category of 'anticancer' and should be simultaneously accompanied with blood moving, tonic and qi regulating digestive herbs. Based on research and practice in China, the integration of herbal medicine should precede or follow for at least a week or so more aggressive treatments such as chemotherapy and radiation.

The basic evaluation of constitutional strength should determine the balance of tonification and eliminative therapies that are appropriate for each patient.

Immune tonics such as reishi mushroom and astragalus can be given in higher dosage during the early stages of disease or to prevent recurrence. In the more advanced stages, tonics are also used but to a lesser extent, with greater emphasis on the use of eliminative, heat clearing herbs. In the middle stages of cancer one combines tonification and elimination substances equally.

Despite classifications, the difference between tonification and elimination is to some extent embodied in the use of all herbs. To eliminate excess in one whose system is congested is to achieve new levels of strength and vitality. However, the same eliminative diet or herbal program in an individual who is already deficient can only achieve further weakness and debility.

In a similar way, one hears of an herbal formula or a particular diet, for instance, one based on the exclusive use of raw foods, as having a profound effect in the treatment of cancer. For those with an excess conformation, a cleansing diet and herbal formula such as the Hoxsey formula can work miracles. For someone with deficiency these may not only be useless but further debilitating.

If a diet is nutritionally too weak, it can generate toxicity if for no other reason than the body may lack the metabolic strength to detoxify its naturally generated cellular waste products. This is true even with when eating the purest, organic foods. On the other hand someone who is in a nutritionally compromised state can through renewed strength provoke a discharge of stored metabolic wastes accumulated from former deficiency. Eliminative anticancer herbs such as coptis and sophora root can have a strengthening or tonic effect by assisting in the elimination through the liver, urine, skin and colon of the toxic burden.

In many instances, only by applying the principles of TCM diagnosis is it possible to discern a deficiency in one or a combination of blood, qi, yin or yang. The type of tonics one chooses should be based on this diagnosis.

Finally, even if a cancer is successfully treated either with diet and herbs or surgery, chemotherapy and radiation, one should continue the use of therapeutic herbs and diet probably for the remainder of one's life. In order to prevent recurrence, ongoing and periodically varied dietary and herbal treatment of cancer should be the rule. After the critical stages are passed through integrative treatment, this may be continued at a somewhat lesser degree of intensity. The basic idea is to lessen anything that places stress on the immune system and use herbs and supplements to try to maintain as much of a margin of immune strength as possible. To this end, having three or four formulas with which to alternate over the course of a year is a good practice. For instance, one might use a liver formula such as the Bupleurum Liver Cleanse or Shiitake Mushroom supreme with roasted dandelion root tea during the spring season. During the hotter climates, a blood purifier such as Red Clover Cleanser with red clover tea with chrysanthemum flower tea can be taken. During the drier months of autumn one might use more lubricating yin tonic herbs such as Rehmannia Endurance, again with chrysanthemum flower tea. During the colder seasons one might use more warming tonics containing astragalus, ginseng, codonopsis and dang quai in a formula such as Ginseng Revitalizer formula. Throughout the year one would alternate use of Reishi Mushroom Supreme or Shiitake Mushroom Supreme. Triphala and Bupleurum Liver Cleanse are useful to take periodically throughout the year as well.

As much as possible, based on palatability and taste, herbs can be integrated with food throughout the year. Turmeric, for instance, has powerful anticancer and liver detoxifying properties and is used alone or combined with other herbs to form a curry mixture. Garlic is regularly consumed in Mediterranean cultures not only for flavor but to promote health. In China, tonic herbs such as codonopsis and astragalus roots, together with various seeds such as lotus, Euryale seed and coix (pearl barley) seeds and fungi including shiitake mushrooms and various other mushrooms with known therapeutic properties are cooked with food. These may be prepared with the morning rice porridge (congee) or in soups.

It is more effective to take the more tonic herbs 20 to 30 minutes before meals and the more eliminative herbs after meals. The tonic herbs may potentiate digestion and assimilation while the eliminative herbs tend to be more harmonious after meals. However, for convenience, a single formula combining both can be taken at once.

Individuals should be encouraged to purchase the herbs they are likely to use regularly by the pound. They may also be purchased in the form of 5 to 1 concentrated dry granules. These are then cooked or added to morning cereals, soups and stews.

Many of the qi regulating herbs such as orange or tangerine peel serve as digestive carminatives and can be combined to aid digestion. Cardamon seed, ginger, garlic and many of the other spices can be used in a similar way to aid digestion of both food and the heavier, hard to digest tonic herbs. Sea vegetables can certainly be added to soups or toasted and crushed as a delicious, mildly salty condiment.

All of the more eliminative anticancer herbs can be taken together with the blood moving, phlegm clearing, qi regulating and tumor softening herbs after meals. The calm spirit or sedative herbs can be taken sometime between meals, especially a half hour or so before retiring to bed in the evening.

The most important categories to be represented for the treatment of all types of cancers are 1) the immune tonics, 2) the anticancer herbs and 3) the blood moving herbs. The other categories may be represented to greater or lesser degree according to each patient.

Finally, there are various herbs that seem to have a particular affinity for specific cancers associated with specific internal organs and/or bodily areas. Some of these are as follows:

Lungs – Black nightshade, Mullein, Herba solani lyrati, Fructificatio lasiopherae seu calvatae

Spleen-pancreas – Radix sophorae

Liver – Calculus bovis, Radix sophorae, Herba solani lyrati

Urinary system – Chapparal, coix, cleavers, houttuyniae, leonurus, lindera

Stomach – Radix sophorae, Radix paridis, Herba oldenlandiae, Herba solani lyrati

Large intestine – Rhubarb, coix, coptis, goldenseal, lonicera, partriniae

Esophagus – Rhizoma balamcandae, Radix sophorae, Herba scutellariae barbatae, Rhizoma paradis, Fructificatio lasiopherae seu calvatae

Nasopharyngeal – Fructus xanthii, Rhizoma paradis

Brain – Rhizoma paridis

Lymphoma – Rhizoma paridis

Pharyngeal – Fructificatio lasiopherae seu calvatae

Tongue – Fructificatio lasiopherae seu calvatae

Various cancers – Herba scutellariae barbatae, flos lonicera, spica prunella

Following are some examples of the use of the Six Methods for the treatment of specific cancers. Choose one to three herbs in each category:

Lung Cancer

Tonics	Astragalus root Cordyceps Ophiopogon Coix
Anticancer Herbs	Black Nightshade Agrimony Garlic or apricot seed Houttuyniae or Lonicera
Moving Blood	Salvia Tienchi ginseng
Regulating Qi	Lindera Bupleurum Nux vomica 30X
Clearing Phlegm	Pinellia or arisaematis
Dissolving Lumps	Seaweeds Bombyx Prunella

Liver Cancer

Tonics	Milk thistle seeds Lycii berries Shiitake mushroom Reishi Mushroom
Anticancer Herbs	Bupleurum Dandelion Andrographis
Moving Blood	Salvia Sparganium
Regulating Qi	Nux vomica 30X Turmeric Qing Pi Citrus Bupleurum
Clearing Phlegm	Arisaematis or pinellia
Dissolving Lumps	Seaweeds Bombyx Prunella

Prostate Cancer

Tonics	Saw Palmetto Poria Reishi Mushroom Maitake Mushroom
Anticancer Herbs	Andrographis Burdock Dandelion Coptis
Moving Blood	Corydalis Tienchi ginseng Zedoaria
Regulating Qi	Cyperus Turmeric Nux vomica 30X potency
Clearing Phlegm	Pinellia or Arisaematis
Dissolving Lumps	Seaweeds Violet Bombyx

Breast Cancer

Tonics	Cordyceps Reishi Mushroom Coix Asparagus root
Anticancer Herbs	Bupleurum or Dandelion Burdock root Red clover Andrographis
Moving Blood	Salvia Leonurus Tienchi
Qi Regulating	Bupleurum Turmeric Nux vomica 30X
Clearing Phlegm	Pinellia Fritillaria

Breast Cancer (continued)

Dissolving Lumps	Seaweeds Prunella Violet

Endnotes

[1] Meyer F., "Dietary fat and prostate cancer survival." Cancer Causes Control 1999 Aug;10 (4):245-251

[2] Djuric, Z., "A clinical trial to selectively change dietary fat and/or energy intake in women: the women's diet study." Nutr Cancer 1999;34(1):27-35 Barbara Ann Karmanos Cancer Institute, Wayne State University, Detroit, MI 48201, USA. djuricz@karmanos.org.

[3] De Stefani, E.; Mendilaharsu, M.; Deneo-Pellegrini, H.; Ronco, A., "Influence of dietary levels of fat, cholesterol, and calcium on colorectal cancer." Nutr Cancer 1997;29(1):83-9

[4] Millet, J.; Jouault, S.C.; Mauray, S.; Theveniaux, J.; Sternberg, C.; Boisson, Vidal C.; Fischer, A.M., "Antithrombotic and anticoagulant activities of a low molecular weight fucoidan by the subcutaneous route." Laboratoires Fournier, Dijon, France. j.millet@fournier.fr, Thromb Haemost 1999 Mar;81(3):391-5

[5] Zhuang, C., Itoh, H., Mizuno, T., Ito, H., "Antitumor active fucoidan from the brown seaweed, umitoranoo (Sargassum thunbergii)." Biosci Biotechnol Biochem 1995 Apr;59(4):563-7 United Graduate School of Agricultural Sciences, Gifu University (Shizuoka University), Japan.

[6] Jimenez-Escrig, A.; Goni Cambrodon, "Nutritional evaluation and physiological effects of edible seaweeds." Departamento de Metabolismo y Nutricion, Instituto del Frio, CSIC, Universidad Complutense de Madrid, Espana. Arch Latinoam Nutr 1999 Jun;49(2):114-20.

[7] Yan, X.; Nagata, T.; Fan, X., "Antioxidative activities in some common seaweeds." National Food Research Institute, Tsukuba, Ibaraki, Japan, Plant Foods Hum Nutr 1998;52(3):253-62

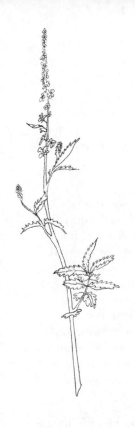

CHAPTER SIX

MATERIA MEDICA

Agrimonia eupatoria / Xian He Cao
Common Name: Agrimony

Family:	Rosaceae
Part used:	Aerial portions and the root
Energy and flavor:	Neutral to warm and slightly bitter
Organ meridians affected:	Lung, liver and spleen
Type of cancer:	For various types of cancer including cancer of the liver, lungs, breast, abdomen, esophagus and bone
Actions:	It is alterative, detoxifying, astringent, analgesic, anti-parasitic, hemostatic and is useful for all types of abnormal bleeding as well as diarrhea and dysentery. The ashes are particularly effective for bleeding.
Indications:	For hemorrhage, low blood pressure, abdomi-

nal distention, regurgitation, dysphagia, throat inflammation, pulmonary abscess, hemorrhoid, hematemesis, and dissolving abdominal mass.

Contraindications: Not for an individual with acute inflammatory symptoms.

Dose: 10-15g

Biochemical constituents: Tannins, bitter glycosides, coumarins, flavonoids, nicotinic acid amide, silicic acid, polysaccharides, vitamins B and K, iron and essential oil. Agrimony has at least six biochemical constituents that have demonstrated anticancer properties. These include catechin, which is antileukemic, cancer preventive and immuno-stimulant, quercitin which is antioxidant, antimutagenic, and anti-tumor and ursolic acid which is antileukemic, anti-lymphomic, anti mutagenic and anti-tumor for the breast, lung, stomach and colon.

Other information: It was reported in the Japanese Journal of Pharmaceutics (Vol. 2, 1980) and later confirmed with Chinese research that the root contained 11 antineoplastic constituents. Research on mice has found it to be effective for sarcoma-180 and Ehrlich's ascites carcinoma. It promotes the growth of normal cells and generally strengthens the body's immunity. It is highly esteemed by the Chinese and Japanese as a treatment of tumors of cancer, though not for leukemia. It dissolves tumors, normalizes circulation, promotes the growth of healthy cells and relieves pain. It also enhances the anti-tumor properties of other herbs such as black nightshade.

For cancer of all types, especially bone cancer:

Ping Xiao Dan Formula

Make pills of the following: Herba agrimoniae, semen strychni, alumen, curcumen root, faeces trogopterori, immature bitter orange, Lacca sinica exsiccata (*Shaanxi Traditional Chinese Medicine* Vol. 6, 1983). Take 4 to 8 pills (0.5g each) three times daily.

For various types of cancer except leukemia:

Herba agrimoniae:	30g
Herba solani lyrati: (or black nightshade)	25g
Semen arecae:	9g
Licorice:	3g

Slowly simmer everything in four cups of water down to two cups. Consume one cup morning and evening.

Akebia trifoliata / Ba Yue Zha
Common Name: Akebia vine fruit

Family:	Lardizabalaceae
Part used:	The fruit
Energy and flavor:	Neutral and bitter
Organ meridians affected:	Liver and stomach
Type of cancer:	Breast and digestive tract tumors
Actions:	Diuretic, opens the liver, dissolves lumps and nodules, and promotes urination.
Indications:	Used for chest pains and hernia pain as well as swollen glands and tumors.
Contraindications:	Not for pregnant women or individuals with a tendency to frequent urination or lack of energy. Aristolochic acid found in akebia has been found to cause pulmonary-cardiac arrest so that it should be used starting with a small dose and gradually increasing to the full-indicated dose according to the patient's tolerance.
Dose:	6-12g
Biochemical constituents:	Akebin, hederageanin, oleganolic acid, aristolochic acid, oleanolic acid, hederagenin, calcium, tannic acid

Other information: Aristolochic acid is the first nitro-compound from the plant kingdom that has demonstrated anti-tumor properties. It is often used in combination with chemotherapy and radiation for the treatment of cancer. It also increases white blood cell count.

Allium sativum / Da Suan
Common Name: Garlic

Family:	Liliaceae
Part used:	The bulb
Energy and flavor:	Warm and spicy
Organ meridians affected:	Lungs, spleen, large intestine and stomach
Type of cancer:	Lungs and gastrointestinal
Actions:	Relieves food poisoning, digestive, expectorant, moves blood and is a parasiticide.
Indications:	1) For all kinds of intestinal parasites as well as parasites in other areas of the body including the vagina and skin; 2) for food poisoning from shellfish; 3) improves appetite; 4) decongests the lungs; 5) removes parasites; 6) promotes circulation, clears the veins and arteries and assists the heart.
Contraindications:	Those with yin deficiency and heat signs should not use this herb. It should not be applied topically for long periods of time as it destroys tissue.
Dose:	6-15g
Biochemical constituents:	Alicin and various sulfur compounds

Other information: Garlic has powerful digestive, antiinflammatory and moving properties. Because of its moving properties, it aids the digestion of all foods and helps to break up the formation of boils, furuncles, other nodules and tumors. The same circulatory properties of garlic help to relieve all types of pains and stop bleeding. Garlic is also effective in improving cardiac function and lowering cholesterol.

A garlic suppository may be made by bruising a fresh clove of garlic and wrapping it with a thin cotton cloth saturated with olive oil. When inserted into the rectum each night it may be used for constipation, parasites and intestinal cancer. When inserted into the vagina, it may be used for various abnormal conditions including cervical dysplasia and uterine cancer. Be sure to leave a portion of the cloth extruding from the orifice for easy removal each morning. Be careful to use enough olive oil to prevent irritation from the garlic. Many Chinese clinical experiments have attested to the anticarcinogenic properties of garlic for many types of cancer. In one experiment, female rats who were fed fresh garlic were immune to breast cancer.

For lung cancer and various other cancers: Take 10 to 30 ml of fresh squeezed garlic juice daily with finely chopped fresh parsley leaves, beer yeast and a drop of peppermint oil.

For leukemia as well as lung cancer: The sublingual vein (under the tongue) is pricked and fresh garlic is rubbed directly on it.

For cancer prevention: Take fresh garlic daily (*Bulletin of Traditional Chinese Medicine, Vol. 6, 1974*).

Lip cancer: In 1958, Russian doctors reported treating 194 patients with lip cancer of which 184 were cured. One method is to simply rub fresh garlic on the affected area several times each day. Garlic may be steamed or fermented to help neutralize the enzyme responsible for the smell. Fermented and deodorized garlic is widely sold by the Japanese as Kyolic and has been proven to be as effective as the fresh variety. One study done by a Japanese researcher involved injecting millions of cancer cells into mice. Absolutely no tumors developed thus resulting in a 100% effectiveness-rate against the development of cancer.

Aloe Vera
Common Name: Aloe

Family:	Aloeceae, Liliaceae
Part used:	The gel of the leaf
Energy and flavor:	Cold and bitter
Organ meridians affected:	Liver, heart and spleen
Type of cancer:	Gastrointestinal and adjunctively for other cancers
Actions:	Vulnerary, laxative and cholagogue
Indications:	Externally for burns, abrasions; internally for ulcers, hepatitis and constipation
Contraindications:	None noted
Dose:	Of the gel and liquid – two tablespoons three times daily in juice
Biochemical constituents:	Polysaccharides, emodin, two aloins, glucomannans, anthraquinones, glycoproteins, sterols, saponins and organic acids

Other information: Even though the direct effects of aloe against cancer seem to be inconclusive, it is useful indirectly to support the immune system and counteract inflammation. It is widely used both internally and topically to offset the negative effects of radiation.

Alumen / Ming Fan
Common Name: Alum

Energy and flavor:	Cold, sour and astringent
Organ meridians affected:	Lung, liver, spleen and large intestine
Type of cancer:	Stomach and abdominal cavity
Actions:	1) Stops itching, relieves damp-heat inflammation and kills parasites; 2) stops bleeding; 3) relieves diarrhea, leukorrhea, anal prolapse; 4) clears heat and relieves wind-phlegm.
Indications:	Hemafecia, serious productive cough, laryngeal and nasal infections, hemorrhoid, tinea, polyps of ear and nose, otitis media, fester of the eye, hepatitis and cancer. 1) Applied topically for damp-heat itching and rashes and infestation of parasites; 2) for blood in the stool, uterine bleeding as well as applied topically for all kinds of bleeding; 3) for chronic diarrhea; 4) for wind-phlegm conditions with symptoms such as convulsions, irritability and difficulty in expectorating sputum.
Contraindications:	This herb should only be used when there is dampness or heat, and used with caution when taken internally.
Dose:	1-3g internally, taken with boiled water
Biochemical constituents:	It is derived from natural alum, namely potassium aluminium sulfate, extracted in Hubei, Anhui, Zhejian and Fujian Provinces.

Other information: Chinese research has found it to have a 90% inhibition rate on JTC-26 type of cancer.[1] For stomach cancer 9g of alumen powder is boiled with 180g of white vinegar for 5 minutes. This is taken internally for the treatment of stomach cancer.[2] For external tumors combine equal parts powder of alumen and Realgar with enough flour and water to make a paste and apply externally (this should never be taken internally).

Andrographis Paniculata / Chuan Xin Lian
Common Name: Andrographis, Green chiretta

Family:	Acanthaceae
Part used:	The aerial portions
Energy and flavor:	Cold and bitter
Organ meridians affected:	Lung, stomach, large and small intestines
Type of cancer:	Gastrointestinal, prostate and breast cancer, Hodgkin's disease, leukemia, melanoma and non-Hodgkin's lymphoma
Actions:	Clears heat, reduces fever, detoxifies, reduces inflammations, relieves pain, reduces swelling. This is one of the more important Chinese anti-cancer herbs, as it promotes phagocytosis, helping break down tumors as well as preventing metastasis.
Indications:	It is used for asthma, lung abscess, sore throat, clears purulent sputum, gastrointestinal inflammations and genito-urinary tract infections. It is used for bacillary dysentery, gastroenteritis, common cold, tonsillitis, pneumonitis, wound infection, pulmonary tuberculosis, and snakebites.
Contraindications:	Because it is very cold and bitter, it can injure stomach qi. For this reason it is best used in formulas with herbs that help protect stomach qi. It is abortive so should not be used by pregnant women.
Dose:	9-15g or 1 to 2g in powder form
Biochemical constituents:	Andrographalide, 14-deoxyandrographolide, neoandrographalide, 14-deoxyandrographolide, b-sitosterol, and other flavonoid type of compounds.

Other information: This is one of the most popular herbs for treating a wide variety of inflammatory conditions in China, India and Thailand. It has broad-spectrum anti-bacterial and anti-viral properties and at the same time has liver protecting properties. For the treatment of infections it promotes phagocytosis. Thus far, animal studies reveal its ability to prevent the proliferation of cancer. For trophoblastic tumors, andrographis has shown the ability to solidify the cytoplasm and nucleus of cancer cells and induce retrograde variations such as breaking down and dissolving. Despite all of this, it is very low in toxicity.

A study in January of 1999, initiated by Paracelsian, Inc., conducted at Roswell Park Cancer Institute in Buffalo, New York, confirmed andrographalide from andrographis to have significant anti-cancer activity against a human breast cancer cell line. Most interesting, it was found to be even more effective than the well-known anti-cancer drug Paclitaxel (tamoxifen) and to have a strong effect against multi-drug resistant tumors (Minyi). Andrographis has selective cytotoxic effects against cancer cells that further inhibit the proliferation of various types of cancers.

Arca granosa / We Leng Zi
Common Name: Clam shell

Family:	Arcidae
Part used:	The shells
Energy and flavor:	Neutral, sweet and salty
Organ meridians affected:	Liver and spleen
Type of cancer:	Various types including cervical cancer and hysteromyoma
Actions:	Moves blood, regulates and moves qi, dissolves phlegm, and dissipates nodules including immobile and mobile abdominal masses such as fibroids. It is also anti-acid and relieves ulcer pains and acid regurgitation.
Indications:	It is used for fibroids, gynecological and abdominal tumors as well as gastrointestinal ulcers.
Contraindications:	None noted
Dose:	9-15g of the decoction of the crushed shells. For stomach acidity calcine the powdered shells.
Biochemical constituents:	Calcium carbonate, trace amounts of magnesium, iron, and sodium phosphate

Arctium lappa / Niu Bang Zi
Common Name: Burdock

Family:	Compositae
Part used:	The root and seeds
Energy and flavor:	Cold, bitter and acrid
Organ meridians affected:	Lungs, pharynx and stomach
Type of cancer:	Various types of cancers including breast, lungs and gastrointestinal
Actions:	Detoxifying, diuretic, nutritive and des-mutagenic (prevents cellular mutation). Anti-pyretic resolving masses and lumps, removing the stagnation of qi in the viscera. It is used to clear fever and dispel wind (spasms and the proliferation of pathogenic influences).
Indications:	For sore throat, skin rashes, eczema, other skin diseases, swelling, constipation and fever.
Contraindications:	Not for a person with diarrhea
Dose:	3-9g. For cancerous edema 60g is fried and pulverized for the oral administration or 6g taken three times daily. Doses of the root often combined with the seed range from 9 to 30g daily.
Biochemical constituents:	Among its constituents are arctiin, fatty oil, sterol and vitamin A and B in the seeds and leaf. The root has proteins, mucilage and inulin. The leaf contains 5% inulin, mucilage and tannins.

Other information: This is a common herb distributed widely throughout diverse areas of the world. The whole plant is used, but predominantly the root and seed. In Japan the root is cultivated and prized as a vegetable called "gobo." The saponins that naturally occur in burdock help to regulate blood sugar, suggesting that the herb has a deeper endocrine activity. Because of its diuretic properties, it is used for edema associated with cancer and lymphoma. For cancerous edema 60g of the seeds are fried and pulverized for oral administration, 6g taken three times daily.

A constituent of both the Hoxsey and the Essiac formula, in 1984 Japanese researchers at Kawasaki Medical School in Okayama discovered an antimutagenic factor that was resistant to both heat and protein digesting enzymes that they called the "burdock factor." It was also found to be effective in the test tube against the HIV virus. Benzaldehyde, one of the constituents of burdock, demonstrated anticancer effects in humans. Some animal studies have confirmed the effectiveness of burdock on various cancers while others have shown none.

The root was official in the United States Pharmacopoeia in 1830 and from 1850-1900. The Eclectics used it as an alterative, diaphoretic, diuretic and laxative. As an alterative, anti-cancer and anti-arthritic and anti-rheumatic herb, a decoction is made by boiling an ounce of the dried root in a pint of water. Three cups are taken regularly each day. The most active properties of burdock are best extracted in water. While the root is effective for skin complaints, the crushed seeds that have diaphoretic properties to aid in discharging toxins through the pores of the skin are more commonly used for practically all chronic and acute skin affections.

A patient, who at the time of my meeting her was in her early 90's, reported how she had been diagnosed with cancer (unspecified) over 25 years previous. It had evidently metastasized at least several times over the last 25 years. Whenever she would suspect or notice tumors coming up she would drink a quart of strong burdock root tea daily until the tumor disappeared.

Arisaematis, Arisaema consanguineum / Tian Nan
Common Name: Jack in the pulpit

Family:	Araceae
Part used:	The rhizome (Rhizoma)
Energy and flavor:	Warm, toxic, bitter and acrid
Organ meridians affected:	Lung, liver and spleen
Type of cancer:	Mainly for cancer of the liver and breast.
Actions:	1) Dries and expels phlegm in the lung; 2) clears wind and phlegm in the channels and stops convulsions and spasms; 3) used topically it reduces inflammation and pain.
Indications:	1) For cough and stifling sensation in the chest with excessive phlegm; 2) for phlegm and wind in the channels with symptoms of high fever, convulsions, paralysis, stroke and lockjaw; 3) for topical application on abscesses, traumatic injuries and tumors.

Contraindications:	This herb should not be used during pregnancy or by those with yin deficient cough with dry phlegm. Its raw, unprepared form is very toxic.
Dose:	4-9g internally of the prepared rhizome. In this dose it should only be used when it is prepared with alum and ginger to detoxify it. Otherwise in raw form only take 0.3 to 1.0g daily.
Biochemical constituents:	Triterpenoid saponin, benzoic acid, starch, amino acid

Other information: Chinese research has demonstrated that it has a 50% to 70% inhibition rate against JTC-26 cancer cells. In mice it inhibits sarcoma-180 and sarcoma-37.[3]

Asparagus cochinensis / Tian Men Dong
Common Name: Ornamental asparagus root

Family:	Liliaceae
Part used:	The root
Energy and flavors:	Cold, sweet and bitter
Organ meridians affected:	Lung and kidneys
Type of cancer:	Breast, lung and leukemia
Action:	It nourishes yin fluids, especially of the lungs and expectorates phlegm and dampness.
Indication:	For yin deficiency, night sweats, muscular degeneration, dry throat, blood in the sputum and constipation.
Contraindications:	Not for symptoms of diarrhea or symptoms of cold and dampness.
Dose:	6-24g

Other information: Research has shown it to inhibit sarcoma-180 and leukemic cells in mice. It also supports and prolongs the cancer antibody to counteract cancer and inhibit the growth of human cancer cells. It is particularly useful for lung and breast cancer.

Astragalus membranicus / Huang Chi
Common Name: Astragalus

Family:	Leguminosae
Part used:	Root (Radix)
Energy and flavor:	Warm and sweet
Organ meridians affected:	Lung and spleen
Type of cancer:	It is used to tonify the immune system for all types of cancers and for patients undergoing conventional Western medical treatment.
Action:	1) Tonifies the wei qi and stops perspiration; 2) tonifies the spleen qi and the yang qi of the Earth element; 3) tonifies the qi and blood; 4) expels pus and assists in the healing of wounds; 5) helps to regulate water metabolism in the body and reduces edema.
Indication:	1) For deficiency of the wei qi and the lungs (since the wei resides in the lungs) with symptoms of frequent colds and flus, shortness of breath, spontaneous sweating and night sweats; 2) for deficiency of the Earth element with symptoms such as lack of appetite, prolapse of internal organs, diarrhea, fatigue and uterine bleeding; 3) for recovery from severe blood loss and postpartum bleeding; 4) for chronic abscesses and ulcers resulting from deficiency; 5) for chronic damp-heat in the kidneys due to deficiency with associated edema.
Contraindications:	This herb should not be used for cases of excess or deficiency of yin with heat signs and should not be used when there is stagnation of qi or dampness, especially when there is painful obstruction.
Dose:	9-30g, although much more can be used when indicated.
Biochemical constituents:	Choline, folic acid, beta sitosterol, polysaccharides, trace elements and iodine.

Other information: While astragalus fails to destroy cancer cells directly, it has been proven to stimulate the production of interferon. It is specific to counteract the immune damaging effects of chemotherapy and is an important ingredient in cancer formulas requiring tonification of energy, stimulation of the immune system and many other conditions.

The alkaloid "swainsonine" is derived from a form of astragalus oxyphysus and has been found to inhibit metastasis of melanoma in mice. Scientists at Howard University's Cancer Center added swainsonine to the drinking water of mice with lung tumors. Within 24 hours it had inhibited 80% of the tumor colonies in their lungs. It was concluded that this was caused by the effect of the alkaloid increasing Natural Killer (NK) cells that fight cancer. Swainsonine has also been found to stimulate spleen cells to exercise an anti-metastatic effect.

Admittedly the astragalus membranaceus is a different species but the overall effect between this and A. oxyphysus in stimulating and modulating the immune system to indirectly fight cancer is similar.

Atractylodes macrocephela / Bai Zhu
Common Name: White atractylodes

Family:	Compositae
Part used:	The root
Energy and flavors:	Warm, sweet and bitter
Organ meridians affected:	Spleen and stomach
Type of cancer:	It is useful for all types of cancer associated with dampness, poor appetite and low energy.
Actions:	1) Tonifies the spleen qi; 2) fortifies the spleen yang and dispels damp; 3) tonifies qi and stops sweating; 4) calms restless fetus when due to deficiency of spleen qi.
Indications:	1) For spleen qi deficiency with symptoms of lack of appetite, chronic diarrhea, fatigue, vomiting and abdominal distention; 2) for edema caused by retention of fluids and lack of urination; 3) for spontaneous sweating caused by deficiency of qi; 4) for restless fetus when caused by deficiency of spleen.
Contraindications:	This herb should not be used by those with yin deficiency with heat signs or with extreme thirst.
Dose:	3-9g

Atractylodes macrocephela (continued)

Biochemical constituents: Atractylone, atractylol and vitamin A

Other information: It tonifies qi, promotes appetite and clears dampness. Research has found it to inhibit cancer growth, increase white blood cell count and promote phagocytosis.

Baptisia Tinctoria
Common Name: Baptisia, Wild indigo

Family:	Leguminosae
Part used:	The bark
Energy and flavor:	Extremely cold, toxic and bitter
Organ meridians affected:	Liver and blood
Type of cancer:	Many types, but especially breast cancer
Actions:	Clears heat, antiinflammatory, antipathogenic, antiseptic, emmenagogue, emetic.
Indications:	Putrid infections, blood poisoning, meningitis, sore throat, swollen glands and malignant sores.
Contraindications:	Not to be used during pregnancy, or in acute conditions of coldness and deficiency.
Dose:	Of the powdered bark, 1-4g; of the 1:5 tincture, 10-20 drops
Biochemical constituents:	Baptitozine (baptisine), two glucosides, baptin, a cathartic and a yellowish resin.

Other information: Eli Jones recommends it during the last stage of cancer when there is great prostration, fetid smell, and the tongue is a dirty yellow color, dry and cracked. He recommends five drops of the tincture every two hours. It is commonly combined with echinacea for infections and inflammations. For cancer it can be combined with poke and thuja.

Belamcanda chinensis / She Gan
Common Name: Blackberry lily

Family:	Iridaceae
Part used:	Rhizome
Energy and flavor:	Cold, bitter

Organ meridians affected:	Lungs
Type of cancer:	Cancer of the pharynx and lungs
Actions:	It clears heat, treats acute sore throat, clears phlegm and lowers the qi.
Indications:	Especially useful for sore throat, acute tonsillitis, acute laryngitis, cough with thick yellow phlegm.
Contraindications:	Not for pregnant women or individuals with weak digestion.
Dose:	6-9g
Biochemical constituents:	Belamcandin, iridin, tectoridin, tectorigenin and mangiferin.

Berberis vulgaris, Mahoniae, folium / San K'e Chan
Common Name: Barberry

Family:	Berberidaceae
Part used:	Rhizomes and stems as well as the dried leaves
Energy and flavor:	Cold and bitter
Organ meridians affected:	Liver, stomach and colon
Types of cancer:	Liver, pancreas, gallbladder, stomach, reproductive organs, intestines and lungs
Actions:	Antipyretic, detoxifying, anti-inflammatory, anti-bacterial and stimulates digestion
Indications:	For acute gastroenteritis, gingivitis, laryngitis, conjunctivitis, boils, jaundice, hepatitis, diabetes, abscesses, ulcers, burns, inflammatory arthritic and rheumatic complaints, traumatic injuries and as a treatment and cure for pulmonary tuberculosis. It is used similarly to another berberine containing Chinese herb, phellodendron amurense (Huang Bai) in that it is anti-inflammatory and can be used for fever caused by weakness and deficiency (yin deficiency).
Contraindications:	Caution with conditions of cold deficiency.
Dose:	The average dose is 15 to 30g taken in two or three divided doses daily.

Berberis vulgaris (continued)

Biochemical constituents: It contains palmatine and berberine, both chemical constituents known to have anti-neoplastic properties.

Bombyx Batryticatus / Jiang Can
Common Name: Silkworm

Family:	Bombycidae
Part used:	Dried larvae of the silkworm
Energy and flavors:	Neutral, acrid and salty
Organ meridians affected:	Liver and lung
Type of cancer:	Cancer of the throat, lungs and liver.
Actions:	1) Antispasmodic, subdues internal wind; 2) expels wind and stops pain; 3) clears toxins and dissipates nodules.
Indications:	1) It is used for childhood convulsions, Bell's palsy, epilepsy and tetanus; 2) effective for migraine headaches, sore throat, conjunctivitis and eye pains as well as rheumatic pains; 3) can be used for toxic swellings and swollen glands.
Contraindications:	Traditionally it is contraindicated with platycodon (Jie Geng), poria (Fu Ling), dioscorea hypoglaucae (Bei Xie), and Ootheca mantidis (Sang Piao Xiao).
Dose:	3-10g; as a powder only 0.9 to 1.5g are taken
Biochemical constituents:	Fat, protein, destruxin, organic acids, chitinase, bassianins, fibronolysin and beauverician

Other information: It has been found to inhibit sarcoma 180 in mice and also to inhibit the growth of human liver cancer cells in vitro.[4]

Brucea javonica / Ya Dan Zi
Common Name: Brucea

Family:	Simarubaceae
Part used:	Fruit and seeds
Energy and flavor:	Cold, bitter and toxic in high sustained dosage
Organ meridians affected:	Liver and large intestine
Type of cancer:	It is especially useful for rectal cancer and leukemia.
Actions:	1) Reduces fever and clears toxins; 2) clears amoebic dysentery and chronic dysentery caused by cold; 3) treats malaria 4) applied externally for warts.
Indications:	1) For fever due to toxic buildup; 2) for chronic dysentery caused by stagnation and cold, also for dysentery caused by amoebas and protozoas; 3) for malaria where there is alternating chills and fever; 4) apply as an ointment for warts, corns; 5) for vaginal parasites use as a douche or wash.
Contraindications:	This herb should not be used during pregnancy. It is a gastrointestinal irritant and contraindicated for individuals with digestive weakness, nausea or vomiting. It should not be used for extended periods of time, and should be used with great caution for children.
Dose:	10 to 30 fruits
Biochemical constituents:	It contains dosamine, formic acid, bruceoside, fatty acid, brusatol and bruceine A, B, C, and GMS.

Other information: The seeds can be crushed and mixed with sesame oil or water and topically applied to papillomas, melanomas and other types of external cancers. A hot water preparation is the most effective. For colorectal cancer the seeds can be pounded and decocted for use as an enema (*Zhejiang Journal of Traditional Chinese Medicine*, Vol. 2, 1980). For squamous epithelial cancer of the external auditory meatus the brucea fruits are wrapped in longan berries and 9 grains are taken 3 times the first week, 10 the second, 11 the third, 12 the fourth and 15 the fifth week. At the same time it is ground and mixed with vaseline and applied over the affected area daily.

Bupleurum chinensis / Chai Hu
Common name: Bupleurum, Hare's ear

Family:	Umbelliferae
Part used:	The root (Radix)
Energy and flavor:	Cool, acrid and bitter
Organ meridians affected:	Liver, gallbladder, pericardium and triple warmer.
Type of cancer:	Liver, spleen, lungs, reproductive organs and abdomen.
Actions:	1) Relieves fever associated with lesser yang diseases; 2) moves the liver qi and relieves liver qi stagnation; 3) lifts the yang qi of the spleen and stomach.
Indications:	1) For successive fever and chills associated with lesser yang diseases accompanied by a bitter taste in the mouth, irritability, vomiting or congested feeling in the chest; 2) for liver qi stagnation with symptoms of menstrual difficulties, mood swings, dizziness or pain in the chest or flanks; 3) for prolapse of anus or uterus due to deficiency of the yang qi of the spleen or stomach; 4) for diarrhea due to deficient spleen qi.
Contraindications:	Those with yin deficiency should not use this herb nor should it be used with symptoms of extreme headaches or inflammatory eye diseases such as conjunctivitis caused by liver fire.
Dose:	3-12g
Biochemical constituents:	Saikosaponins

Other information: Bupleurum saponins have shown the ability to lesson cell-adhesive ability in the proliferation and development of cancer cells.[5,6]

Buthus Martensi / Quan Xi
Common Names: Scorpion

Family:	Buthidae
Part used:	The whole insect
Energy and flavors:	Neutral, pungent, sweet and toxic in higher doses
Organ meridians affected:	Liver
Types of cancer:	Wide variety of cancers but especially brain, liver, lung, breast and intestines
Actions:	1) Antispasmodic, subdues internal wind; 2) clears toxins; 3) stops pain.
Indications:	1) Stops tremors and convulsions in conditions such as opisthotonos, tics, and epilepsy; 2) detoxifies sores, swellings and swollen glands; 3) opens the channels and stops pain for the treatment of stubborn headaches such as migraines and other wind damp pains.
Contraindications:	It is toxic and overdose should be avoided. It should not be used in patients with blood deficiency. It is contraindicated during pregnancy.
Dose:	2 to 5g or 0.6-1g of the powder
Biochemical constituents:	It contains buthotoxin, a sulfurous toxic protein similar to the neurotoxin of snakes; lecithin, trimethylamine and taurine.

Other information: 1) For spasms, rigidity, muscle twitches throughout the body and convulsions, combine with centipede (Wu Gong) and uncaria (Gou Teng); 2) for stubborn or migraine headache and rheumatic pain combine with Silkworm (Jiang can), centipede (Wu Gong) gastrodia (Tian Ma) and ligusticum (Chuan Xiong); 3) for cancer and tumors make into a powder and combine 2g each of buthus (Quan Xie), Silkworm (Jiang Can) and scolopendra (Wu Gong) in a cloth bag suspended in water while cooking an egg. The egg is eaten and the broth is taken as a tea.

Celandine (Chelidonium majus)
Common Name: Greater celandine

Family:	Papaveraceae
Part used:	The aerial portions
Energy and flavor:	Cold and bitter
Organ meridians affected:	Liver, gall bladder and large intestine
Type of cancer:	Liver and gastrointestinal type cancers
Actions:	Alterative, diuretic, purgative, antispasmodic, diaphoretic, anodyne, antitussive, narcotic and mildly toxic
Indications:	Liver congestion, hepatitis, gall bladder disease and candida (tea from the dried herb)
Contraindications:	Not for an individual with a cold condition and diarrhea.
Dose:	Of the dried herb take 1 or 2g three times daily. Of the 20% tincture take 5 to 15 drops three times daily. Overdose can be toxic.
Biochemical constituents:	Various alkaloids, including berberine, coptisine, choline, dihydrosanguinarine, histamine, sanguinarine, formic acid, nicotinic acid, citric acid, malic acid, succinic acid and flavonoids. It has at least six biochemical constituents known to be anticancer.

Other information: One of the most common European folk treatments for various types of cancers. In the late 20th century it was one of two ingredients in the anticancer remedy called Ukrain. The other substance in Ukrain is a chemotherapeutic drug called thiotepa (thiosphosphoric triazidine). When the alkaloids of chelidonium are purified and combined with thiotepa it creates a unique and effective substance that has a strong affinity to selectively kill cancer cells. Ukrain is an important, relatively non-toxic drug that has been shown to be medically effective for a wide variety of solid and non-solid cancers. In one study on 70 cancer patients (age 14 to 80 years) conducted by the Ministry of Science and Research in Austria, Ukrain was highly effective in even advanced metastatic cancers. It seemed to induce cell death (apoptosis) of cancer cells by degrading the permeability of the cell surface. It was also found to fragment the DNA of cancer cells. These findings have been confirmed by the NCI (National Cancer Institute).

While Ukrain is extremely safe, patients with cancer tend to experience a temporary reaction of an increase of pain, rise of body temperature (between 102.2 to 104.4 degrees) tiredness and fatigue, swelling over the tumor area, hot and cold bodily reactions. When this occurs it is considered a favorable reaction. Ukrain is indeed one of the most promising and effective western chemotherapeutic drugs for a variety of cancers and represents a unique example of integrative medicine at its best. For more on Ukrain, I recommend reading Ralph Moss's excellent book, *Herbs Against Cancer* (Equinox Press, 1998).

For stomach cancer: Make a Decoct of 2.5g each of the aerial portion of the dried chelidonium herb, rhubarb root and slippery elm bark in water. This is taken three times daily.

Other uses for Greater celandine include:

1) The fresh juice applied topically is a well-known treatment for warts and other excrescences on the skin; 2) has been found to inhibit sarcoma-180 and Ehrlich's ascites carcinoma of mice but with a high level of toxic side effects; however, a 40% alcoholic extract of the whole herb is anticarcinogenic with little toxic reactions; 3) effective for gastrointestinal ulcers and pain; 4) effective when topically applied for the treatment of tinea and scabies.

Centella Asiatica
Common Name: Gotu Kola

Family:	Umbelliferae
Part used:	The aerial portions
Energy and flavor:	Cool energy, mildly bitter and sweetish
Type of cancer:	Various types
Actions:	Alterative, antipyretic, antiinflammatory, vulnerary, immuno-modulatory tonic
Indications:	Used for skin diseases including leprosy, wound healing, burns, ulcers and improving mental function. A recent in vitro study[7] has found that an extract of Centella exhibited anticancer, antiinflammatory and long-term immuno-modulatory effects. In addition, long term use is indicated for wound healing, radiation burns (may also be topically applied), to relieve pain, counteract ulcers and hepato-protection.
Contraindications:	None noted

Centella Asiatica (continued)

Dose: Steep 1–2 U.S. teaspoons (5–10g) in 1 cup of boiling water for ten to fifteen minutes. Drink three cups per day. Tincture is approximately 1 teaspoon three times daily. Standardized extracts of Gotu kola containing up to 100% total triterpenoids are generally taken as 60 ml once or twice per day.

Chaparral / Larrea tridentata
Common Name: Creosote Bush, Gobernadora, Hediondilla

Family:	Zygophyllaceae
Part used:	Leaves and terminal stems
Energy and flavor:	Cool, bitter, acrid and slightly salty
Organ meridians affected:	Liver
Type of cancer:	Various types of cancers
Actions:	Alterative, antibacterial, anti-bilious, anticancer, antifungal, antimicrobial, antiparasitic, antiseptic, antispasmodic, anti-tubercular, antitumor, carminative, diuretic, emetic, expectorant, lymphatic alterative, powerful antioxidant, radiation damage preventative, reduces LDL levels, respiratory alterative and tonic properties.
Indications:	Used as a blood purifier, for cancer and tumors, antioxidant, for arthritic and rheumatic conditions, sciatica, colds, flu, skin conditions including abscesses, boils, acne, psoriasis, eczema, diarrhea, and various infections including genito-urinary tract infections.
Contraindications:	Lactation, liver conditions (cirrhosis, hepatitis), pre-existing kidney disease and pregnancy.
Dose:	3-6g in decoction, of the 1:5 in 75% alcohol, dose; 20-60 drops up to 3x/day
Biochemical constituents:	Its most characteristic constituent is NDGA (Nordihydroguaiaretic Acid).

Other information: Studies seem to be mixed regarding its antioxidant and antitumor properties. However, numerous anecdotal reports substantiate the value of chaparral for the treatment of cancer.

The natives of southern California traditionally use chaparral tea to prevent and treat a wide variety of diseases including cancer. Researchers experimented by applying benzyl peroxide (BPO), a powerful carcinogen, to the skin of mice that were prone to developing cancer. They found that NDGA was effective in preventing the development of cancer cells. It was concluded that the potent antioxidant properties of chaparral were responsible for inhibiting the generation of cancer cells that would arise as a result of exposure to BPO. The well-documented and dramatic anticancer effect from the use of chaparral was that of an 85-year-old man who had undergone four operations for malignant melanoma of the right cheek. Each time after the operation the cancer would reappear. Dr. Charles Smart of the University of Utah, who documented that the tumor was 3 to 4 centimeters, attended him. Because the previous operations failed to fully prevent the recurrence of the melanoma, the patient returned home and decided to take chaparral tea. He brewed 7 to 8g of the leaves to a quart of hot water and drank 2 to 3 cups daily. He began taking chaparral tea in November of 1967 and by February 1968 the facial lesion had reduced to a fraction of its original diameter. In September 1968, the lesion shrank to 2-3 millimeters and the masses in his neck were completely gone. Further, his general health improved and he gained 25 pounds. Dr. Smart and his colleagues decided to study 59 cancer patients who were given chaparral tea. Of these, 45 completed the study and four showed significant tumor regressions while two others had striking degrees of tumor regressions. Some, however, had an acceleration of tumor growth. As a result, while the report of the 85-year-old man with melanoma is of significance, the subsequent study with various types of cancers was essentially inconclusive. From an herbalist's perspective, this is not surprising since the use of one herb to treat a condition such as cancer, which has a wide degree of constitutional and individual manifestations, is "shotgun" herbalism and would be inconclusive. It is only when chaparral is combined with other herbs based on individual characteristics of each patient that its anticancer properties would be realized.

There are a handful of seemingly idiosyncratic reports of chaparral causing liver damage. This would suggest that patients who are at risk for liver disease, perhaps from prior alcohol and drug use or exposure to hepatitis viruses, should avoid the use of chaparral.

Citrus aurantium / Chen Pi
Common Name: Orange peel, Citrus peel

Family:	Rutaceae
Part used:	The peel
Energy and flavor:	Warm, spicy and bitter
Organ meridians affected:	Lungs and spleen
Type of cancer:	Most types of cancers
Actions:	It regulates qi and as such acts as a carminative, clears dampness in the lungs and reverses the upward flow of qi.
Indications:	It treats gastrointestinal fullness and is used for coughs caused by phlegm. It also treats hiccup, nausea and vomiting.
Contraindications:	Not for a person who is spitting blood or has symptoms of extreme dryness.
Dose:	3-9g
Biochemical constituents:	Essential oil (limonene, linalool, perpineol), hesperidin, carotene, cryptosanthin, vitamins B1 and C

Other information: The best quality is well aged. D-limonene, found as part of the oil of orange and other citrus fruits, is known to destroy and inhibit cancer cells and increase the beneficial effects of chemotherapy.

Modified citrus pectin is a water-soluble carbohydrate found in ripe fruits such as apples, grapefruits, and plums. It is most concentrated in citrus fruits and has many commercial uses.

In modified citrus pectin (MCP), the pH and polysaccharides have been altered to form groups of the simple sugar galactose. In making MCP, the carbohydrate chains are split into smaller pieces. MCP's source is the peel and membrane of citrus fruits. Studies have shown that rhamnogalacturonan found in MCP has a powerful effect in enhancing the cytotoxic ability of T-cells and Natural Killer (NK) cells in their ability to prevent metastasis. [8],[9],[10] In another study it was found that tangeretin and other flavonoids from tangerine peel neutralized the effect of tamoxifen. Tangeretin, on the other hand, showed no tumor inhibiting properties. This strongly suggests that tangerine, citrus peel extract and other flavonoids commonly found in herbs should not be used if one has decided to undergo tamoxifen therapy.

Citrus aurantium immaturus / Zhi Shi
Common Name: Immature bitter orange

Family:	Rutaceae
Part used:	The fruit
Energy and flavor:	Slightly cold, acrid, bitter and sour
Organ meridians affected:	Large intestine, spleen and stomach
Type of cancer:	Esophagus and stomach
Actions:	1) Stimulates digestion and breaks up stagnation through the gastro-intestinal tract; 2) moves qi downward and helps constipation; 3) reduces stagnant phlegm and lessens distention and pain.
Indications:	1) For pain and distention in the abdominal region, indigestion and gas; 2) for constipation caused by stagnation of qi; 3) for stifling sensation with fullness in the chest and epigastrium with a thick, sticky, yellow coat on the tongue caused by phlegm; 4) for prolapse of the stomach, rectum or uterus, only when in combination with the appropriate herbs.
Contraindications:	This herb should be used with caution during pregnancy, when there is qi deficiency or when there is cold in the stomach.
Dose:	3-9g
Biochemical constituents:	Volatile oils and resins

Other information: It dries and transforms congealed phlegm that obstructs the circulation of digestive qi. It is therefore important to use this herb with tonics that tend to contribute to damp stagnation.

Codonopsis lanceolata / Dang Shen
Common Name: Codonopsis

Family:	Campanulaceae
Part used:	The root
Energy and flavor:	Warm and sweet
Organ meridians affected:	Lungs and spleen

Codonopsis lanceolata (continued)

Type of cancer:	All types when there is qi deficiency
Actions:	Tonifies the spleen and lungs and assists in the production of fluids.
Indications:	Used for low energy, fatigue, poor appetite, weak digestion, chronic cough, shortness of breath, wasting and thirsting diseases and injury of bodily fluids. It generally is used like ginseng to enhance digestive metabolism and support the immune system.
Contraindications:	Caution for acute febrile conditions.
Dosr:	9-30g
Biochemical constituents:	Saponins, sacharides, protein and vitamin B

Other information: As a tonic, codonopsis is considered approximately half the strength of ginseng. Because of this, it is often substituted for ginseng in formulas. Its main indications are for digestive weakness, lung weakness and low energy. Two species are usually used for the formula, C. lanceolata and C. pilosulae. Both have been found to decrease leukocytes and increase erythrocytes (red blood cells) and hemochrome, which accounts for their tonic properties. However, C. lanceolata has been found to be the superior tonic for treating patients with qi deficiency. Generally, since both are sold interchangeably, it is not possible to specify a preference for a particular species.

The special area of use for codonopsis, or ginseng, for the treatment of cancer is when the disease is associated with a deficiency of qi and/or blood. For this indication, codonopsis is given in large doses, 30g with 20 to 30 jujube dates. For this purpose, other herbs such as astragalus and angelica sinensis (Dang Gui) are also used with it. One can add codonopsis to any formula for cancer when there is associated qi or blood deficiency.

Since it is a tonic, one might ask how it can contribute to any detoxifying effect? Toxicity can be a matter of either excess or deficiency. When the condition is one of excess, one would not use a tonic to promote detoxification. However, many individuals with cancer, because the condition is chronic, have associated chronic deficiencies. The body lacks the energy or reserves to maintain appropriate levels of detoxification. This is when codonopsis is to be considered. In such a depleted state, the individual may further lack sufficient capacity to utilize the active eliminative and detoxifying properties of other herbs in a formula. This is another use for codonopsis, to act as a catalyst to optimize the effects of other herbs. A third use for codonopsis, or nutritive tonics generally, is to offset the predominantly eliminative and therefore weakening effects of the primary therapy. Since weight loss and muscle atrophy is associated with advanced stages of cancer, codonopsis with jujube dates taken as a tea, or more effectively, cooked with nourishing foods such as grains or soups, is of great value.

Coix/Coicis lachryma-jobi / Yi Yi Ren
Common Name: Job's tears

Family:	Gramineae
Part used:	The seeds
Energy and flavors:	Slightly cool, sweet and bland
Organ meridians affected:	Spleen, stomach, kidney, lung and large intestine
Type of cancer:	Most types but especially the lungs, breast, stomach and large intestine
Actions:	1) Regulates water and encourages urination; 2) tonic to the spleen and stops diarrhea caused by spleen deficiency; 3) reduces inflammation and eliminates pus; 4) treats arthritic and rheumatic conditions, increasing joint mobility; 5) Expels damp-heat.
Indications:	1) For improper water metabolism with symptoms of edema, urinary difficulty, ascites and damp leg qi; 2) for spleen deficiency with diarrhea; 3) for abscesses of the lung and intestines as well as pus filled inflammations of the exterior; 4) for painful obstruction associated with wind and damp with symptoms of lack of mobility, inflammation and spasms; 5) for any kind of damp-heat with symptoms of digestive difficulty with a thick greasy tongue coating and a slippery rapid pulse; 6) for treatment of plantar warts.
Contraindications:	Pregnant women should not use this herb.
Dose:	9-30g
Biochemical constituents:	Coixol, coixenolide, vitamin B1, leucine, lysine and arginine.

Other information: Coix in Chinese is called Yi Yi Ren and is closely related to pearl barley, which is often substituted for it. Coix or pearl barley along

Coix/Coicis lachryma-jobi (continued)

with rice and various beans should form an important part of the diet of cancer patients. Coix has been found to change the nature of oncocytoplasm and stop the nucleodivision of the middle stage. The ester of coix has been synthesized to resist cancer. Extracts of the herb and seed have been found to inhibit ascites cancer and Yoshida's sarcoma.

For stomach and lung cancer: Yoshida's sarcoma and malignant reticular cellular hyperplasia: cook 30 to 59g of coix with glutinous rice and take once or twice daily throughout the year.

For uteromyoma: Grind 500g of coix with 150g of tienchi ginseng. Take 15g three times daily with boiled water.

For breast cancer: Decoct 15g of coix with 15g of corydalis in millet or rice wine and take on an empty stomach.

Stomach cancer:

Coix seed	15g
Wisteria stems	6g
Chebula fruit	6g
Trapae bispinosae	6g

Slowly simmer all ingredients in 4 cups of water down to two. Drink two cups daily.

Coptis chinensis / Huang Lien
Common Name: Coptis

Family:	Ranunculaceae
Part used:	The rhizome (Rhizoma)
Energy and flavor:	Cold and bitter
Organ meridians affected:	Heart, liver, stomach and large intestine
Type of cancer:	Most types of cancers, especially liver, pancreas, esophagus, breast, and large intestine
Actions:	1) Expels damp-heat especially in the lower burner; 2) eliminates fire toxicity especially when there is associated dampness; 3) as a sedative by eliminating heart fire; 4) eliminates stomach fire; 5) applied topically for damp-heat sores.

Indications:	1) For damp-heat in the lower burner, especially in the stomach and intestines, with symptoms of diarrhea, dysentery or vomiting associated with heat; 2) for patterns of fire toxicity with symptoms of high fever, conjunctivitis, irritability, a red tongue and a big rapid pulse; 3) for heart fire because of poor communication between the heart and the kidney with symptoms of insomnia, high fever, irritability and restlessness; 4) for stomach fire with symptoms of poor digestion with associated bad breath; sores and inflammation of the mouth and tongue; dental decay; 5) for damp-heat sores of the skin such as carbuncles, abscesses, sores of the mouth and tongue and red, swollen and painful eyes.
Contraindications:	This herb should not be used by those with stomach or spleen qi deficiency especially when there is diarrhea. It should not be used by those with yin deficiency when there is vomiting or nausea and cold.
Dose:	1-9g
Biochemical constituents:	Berberine, coptisine, columbamine, obakunone, obakulactone, jatrorrhizine, palmatrine, worenine, magnoflorine, and ferulic acid.

Other information: It expels damp heat, detoxifies the blood, has sedative properties, clears stomach fire and can be applied topically for oozing sores with pus. Its action is to inhibit the respiration of cells especially with a yellow enzyme (pus), which is also present to an extent in cancer cells. Its most prominent constituent is from 7 to 9% berberine, which has been found to inhibit the respiration especially of the more sensitive cancer cells and thus inhibit their growth. It inhibits JTC-26 in a culture medium as well as fibroembryocytes at the same rate.

This is one of a number of berberine-rich herbs that have anticarcinogenic properties. These include: Phellodendron (Huang Bai), barberry root and golden seal (Hydrastis).

Cordyceps sinensis / Dong Chong Xia Cao
Common Name: Cordyceps, Winterworm, Caterpillar fungus

Family:	Polyporaceae
Part used:	The fungus growing on the larva of a caterpillar and the mycelia
Energy and flavor:	Warm and sweet
Organ meridians affected:	Lungs and kidneys
Type of cancer:	Lungs, liver, breast, leukemia & other cancers
Actions:	Tonifies lungs and kidney-adrenals, stops cough and is anti-asthmatic. It is both immuno-stimulant and immuno-modulatory.
Indications:	Impotence, lumbago, night sweats, nocturnal emission, TB, chronic cough, spitting of blood and lung cancer.
Contraindications:	Because it is a tonic, it should not be used for someone with a cold, flu or fever.
Dose:	6-15g
Biochemical constituents:	Cordycepic acid, protein, cellulose, starch, saturated and unsaturated acid, vitamin B12

Other information: It has anti-inflammatory properties and at least three anti-tumor protein polysaccharides have been identified. It has been found to be useful for heart arrhythmias, lung cancer, chronic nephritis and kidney failure. Numerous studies have shown positive effects of cordyceps in increasing immune function, NK (Natural killer) cells against cancer and in inhibiting various types of cancer especially cancer of the lungs[11] and liver metastasis.[12] Studies have also exhibited its ability to treat the proliferation and differentiation of leukemic cells. Its tonic properties seem to be increased when it is cooked with duck.

Coriolus versicolor, Trametes versicolor / Yun-Zhi
Common Name: Turkey tails

Family:	Polyporaceae
Part used:	The fruiting body
Energy and flavor:	Slightly cold and sweet
Organ meridians affected:	Spleen and pancreas

Type of cancer:	For various cancers including leukemia
Actions:	Drains dampness, clears heat and detoxifies
Indications:	Edema and weak digestion
Contraindications:	None noted
Dose:	3-9g divided in two doses daily
Biochemical constituents:	One of the highest known sources of polysaccharides. Its two principle constituents are PSK or Krestin and a polysaccharide-peptide consisting of 10% peptides and 90% polysaccharides.[13]

Other information: This mushroom, common throughout the world, has been shown to resist cancer by strengthening the immune system. At the same time it has the ability to inhibit the growth and spread of various cancers. For a malignant tumor take 3 to 6g of the powder twice daily. PSK has powerful antioxidant properties and patients given 3g of PSK per day were shown to have increased interferon production.[14]

The Polysaccharide-peptide (PSP) of Coriolus versicolor extracted from the mycelia has been shown to be effective against cancer in both animal and human patients. Results of recent experiments suggest that PSP may act by 1) potentiating T-cell mediated cytotoxicity; 2) definite concentration of PSP produced direct cytotoxic activity in vitro; 3) Induction of tumorcidal macrophages killed more cancer cells.[15]

Corneum gingeriae galli, C. stomachichum galli / Ji Nei Jin
Common Name: Inner lining of the chicken gizzard

Family:	Phasianidae
Part used:	Gizzard lining
Energy and flavor:	Neutral and sweet
Organ meridians affected:	Small intestine, bladder, spleen and stomach
Type of cancer:	Esophagus, stomach and heart
Actions:	Removes food stagnation, aids digestion and dissolves urinary stones
Indications:	Counteracts the negative effects including nausea, vomiting, indigestion and malnutrition caused by the use of strong aggressive drugs, herbs and other substances.
Contraindications:	None noted

Corneum gingeriae galli (continued)

Dose:	1.5 to 3g as often as needed
Biochemical constituents:	Ventriculin, keratin, bilatriene and vitamins B1 and B2

Other information: Best when combined with other digestive herbs including radish seed, cardamon, hawthorn berry and ginger. For cardiac cancer, burn corium stomachichum galli and take 3g each time with rice wine (*Prescriptions Worth a Thousand Gold*). It benefits the transportive function of the spleen and promotes digestion, appetite and the growth of new tissues including the muscles and bones. Patent formula with similar effects.

Curcuma Aromatica / Yu Jin
Common Name: Yu Jin Turmeric

Family:	Zingiberaceae
Part used:	The tuber
Energy and flavor:	Cold, acrid and bitter
Organ meridians affected:	Liver, lung, heart and gallbladder
Type of cancer:	Liver, gall bladder and pancreas
Actions:	Moves blood, relieves stagnation, especially of the liver and heart and cools the blood.
Indications:	Pain from trauma, chronic sores, anxiety, seizures and jaundice
Contraindications:	Caution during pregnancy
Dose:	3-9g
Biochemical constituents:	Curcumin, demethoxycurcumin, turmerone and carvone

Other information: Has been used successfully to treat viral hepatitis. Studies on humans at risk of palatal cancer due to smoking tobacco showed that turmeric (1 gram/day) for 9 months had a significant impact on the regression of precancerous lesions. Previous studies have shown that curcumin causes an increase in glutathione S- transferase (GST) activity in rodent liver, which may contribute to its anti-cancer and anti-inflammatory activities.

Curcuma longa, Radix Curcumae / Jiang Huang
Common Name: Turmeric

Family:	Zingiberaceae
Part used:	The rhizome
Energy and flavor:	Acrid and bitter. Depending on its use this herb can be classified as both warm and cool.
Organ meridians affected:	Liver and spleen
Type of cancer:	Liver, gall bladder, pancreas and reproductive organs
Actions:	Activates the circulation of vital energy, dispels stasis, promotes the function of liver and lung and brightens the mind.
Indications:	Poor liver function, chest pain and pain along the ribs, stomach distension, jaundice, fever, hematemesis, hematuria, epilepsy, menorrhagia, menoxenia, carbuncle and productive cough with low fever.
Contraindications:	Do not use during pregnancy, or if there is blood deficiency with no symptoms of blood and qi stagnation.
Dose:	Each decoction consists of 4.5 to 15g
Biochemical constituents:	Essential oil, curcumin, arabinose, fructose, glucose, fatty oil, starch and camphor

Other information: Its volatile oil exerts a beneficial effect by causing the gall bladder to contract and secrete. It has also been found to inhibit fungi, which cause skin diseases. Both curcumin and genistein have been shown to exert synergistic inhibitory effects on the growth of human breast cancer MCF-7 cells induced by estrogenic pesticides.[16] Mechanism of inhibition of benzo[a]pyrene-induced for stomach cancer in mice by dietary curcumin[17]. Turmeric as part of one's diet has demonstrated effective antioxidant properties useful for the prevention and treatment of various types of cancer.[18]

Curcuma Zedoaria / E Zhu
Common Names: Zedoaria

Family:	Zingiberaceae
Part used:	The rhizome

Curcuma Zedoaria (continued)

Energy and flavors:	Warm, spicy and bitter
Organ meridians affected:	Liver and spleen
Types of Cancer:	Abdomen, cervix, uterus, breast, testicles, liver and pancreas
Actions:	Promotes blood circulation, emmenagogue, relieves pain, helps digestion and is an anti-carcinogenic.
Dose:	4-9g
Contraindications:	Not for someone with deficiency of qi and blood, spleen and stomach.
Biochemical constituents:	Includes zedoarone, curcumin, curcumol and curdione

Other information: Zedoaria has shown an inhibitory effect on sarcoma 180 in mice. It has also been used to treat early stage cervical cancer.[19] The Chinese have injected the volatile oil directly into tumors, which resulted in their necrosis eventually sloughing off. Zedoaria has also been found to increase phagocytosis and the immune system generally.

Cyperus rotundus / Xiang Fu
Common name: Nutgrass

Family:	Cyperaceae
Part used:	The root
Energy and flavor:	Neutral, acrid, bitter and sweet
Organ meridians affected:	Liver, triple burner and stomach
Type of cancer:	Cancer of the digestive tract, uterus, ovary and for the relief of pain
Actions:	1) Unblocks stagnant liver qi and relieves pain; 2) regulates the liver and spleen; 3) assists the regulation of menses and relieves pain.
Indications:	1) For stagnant liver qi causing pain and distention in the epigastic region; 2) for aggressive liver qi that attacks the spleen with symptoms of abdominal distention and acid and food regurgitation; 3) for painful menstruation as well as lack of menstrual flow and irregular menstruation; 4) breast masses,

swollen breasts, especially around the time of menstruation.

Note: Because of the neutral property of this herb it is very widely used.

Contraindications: This herb should not be used when there is yin or qi deficiency especially when there is heat associated with the condition.

Dose: 4-12g

Biochemical constituents: Essential oils (B-pinene, camphene, limonene, 1, #9-cineole, p-cymene, cyperene, selinatriene, B-selinene, patchoulenone, A-cyperone, B-cyperone, A-rotunol, B-rotunol, cyperol, isocyperol, copadiene, epoxyguaine, cyperolone, rotundone, kobusone, isokobusone, glucose, fructose and starch.

Dionae muscipula
Common Name: Venus flytrap, Carnivora®

Dr. Helmut Keller, M.D., an oncologist and medical director of the Chronic Disease Control and Treatment Center in Bad Steben, Germany, first studied the Venus' flytrap at Boston University in 1980. In order to find more support and freedom for his research he moved to Germany a year later. Carnivora® is a drug derived from the sterilized fresh juices of the Venus flytrap, which is native to the wet pinelands and sandy bays of North and South Carolina. Dr. Heller claims promising therapeutic results from its use for a variety of conditions including various types of cancer. Proponents of Carnivora® claim that it works to shrink solid tumors, but has no effect on non-solid cancers such as leukemia. It also stimulates the immune system to assist its anticancer properties. They also believe that it works best for those individuals who have not undergone chemo or radiation therapy.

In one study of 210 cancer patients who had failed conventional treatments and were given 50-60 drops of Carnivora® orally 5 times a day plus one injection, 16% showed tumor remission, 40% had no further tumor progression, and 43% showed no improvement in tumor size but about 25% had a palliative response, such as subjective relief of pain, increase in appetite, vitality, and positive attitude.

Another study of 57 patients with an average age of 51 and malignancies or chronic immune disorders took 2ml of Carnivora® daily for 116 days; 57% reported improvement in their condition, 25% showed no change,

Dionae muscipula (continued)

and 18% worsened.

President Ronald Reagan, following the surgical removal of malignant polyps from his colon used Carnivora®. The purpose was prophylactic against the cancer's spread. He drank the recommended 30 drops of Carnivora® extract in a glass of purified water or herb tea four times a day.

Besides its use for cancer, Dr. Keller has found that Carnivora® is effective in treating a variety of other immune deficient conditions including ulcerative colitis, Crohn's disease, rheumatoid arthritis, multiple sclerosis, neurodermatitis, chronic fatigue syndrome, HIV infection, and certain kinds of herpes. It is also recommended as an adjunct to strengthen the effects of antibiotics.

Carnivora® can be administered as drops orally, by inhalation or by injection. Laboratory studies indicate that purified Carnivora® is safe, and its new drug application is pending approval by the German Food and Drug Administration. It is readily available for application to patients by physicians in Germany and other European countries. It remains unapproved by the U.S. Food and Drug Administration (FDA), however, and cannot be imported or used legally except by people suffering from life-threatening illnesses such as cancer and AIDS.

Side effects: Taken orally without dilution, Carnivora® can sometimes produce nausea or vomiting; when injected, it can produce a temporary increase in body temperature. Ninety-day studies with rats in which the rodents received doses 30-60 times higher than the recommended human dose reported no toxic reactions.

Carnivora® is available as drops or injectable ampules from Carnivora-Forschungs-Gmbh®, Postfach 6, Lobensteiner Strasse 3, D-96365, Nordhalben, Germany; Tel: 09267-166; Fax: 09267-1040.

Other information: According to Donny Yance,[20] it apparently contains the same active constituents as sundew (Drosera rotundiflora), which is easier to find and less expensive.

Duchesnea indica / She Mei
Common Name: False strawberry

Family:	Rosaceae
Part used:	The whole herb
Energy and flavor:	Cool, slightly toxic, sweet and sour
Organ meridians affected:	Liver and gastrointestinal

Type of cancer:	Cancer of the vocal cords, thyroid, lungs, stomach, nasopharynx, cervix, liver & chest
Actions:	Antipyretic, anti-inflammatory, antibiotic, anti-swelling and dispels blood stagnation.
Indications:	It is used for a wide variety of inflammatory conditions ranging from influenza, fever, cough, to sore throat, hepatitis, bacillary and amebic dysentery and menorrhagia. It is also used for a wide variety of cancers.
Contraindications:	Not for pregnant women, or individuals with a cold and deficient tendency.
Dose:	30g in decoction
Biochemical constituents:	Not known

Other information: For cancer of the stomach, nasopharynx, lungs, cervix and breast combine duchesnea 30g, scutellaria barbata 30g and Livistonia chinensis 30g in decoction. Divide into two or three doses and take daily.

Chinese research has found it to inhibit various types of cancers and it also increases white blood cell count.

Echinacea species (E. angustifolia, E. purpurea, E. pallida)
Common Name: Echinacea, Black sampson, Prairie coneflower

Family:	Compositae
Part used:	The root and aerial portions
Energy and flavor:	Cool, bitter and pungent
Organ meridians affected:	Lungs and liver
Type of cancer:	Various types of cancers
Actions:	Immune-modulatory, detoxifying, antiinflammatory, and analgesic
Indications:	Infections, inflammations and to relieve pain
Contraindications:	None noted
Dose:	For acute conditions, 30 to 60 drops of the liquid extract (1:1 or tincture 1:5) every two hours, tapering off as symptoms subside. For chronic conditions as an immune stimulant, 15 to 30 drops three times daily.
Biochemical constituents:	Essential oil, polysaccharides, echinacoside, (a triglycoside of caffeic acid derivative only

found in E. angustifolia and E. pallida), echinacein and other constituents.

Other information: Echinacea is primarily effective for infections and inflammations that occur secondary to many cancers. Since these can present serious life-threatening complications with cancer, this can be a significant benefit. The other use for echinacea is as an immune modulatory agent. It is known to stimulate T-cell activity, interferon, natural killer cells and tumor killing phagocytotic macrophages. Topically it can be applied as a poultice, fomentation or powder directly to promote healing of infections and inflammations.

One study found that a combination of echinacein, an extract from E. purpurea, with cyclophosphamide and thymostimulin to be of benefit to patients with far advanced colorectal cancers.[21]

Eleutherococcus Senticosus
Common Name: Siberian ginseng

Family:	Araliaceae
Part used:	The root bark
Energy and flavor:	Warm and sweet
Organ meridians affected:	Liver and kidneys
Type of cancer:	All types
Actions:	Adaptogenic, energy tonic, antirheumatic and antispasmodic
Indications:	Low energy and increasing endurance
Contraindications:	None noted
Dose:	3-15g; of the 1:5 tincture, use 15 to 30 drops two or three times daily.
Biochemical constituents:	Eleutherosides, essential oil, resin, starch and vitamin A

Other information: It increases endurance and strengthens the immune system specifically by increasing T-cell lymphocytes.[22] It has also shown anti cancer activity in experiments on mice. [23,24,25]

Emblica officinalis (Phyllanthus emblica)
Common Name: Amla or Amlaki

Family:	Combretaceae
Part used:	The fruit
Energy and flavor:	Cool, sour and astringent
Organ meridians affected:	Liver and lungs
Type of cancer:	Liver, lung and other cancers
Actions:	Detoxifying, nutritive tonic, astringent, cholagogue and a mild laxative
Indications:	Detoxifies and protects the liver and gastrointestinal tract; skin diseases, diabetes, anemia, loss of appetite, inflammatory conditions, hemorrhage, diarrhea, jaundice, bronchitis, asthma, stimulates libido and dries mucus.
Contraindications:	None noted
Dose:	6-30g
Biochemical constituents:	Vitamin C and tannins

Other information: Much more research is warranted with this wonderful herb, which is the highest known natural source of non-degradable vitamin C. In the system of East Indian Ayurvedic medicine, it is considered a supreme tonic, especially for the liver. It is one of the three fruits in Triphala preparation. The other two include chebulic myrobalan, discussed in this section for its anticarcinogenic properties, and beleric myrobalans. One study found that emblica officinalis, phyllanthus amarus and picrorrhiza kurroa had an anticarcinogenic effect on rats with induced liver cancer.

Faeces Trogopterorum / Wu Ling Zhi
Common Names: Trogopterus dung, Pteropus excrement

Family:	Pteropodidae
Part used:	The excrement
Energy and flavor:	Moderate, bitter, sour, pungent, sweet, and poisonless
Organ meridians affected:	Liver and spleen
Type of cancer:	Liver, spleen, reproductive organs, pancreas and abdomen

Actions:	Promotes circulation of blood and qi, removes blood stasis and relieves pain.
Indications:	For amenorrhea, dysmenorrhea, abdominal pain and retention of the placenta, infant maldigestion, hernial pain, stabbing pain, pain caused by stagnation or obstruction, scabies and bites by insects and snakes.
Contraindications:	Not for those with symptoms of anemia with blood stagnation. Traditionally ginseng is claimed to counteract it, though this may not be true according to contemporary research.
Dose:	3-9g
Biochemical constituents:	Resin, urea, uric acid and vitamin A

Other information: It relaxes spasms of smooth muscle and destructs tubercle bacillus and fungus that causes skin diseases.

Foeniculum vulgare / Xiao Hui xiang
Common Name: Fennel seeds

Family:	Umbelliferae
Part used:	The seeds
Energy and flavor:	Warm and pungent
Organ meridians affected:	Spleen, stomach, liver and kidney
Type of cancer:	Cervical and stomach cancer
Actions:	Analgesic, dispels cold, carminative; regulates qi and relieves pain.
Indications:	It is used for abdominal pain with distension and cold stagnation, nausea, vomiting and loss of appetite. It is also used to relieve testicular pain and the pain of hernias.
Contraindications:	Not for someone with yin deficiency with symptoms of acute inflammation.
Dose:	3-8g
Biochemical constituents:	Essential oil, fatty oils, stigmasterol and 7-hydroxycoumarin

Other information: It increases white blood cell count.

Fritillaria Cirrhosae / Chuan Bei Mu
Common Name: Fritillaria

Family:	Liliaceae
Part used:	The bulb (Bulbus)
Energy and flavor:	Cold, sweet and bitter
Organ meridians affected:	Heart and lung
Type of cancer:	For cervical, breast and lung cancer
Actions:	1) Clears Hot phlegm and stops cough; 2) clears lung heat caused by yin deficiency; 3) clears heat and reduces hard lumps and swellings.
Indications:	1) For thick yellow sputum with or without blood streaks that is difficult to expectorate; 2) for lung yin deficiency with fire where there is dry cough and little sputum; 3) for conditions of phlegm-fire where there is hard swelling, scrofula, or lung or breast abscesses.
Contraindications:	Those with cold-damp phlegm conditions should not use this herb.
Dose:	3–9g
Biochemical constituents:	Fritimene, fritiminine, sonpeimine and sipeimine

Other information: It has a downward dispersing energy and as such eliminates toxicity.

Fritillaria thunbergii / Zhe Bei Mu
Common Name: Fritillaria

Family:	Liliaceae
Part used:	The bulb (Bulbus)
Energy and flavor:	Cold, bitter and sweet
Organ meridians affected:	Lung and heart
Type of cancer:	Lung, breast and liver
Actions:	1) Clear phlegm-heat and stop cough; 2) reduces swellings caused by phlegm-fire; 3) transforms qi.

Fritillaria thunbergii (continued)

Indications:	1) For acute lung heat with symptoms of productive cough with thick yellow sputum; 2) for swelling and abscesses of the neck and lung where there is a pattern of phlegm-fire.
Contraindications:	This herb should not be used when there is cold and damp phlegm.
Dose:	3-9g
Biochemical constituents:	Its main components are alkaloids.

Other information: The fresh herb is toxic and should never be used without first being processed.

Galium aparine
Common Name: Cleavers

Family:	Rubiaceae
Part used:	The aerial portions
Energy and flavor:	Slightly cold, mild, sweet and spicy
Organ meridians affected:	Liver and bladder
Type of cancer:	Lymphomas, leukemia, liver, breast, lung, colon, urinary and reproductive systems cancers.
Actions:	Clears heat, diuretic and promotes blood circulation
Indications:	Used for urinary infections, detoxification and lymphatic congestion.
Contraindications:	Not for cold, deficient conditions
Dose:	45g
Biochemical constituents:	Asperuloside, rubiadinprimveroside, galiosin and 2-2-Dimethyl napthol (1,2b) pyran, coumarins, citric acid and tannins all of which have shown anticancer activity.

Other information: It is particularly used for non-solid tumors such as leukemia and soft lumps such as malignant lymphomas. This is because of its lymphatic detoxifying properties widely acknowledged by both eastern and western herbalists. Research has found that it inhibits the growth of oncocytes as well as sarcoma-180 in mice and leukemia.

For breast cancer: Decoct 30g of the herb in water, add brown sugar and take 3 to 6 times daily. The juice of 250g of the fresh herb can be combined with brown sugar and taken similarly. This method is particularly favored as most potent by western herbalists. The herb can also be steamed and made into a poultice or strong decoction for fomentation and applied topically for cancerous ulceration of the breast, vulva and penis. The decoction can be freely and often used as a gargle for glossocancer and gingival cancer. Research has found that it inhibits the growth of oncocytes as well as sarcoma-180 in mice and leukemia.

For leukemia:

Herba galii aparine	45g
Caulis lonicerae	30g
Herba scutellariae barbatae	30g
Herba solani nigri	30g
Rx salviae miltiorrhizae	30g
Hb dichondrae	15g
Rhz polygonati	15g

For malignant lymphoma:

Hrb galii	60g
Hrb solani nigri	120g
Hrb oldenlandiae	250g

For visceral and mammary cancer: 150g of the herb is pounded into a juice and taken orally, or 30g are taken in decoction.

Topically 120g of the herb can be pounded and mixed with lard and applied topically to cure breast cancer. It should also be taken orally at the same time. Decoct 30g of the herb in water, add brown sugar and take 3 to 6 times daily.

Ganodermum lucidum / Ling Zhi
Common Name: Reishi mushroom

Family:	Polyporaceae
Part used:	The fruiting body
Energy and flavors:	Warm and sweet
Organ meridians affected:	All meridians
Type of cancer:	All cancers

Ganodermum lucidum (continued)

Actions:	Calming, tonifying, sedative and replenishes vital essence and energy
Indications:	Tonifies the immune system, inhibits cancer, vitalizes, calms the spirit, treats altitude sickness and chronic bronchitis.
Contraindications:	None noted
Dose:	9-30g. This herb should be broken and boiled for hours to extract its active properties.
Biochemical constituents:	Contains ergosterol, fumaric acid, aminoglucose, mannitol, and the latter, coumarins, alkaloids, lactone and diverse enzymes.

Other information: As with other medicinal mushrooms, this herb is rich in polysaccharides that increase white blood cells; it serves as a potent free radical scavenger and generally exerts broad anticancer and antitumor properties. Reishi contains the immune stimulating polysaccharide, beta D-glucan, which has been shown to be effective against sarcoma 180.[26] The polysaccharide stimulates macrophage activity to produce tumor-necrosis factor (TNF-a), together with cancer killing interleukins.[27] In another study the polysaccharides (PS) from fresh fruiting bodies of G. lucidum (PS-G) were isolated and used to potentiate cytokine production by human monocytes-macrophages and T lymphocytes. Results demonstrated that the levels of interleukins (IL)-1 beta, tumor necrosis factor (TNF)- alpha, and IL-6 in macrophage cultures treated with PS-G (100 micrograms/ml) were 5.1, 9.8 and 29 fold higher, respectively, than those of untreated controls. In addition, the release of interferon (IFN)- gamma from T lymphocytes was also greatly promoted in the presence of PS-G (25-100 micrograms/ml). Furthermore, these cytokine-containing mononuclear cell-conditioned media (PSG-MNC-CM) suppressed the proliferation of both the HL-60 and the U937 leukemic cell lines. Further, a process of DNA labeling was able to induce cell death (apoptosis) only of cancer cells. [28,29]

Besides its anti-tumor and immuno-modulatory properties, reishi also helps counteract stress.[30] The crude extract of reishi has been found to be more effective in fighting free radical damage than isolated, synthetic compounds. Reishi also contains bitter triterpenes. These strengthen the circulatory and immune systems, tone the liver and protect the body from physical stress. Triterpenes work as adaptogenics, antihypertensives and to control allergic reactions.

Studies done at the Cancer Research Center in Moscow have found reishi to act as a host defense protector. It helps the body to fight cancer and slow down tumor growth. It helps to reinforce the membrane of the cancer cell to help prevent its spreading. It also diminishes the side effects of chemotherapy.

Its major action is to powerfully increase immunological function and raise the quantity of leukocytes. It is especially effective when used with chemotherapy. It both augments the effect of the chemotherapeutic agent and at the same time strengthens the immune system. For various types of cancer 15 to 20g is decocted in three cups of water and taken three times daily.

Fu Zhen Therapy is used before, during or after chemotherapy. The following formula with ganoderma was used to arrest bone marrow cancer and stimulate immunological function following chemotherapy:

Ganoderma	9g
Codonopsis	9g
Astragalus	9g
White peony	9g
Saussurea	9g
Caulis spatholobi	12g
Herba Bidens triparititae	15g

These were made into a powder and taken daily in two separate doses. (*Shanghai Journal of Medicinal Herbs, Vol. 1*, 1980). Combine ganoderma with ginseng, astragalus and lycii berries for Fu Zhen therapy to strengthen the immune system and inhibit the growth of cancer cells.

Ginkgo biloba
Common Name: Ginkgo, Maidenhair tree

Family:	Ginkgoaceae
Part used:	The leaves and nuts
Energy and flavor:	Neutral, bitter and astringent. The nuts are mildly toxic
Organ meridians affected:	Lungs and kidneys
Type of cancer:	All types
Actions:	Promotes blood circulation
Indications:	Used for all circulatory disorders, including memory enhancement, tinnitus, coldness, arthritic and rheumatic conditions, arteriosclerosis, eye weakness and vertigo.
Contraindications:	Care should be exerted on patients who are on other blood thinning medications, includ-

Ginkgo biloba (continued)

	ing aspirin. Other possible but rare adverse reactions include dermatitis, irritability, restlessness, diarrhea and vomiting.
Dose:	This should only be taken in its standard extract form of 50:1 concentration.
Biochemical constituents:	Flavonoids, including quercetin, isorhamnetine and other glycosides, proanthocyanidins and nonflavonoid terpenes, bilobalide and gingkolides A, B and C, lignans; essential oil and tannins.

Other information: Chinese research has found that the use of blood moving herbs such as gingko with either chemotherapy or radiation actually enhances the therapeutic benefit of these therapies.[31] They do this by increasing tumor blood flow generally, which allows for more efficient exposure to the chemotherapeutic agents or radiation. Others herbs in this category include panax pseudoginseng, salvia milthiorrhiza, angelica sinensis, ligusticum wallichii, trifolium pratense etc. and all herbs that would classify as emmenagogue or menses inducing herbs. Chinese theory also believes that promoting circulation diminishes the tendency towards metastasis by making the blood less viscid.

Another study found that ginkgo biloba extract (GBE) exerted a protective effect on cisplatin-induced toxicity in rats. This included various side effects such as hearing loss, hair loss and kidney damage.[32]

Gleditsia sinensis / Xao Jiao Ci
Common Name: Honey locust spine

Family:	Leguminosae
Part used:	Spine or thorn
Energy and flavor:	Warm and pungent
Organ meridians affected:	Lung and large intestine
Type of cancer:	Breast, lung and cancer of the large intestine and nasopharyngeal carcinoma
Actions:	Reduces inflammation and clears purulence. It also alleviates itching.
Indications:	Used for purulent inflammation, skin diseases and tonsillitis.
Contraindications:	Not for use during pregnancy.

Dose: 3-9g

Biochemical constituents: Flavone, phenol and amino acid

Other information: Chinese research has shown that the hot water extract has been able in vitro to exert about a 50-70% growth rate on JTC-26. It has also been shown to inhibit sarcoma in rats. For mammary abscess, administer both topically as well as internally about 3g of the charred herb along with dry fried rhubarb root after each meal.

Glycyrrhiza species / Gan Cao
Common Name: Licorice

Family: Leguminosae

Part used: The root

Energy and flavor: Neutral and sweet

Organ meridians affected: All 12 meridians

Type of cancer: Various types, especially gastrointestinal and lung

Actions: 1) Tonifies the basal qi and nourishes the spleen qi; 2) clears heat and dispels toxicity; 3) moistens the lungs; 4) relieves spasms and alleviates pain; 5) harmonizes and moderates herbs in formulas.

Indications: 1) For deficiency of spleen qi with symptoms of shortness of breath, diarrhea, fatigue, palpitations and irregular pulse caused by either qi or blood deficiency; 2) for fire and toxicity with symptoms of sore throat, carbuncles or sores, it can be used both internally and externally for these symptoms; 3) for either heat or cold in the lungs with symptoms of dry cough and wheezing; 4) mildly relieves spasm and thus pain in the abdomen or legs; 5) used in many formulas to harmonize and moderate the action of the other herbs.

Contraindications: Licorice should not be used when there is excess dampness, nausea or vomiting and generally should be used with caution by those who tend to retain water.

Dose: 2-9g in a decoction

Glycyrrhiza species (continued)

Biochemical constituents: Glycyrrhizin and glycyrrhetinic acid

Other information: As with rehmannia root, licorice is often used in two forms. Unprepared licorice is less tonifying while licorice that has been heated with honey is warmer natured and used more as an energy tonic. It has a neutral to warm energy depending on the form that is used. It is tonic, demulcent, expectorant and alterative. It has similar properties to hydro-cortisone and is often used in formulas and for patients to ameliorate or prevent adverse reactions to the primary herbs in formula. As such it is colloquially called "the peacemaker" herb. Licorice is also an analgesic pain reliever. This gives it a good usage for the non-drug relief of pains associated with cancer.

Because of its protective effects, licorice is used prophylactically to prevent damage to the liver and other internal organs. It can also be taken with stronger and harsher anticancer drugs and therapies to lessen any negative reaction or damage. Licorice has been found to have a 70-90% cancer inhibitive effect on cancer cells with little effect on normal cells. This corroborates closely with its known historical usage as a protective herb.

Both glycyrrhetinic acid and glycyrrhizin have been found to have anticancer properties in various animal studies on mice.

For stomach cancer:

Licorice root	2g
Fresh ginger	4g
White peony root	6g
Jujube dates	15 pieces
Unrefined sugar	20g

Slowly simmer the first four herbs in 4 cups of water, down to three. Then dissolve the sugar into the final liquor. It should be divided in three doses and taken three times daily.

For esophageal cancer:

Licorice root	2g
Ginseng	2g
Ophiopogonis	2g
Pinellia root	5g
Rice	5g
Jujube dates	10 pieces

Slowly simmer in 6 cups of water down to four. Take one cup three times during the day and one at night before retiring.

For tongue cancer: Make a thick decoction of unprocessed licorice and gargle with it several times daily while it is still warm.

For lung cancer: Chang Minyi has found that patients with lung cancer experienced a dramatic improvement with high dosages of 9-12g of licorice taken with other herbs in decoction. He describes a formula published in the *New Edition of Mei's Proved Recipes* for mastocarcinoma:

Trichosanthes fruit (peeled)	2g
Licorice root	15g
Dang gui steamed with wine	15g
Olibanum (Frankincense)	4.5g
Myrrh	4.5g

The herbs are finely powdered and macerated in about 3000 ml of rice wine each night before retiring. One third or 1000 ml of the preparation is simmered and taken warm three times daily.

Contraindications: Licorice has a very low toxicity, however, long-term high dosage use may be associated with edema and hypertension. Patients with hypertension and signs of fluid retention should be carefully monitored when using licorice.

Grifola frondosus
(Boletus frondosus, polyporus frondosus) / Zu Ling
Common Name: Maitake mushroom, Dancing mushroom, Hen of the woods

---

Family:	Polyporaceae
Part used:	The fruiting body
Energy and flavor:	Mild, sweet and bland
Organ meridians affected:	Liver, spleen and lungs
Type of cancer:	Various types
Actions:	Diuretic, sedative and removes damp heat.
Indications:	High blood pressure, high blood lipids,[33] diabetes, depressed immune system.[34]
Contraindications:	None noted
Dose:	9-15g
Biochemical constituents:	Both a- and -D-glucans are present in maitake with D-glucans predominating.[35]

Grifola frondosus (continued)

Other information: It grows on trunks or stumps of trees in deciduous forests in temperate climates. Called the "dancing mushroom", "cloud mushroom" because Japanese folklore tells how Japanese would dance for joy when they found it. Grows in eastern Canada, northeastern and mid-Atlantic regions of the US, also in Japan and parts of Europe. Before 1979 it was not cultivated.

Like other medicinal mushrooms, maitake is rich in polysaccharides. These are complex natural sugars that work by strengthening the immune system to fight disease. Maitake contains beta D-glucan, a particularly powerful substance that stimulates the immune system. There are numerous studies supporting the use of maitake's ability to inhibit cancer. Human studies have found that the D-fraction polysaccharides in maitake may help various types of cancer because the D-fraction component seems to inhibit carcinogenesis and metastasis.[36] A Chinese study using D-fraction of maitake extract treated 63 individuals with lung, stomach, liver cancers and leukemia. There was a demonstrable effect.[37] In Japan a study found that the D-fraction of maitake administered orally exhibited powerful activity against cancers, inhibiting both carcinogenesis and metastasis.[38, 39] The immune stimulating properties of the mushroom enhance the protective properties of interleukin-1, a possible explanation for maitake's antitumor abilities. Patients using maitake often exhibit improvement from the side effects of chemotherapy treatment.

Besides cancer, maitake seems to be effective to reduce blood pressure, treat diabetes,[40] liver protection and HIV.[41]

Houttuyniae cordata / Yu Xing Cao
Common Name: Houttuynia, Fishy smelling herb

Family:	Saururaceae
Part used:	The herb and root
Energy, flavors:	Cool, sweet, acrid and salty
Organ meridians affected:	Liver, lung and urinary bladder
Type of cancer:	Lungs, breast and colon
Actions:	1) Expels heat and toxins; 2) reduce inflammation and expel pus; 3) dispels damp-heat and stimulates urination.
Indications:	1) For any kind of infection; however, it is especially useful for lung infections and abscesses; 2) for boils, carbuncles and other toxic swellings, can be used either internally

or externally; 3) for damp-heat in the lower burner especially when there is inflammation with symptoms of diarrhea, urinary tract infection or colitis.

Contraindications: This herb is contraindicated for those with cold from deficiency symptoms.

Dose: 15-40g only lightly decocted. But it can also be taken freshly juiced or combined with other herbs in decoction. The leaves are sometimes eaten steamed or fresh as a potherb.

Biochemical constituents: It contains a volatile oil, decanoyl acelaldehyde, quericitrin, cordarine, quercetrin, potassium sulfate and hyperin.

Other information: It clears heat and toxins from the lungs, liver and bladder, clears pus and has diuretic properties making it effective for urinary tract infections. It is also used for colitis. Decanoyl acelaldehyde has potent anti-bacterial and antifungal properties. It generally increases phagocytosis of white blood cells and thus tonifies the body's immune system.

It is particularly indicated for lung cancer but also for colon cancer.

For lung cancer:

Houttuyniae	30g
Scutellariae	30g
Scrophulariae	30g
Unprepared rehmannia	30g
Lonicerae	15g
Trichosanthes root	15g
Mullein leaf	15g
Mullein root	15g
Black nightshade	15g
Codonopsis	9g
Astragalus	9g
American ginseng	9g
Agrimony herb	9g
Scolopendra	9g (powder taken separately with the tea)

Slowly simmer all but the scolopendra in a quart of water down to two or three cups of water. Take a half portion of the powdered scolopendra with each dose of the tea.

Hydrastis canadensis
Common Name: Goldenseal

Family:	Ranunculaceae
Part used:	The rhizomes
Energy and flavors:	Cold and bitter
Organ meridians affected:	Liver
Type of cancer:	Liver, breast, lungs, gastrointestinal and various other types of cancers
Actions:	Clears heat, alterative, anti-inflammatory, aperient, hemostatic and astringent.
Indications:	Bitter tonic, clears heat, dries dampness, moves blood and detoxifies.
Used for:	Dyspepsia, gastritis, colitis, duodenal ulcers, menorrhagia, tonic for the female reproductive organs, leucorrhea, penile discharge, rhinitis, inflammations, eczema and various skin disorders.
Contraindications:	Not for acute symptoms associated with cold deficiency. Do not use during pregnancy, or for cases of hypertension, or for yin deficient with symptoms of wasting.
Dose:	6–9g, 1:5 tincture 20-40 drops, powder 1-2g.
Biochemical constituents:	Hydrastine, 3.5-6% berberine, resin, traces of essential oil, chlorogenic acid, fatty oil, ascorbic acid, magnesium, calcium, selenium, albumin and sugar.

Other information: There are a number of herbs that contain berberine that have shown definite anticancer properties. These include the various species of barberry including Oregon grape root, coptis species, and phellodendron species. Each of these is in different families and while having different biochemical profiles they all share the characteristic yellow color associated with the concentration of berberine and beta-carotene. Berberine found in all of these plant species has been found to have definite antineoplastic properties.

Eli Jones[42] says that when the tongue is broad and indented with a very light coating this remedy is indicated. This describes its tonic usage for qi deficient, damp spleen conditions. He further states its use for atonic dyspepsia, constipation and flatulence. He says it is specific for breast tumors when pain is the principal symptom. He recommends hydrastis tincture given ten drops every two hours.

For liver cancer:

Dried leaf and stems of barberry	30g
Black nightshade	30-60g
Dandelion root and herb	15g
Milk thistle seeds and leaf	15g
Agrimony	15g

Crush the seeds or take separately in capsules. Slowly simmer all the herbs in four cups of water, down to three. Take three cups daily.

For lung cancer:

Golden seal root	6 capsules (two taken three times daily with the following tea):
Houttyuniae herb	30g
Red clover blossoms	30g
Scutellariae	30g
Scrophulariae	30g
Lonicerae	15g
Trichosanthes root	15g
Mullein leaf	15g
Mullein root	15g
Black nightshade	15g
Codonopsis	9g
Astragalus	9g
American ginseng	9g
Agrimony herb	9g

Make a decoction by slowly simmering all of the above in six cups of water, down to 3. Take three cups daily with the capsules of golden seal, scolopendra and scorpion described below.

Scolopendra	4.5g
Scorpion	4.5g

(Powder the above substances and put into gelatin capsules and take with the tea)

Hydrastis canadensis (continued)

For cervical cancer:

Phellodendron	15g
Scutellariae root	15g
Coptis root	15g
Golden seal	15g
Alum	30g
Borax	30g

Finely powder and blend with a small amount of fresh garlic juice. Mix into a paste with a little slippery elm powder and apply as a suppository or bolus directly into the vagina. The amount that should be inserted each night is about the length and width of the middle finger. In the morning, douche with tepid water that has been stirred with 3 tablespoons of fresh yogurt.

For skin cancer:

Phellodendron or Golden seal	10g
Yellow dock root	10g
Alum	30g
Gypsum	20g

Finely powder the above ingredients. Mix with olive oil and apply topically over the affected area.

For colo-rectal cancer:

Phellodendron or barberry	15g
Coptis	15g
Scutellaria	15g
Turmeric	15g
Dioscorea vilossa	30g
Tienchi ginseng	60g
Rhubarb root	15g
Citrus peel	9g
Licorice root	9g
Honeysuckle blossoms	9g

Finely powder the above ingredients and place in gelatin capsules. Take two to four capsules three times daily. One may also insert a bruised clove of garlic, wrapped with a cloth saturated with olive oil, into the rectum each night (be sure to leave a portion of the cloth protruding externally for easy removal in the morning).

Indigo naturalis / Qing Dai
Common Name: Indigo

Family:	Made from several plants
Part used:	Blue powder made from baphicacanthus cusia, indigofera suffructicosa, polygonum tinctorium and isatis tinctoria.
Energy and flavor:	Cold and salty
Organ meridians affected:	Liver, lung and stomach.
Types of cancer:	Leukemia and fevers associated with cancer
Actions:	Antiinflammatory, antiviral and detoxifying inhibits leukemic cells.
Indications:	Viral and bacterial inflammation
Contraindications:	Not for use during pregnancy nor for an individual with weak, cold digestion.
Dose:	1.5–3g

Inonotus sciurinus, I. Tabacinus, I. Orientalis, Poria obligua, Polyporus obliquus
Common Name: Chaga, Black birch touchwood, Birch mushroom

Family:	Polyporaceae
Part used:	The fruiting body
Energy and flavor:	Neutral and sweet
Organ meridians affected:	Liver, lungs and spleen
Type of cancer:	Various types of cancers
Actions:	Tonic, blood purifier and analgesic; Chinese medicine states that it regulates qi, strengthens the mind and spirit and removes harmful wind.[43]
Indications:	Widely used as a folk medicine and found growing from Poland, western Siberia and throughout North America. It is used for

Inonotus sciurinus (continued)

	diverse conditions ranging from the common cold, heart disease, worms, T.B., gastric diseases, hemorrhages and skin diseases. There is a respected tradition of use for various types of cancers. Russian folk medicine uses it for inoperable breast cancer, lip cancer, gastric, parotid gland, pulmonary, stomach, skin rectal cancers and Hodgkin's disease.[44]
Contraindications:	No information available
Dose:	The active constituents are empirically believed to be only available after boiling about three-square centimeters of the grated fungus for about 20 minutes and taking it as a tea. Russian clinicians have found that it is effective for some but not all cancers and that it requires long term use for at least a year.[45]
Biochemical constituents:	Inoidiol, oxygenated triterpenes, trametenolic acid, tannins, steroids and alkaloids. Polysaccharide fraction B from inonotus polysacharides showed positive activity against tumors.[46]

Other information: According to Christopher Hobbs "Polish studies with 48 patients having 3rd and 4th stage malignancies found chaga injections with cobalt salts to be the most effective form of preparation. In ten patients, tumors reduced in size, pain decreased, hemorrhaging occurred less often and became less intense, and recovery was attended with better sleep and appetite and feelings of improvement. Most of these patients were women treated with chaga for cancer of the genital organs or breast cancer."[47]

Inula japonica / Xuan Fu Hua
Common Name: Elecampane flower

Family:	Compositae
Part used:	The flower (Flos)
Energy and flavor:	Warm, acrid and bitter
Organ meridians affected:	Lung, spleen, stomach, liver, and large intestine
Type of cancer:	Lungs and breast

Actions:	1) Moves stagnant phlegm in the lungs; 2) reverses the flow of rebellious qi of the lungs and stomach.
Indications:	1) For stagnation of phlegm in the lungs with symptoms such as wheezing and bronchitis with excessive phlegm; 2) for belching and vomiting due to cold and/or damp of the stomach and spleen or excessive coughing or wheezing.
Contraindications:	Those with tuberculosis or cough due to wind-heat or deficiency should avoid this herb.
Dose:	3-9g
Biochemical constituents:	Britanin, inulicin, quercetin, isoquercetin, caffeic acid, chlorogenic acid, taraxasterol and inulin

---

Isatis tinctoria / Ban Lang Gen
Common Name: Isatis

Family:	Cruciferae
Parts Used:	The root
Energy and flavor:	Cold and bitter
Organ Meridians affected:	Lung, heart and stomach
Type of cancer:	All types including non-solid cancers especially leukemia
Actions:	1) Expels heat and fire toxicity; 2) cools the blood; 3) dispels damp-heat in the lower burner.
Indications:	1) For febrile diseases especially infectious diseases such as mumps and others associated with viral infections; 2) for febrile diseases with symptoms of fever, rapid pulse and a red tongue body with a yellow coat; 3) for jaundice and hepatitis.
Contraindications:	Those who are deficient or are without true fire toxicity should not use this herb.
Dose:	10-30g
Biochemical constituents:	Indoxyl-B-glucoside, isatin, kinetin, kaemperferol, linoleic acid, linolenic acid, magnesium, potassium and quercetin

Lacca sinica exsiccata (Rhus vernicifera) / Gan Qi

The dried secretion of Rhus vernicifera De Candolle.
It is used as a drug only when it becomes dry after being stored in a container to dehydrate. Once dried, it is solid and dark brown.

Family:	Anacardiaceae
Part used:	The sap
Energy and flavor:	Cold, slightly toxic and pungent
Organ meridians affected:	Liver and stomach
Type of cancer:	Stomach, intestines and liver
Actions:	Activating the circulation of body fluid, dispelling stasis, subsiding edema and curing parasitosis and rheumatism.
Indications:	Cough, amenorrhea, lumbago, cold, rheumatism, hernia, scabies, spasm, paralysis, stagnation, all cardiac pains, pains in the chest and abdomen, and infant parasitosis
Contraindications:	Do not use during pregnancy and use with caution for those who are very weak.
Dose:	2.4 to 4.5g for each dose
Biochemical constituents:	Laccase, including urushiol, elastin and protein, which is oxidized when exposed to the moisture in the air

Other information: This is one of the four herbs in the WTTC formula used for a variety of cancers in Japanese traditional medicine. It is especially useful for abdominal cancers.

Laminaria japonica (Ecklonia kurome) / Kunbu, Kombu
Common Name: Kombu seaweed, Kelp, Ecklonia

Family:	Laminariaceae
Part used:	The thallus
Energy and flavor:	Cold and salty
Organ meridians affected:	Spleen, stomach, liver and kidney
Type of cancer:	Thyroid tumors, cancer of the neck, digestive tract and lungs
Actions:	Resolves phlegm, softens hard nodules and is

diuretic.

Indications:	It is used for goiter, swollen glands, clearing phlegm, reducing inflammation of the lymph glands and treating edema.
Contraindications:	Use with caution for those with symptoms of coldness and dampness. It is also hard on the digestion, therefore it should not be used with symptoms of weakness and coldness of the digestive system.
Dose:	9-15g
Biochemical constituents:	Alginic acid, laminarin, mannitol, protein, amino acid, vitamin C, iodine, potassium and calcium cobalt

Other information: Kelp and seaweeds in general, when boiled in hot water, contain a high concentration of polysaccharides. Chinese research has demonstrated that injections of the hot water extract in rats that had transplanted carcinomas had over a 90% inhibitory rate. Other studies have shown that it was able to inhibit the growth hormone of tumors.[48]

Lentinus edodes, Tricholomopsis edodes / Hua Gu
Common Name: Shiitake (Japanese), Snake butter, Pasania fungus, Forest mushroom

---

Family:	Polyporaceae
Part used:	The fruiting body
Organ meridians affected:	Liver and spleen
Type of cancer:	Liver and other types of cancer
Energy and flavors:	Mild and sweet
Actions:	It clears dampness, strengthens the immune system, and is tonic and restorative.
Indications:	It has been found to be useful for cancer, heart disease, AIDS, flu, tumors, viruses, high blood pressure, obesity and aging. It is also very beneficial for the cardiovascular system, in the treatment of HIV and the treatment of viral/bacterial infections.
Contraindications:	None noted
Dose:	9-12g

Lentinus edodes (continued)

Biochemical constituents: High in vitamins B1, B2, B12, niacin and pantothenic acid. B vitamins are necessary for cell energy and hormone production. Shiitake also contains protein, enzymes and 8 essential amino acids.

Other information: In Japan, shiitake taken through oral ingestion as an extract has been found to have potent anticancer properties and immuno-stimulatory effects generally.[49] Lentinant is a polysaccharide found in the root and cell wall of shiitake. It has a triple helix structure, a shape considered important for the healing properties of shiitake. It stimulates the production of T-lymphocytes and macrophages that ingest foreign invaders. It also helps the production of interleukins, known to inhibit the growth of cancer and viruses. In general it stimulates the immune system of the body.[50]

In Japan lentinan, the polysaccharide found in shiitake, is an approved drug used together with chemotherapy to treat cancer patients. Studies have shown that it increases the lifespan of cancer patients and may also prevent the recurrence of cancer after surgery.

Leonurus heterophyllus, L.Cardiaca / Yi Mu Cao
Common Name: Motherwort, Chinese motherwort

Family:	Labiatae
Part used:	The aerial portion (Herba)
Energy and flavor:	Slightly cold, acrid and bitter
Organ meridians affected:	Heart, liver and urinary bladder
Type of cancer:	Breast and uterus
Actions:	1) Moves and regulates blood, breaks stasis and regulates menses; 2) Increases the flow of urine and reduces stagnation of water.
Indications:	1) For stagnation of blood with symptoms of pain from blood stasis, late or slow menstruation, infertility, uterine bleeding, post partum pain and masses caused by blood stagnation; 2) For retention of water with symptoms of acute edema with or without heat in the kidney or bladder causing blood in the urine.
Contraindications:	Motherwort should not be used during

pregnancy or by those with blood deficiency or yin deficiency.

Dose: 9-30g

Biochemical constituents: Leonurine, stachydrine, leonuridine, lauric acid, linolenic acid, sitosterol, vit. A, flavonone and stachyose.

Other information: A hot water extract has been shown to be 78% effective in inhibiting sarcoma-180 in mice.

Levistonia chinensis
Common Name: Palm

Family: Palmaceae

Part used: The seeds, root and leaf

Energy and flavor: Neutral, sweet and astringent

Organ meridians affected: Not known

Type of cancer: Various cancers including esophageal, nasopharyngeal cancers and leukemia.

Actions: The seeds are anticancer and they soften tumors. The roots are analgesic.

Indications: The seeds are used for various malignancies. For functional uterine bleeding, calcine the leaves to form an ash. Take 15 to 30g of this with water in decoction.

Contraindications: None known

Dose: Of the seeds, 30 to 60g of the seeds for various types of cancers. 30g can also be cooked with equal amount of lean pork for 1-2 hours.

Biochemical constituents: Phenol, reduced sugar, tannin and triglyceride

Other information: This is still another use for the world's most useful botanical. Chang Minyi states that it has been shown to inhibit encephaloma-22 in mice and also relieves pain. For leukemia and malignant hydatidiform mole cook 30g of the crushed seeds with 6 jujube dates and take twice daily. A course of treatment is 20 days. For lung cancer decoct 60g each of the seeds and scutellariae barbatae and take in one or two doses daily.

Ligustrum lucidum / Nu Zhen Zi
Common Name: Japanese privet

Family:	Oleaceae
Part used:	The fruit
Energy and flavor:	Neutral, sweet and bitter
Organ meridians affected:	Liver and kidney
Type of cancer:	All cancers
Actions:	Tonifies the immune system, replenishes the vital essence (hormones), darkens the hair, improves eyesight, strengthens the knees and waist. It nourishes the liver and kidneys and clears yin deficient heat from wasting.
Indications:	Used for premature graying of the hair, weak eyesight, lower back ache, vertigo, retinitis and cataracts.
Contraindications:	Not good to use as a single agent for someone with symptoms of diarrhea or symptoms of yang (vital energy) deficiency.
Dose:	9-15g
Biochemical constituents:	Oleanolic acid, ursolic acid, mannitol, glucose and fatty oil.

Other information: It is effective for Chinese Fu Zheng (immune protecting) therapy to tonify the immune system and to help counteract the adverse effects of radiation and chemotherapy. A combination of two herbs well known as part of Chinese Fu Zheng therapy, Ligustrum and astragalus was able to inhibit the growth of kidney cell carcinoma in mice. Part of the mechanism was believed to be because of the ability of these herbs to increase phagocytosis.[51] Chinese research found that a decoction of the berries was able to inhibit the growth of certain transplanted tumors in mice.

Lilii, Lilium brownii, L. longiflorum, L. concola, L. lanciflorum / Bai He
Common Name: Lily bulb
(Only the sweet tasting, white-flowered varieties are the best to use.)

Family:	Liliaceae
Part used:	The bulb (Bulbus)

Energy and flavor:	Slightly cold, sweet and bland
Organ meridians affected:	Heart and lung
Type of cancer:	Lungs and breast
Actions:	1) Clears heat and stops cough due to either lung yin deficiency or lung-heat; 2) clears heat from the heart and calms the spirit (shen).
Indications:	1) For heat in the lung with symptoms such as cough, sore throat and blood streaked sputum; 2) for heat in the heart caused by either febrile disease or yin deficiency with symptoms such as insomnia, low-grade fever, irritability or palpitations.
Contraindications:	Those with wind-cold conditions should not use this herb nor should it be used when there are symptoms of phlegm and spleen deficiency with symptoms of diarrhea.
Dose:	9-30g
Biochemical constituents:	Alkaloids including colchicine.

Lindera strychnifolia / Wu Yao
Common Name: Lindera root

Family:	Lauraceae
Part used:	The root (Radix)
Energy and flavor:	Warm and acrid
Organ meridians affected:	Spleen, lung, kidney, urinary bladder and stomach
Type of cancer:	Cancers of the thyroid gland, breast and liver
Actions:	1) Warms and stimulates the flow of qi and relieves pain; 2) disperses cold and warms the kidneys.
Indications:	1) For stagnation of qi caused by cold with symptoms of pain and distention of the abdominal and epigastric region, menstrual pain and bi pain associated with cold; 2) for cold in the kidneys with symptoms of inability to hold urine and frequent urination.
Contraindications:	This herb should not be used by those with qi deficiency or interior heat.

Lindera strychnifolia (continued)

Dose:	3-9g
Biochemical constituents:	Linderol (borneol), linderane, linderalactone, isolinderalactone, lindestrenolide, lindrene, lendene, lindenenone, lindestrene, linderene acetate, isolinderoside, linderaic acid, lindera-zulene, chamazub and laurolitsine.

Lithospermum seu arnebiae seu macrotomia / Zi Cao
Common Name: Gromwell, Lithospermum

Family:	Boraginaceae
Part used:	The root
Energy and flavors:	Cold, sweet and bitter
Organ meridians affected:	Heart, liver and pericardium
Type of cancer:	All types of cancer including leukemia
Actions:	1) Expels heat, moves and cools the blood; 2) helps the incomplete expression of rashes and removes toxins from the blood; 3) applied topically it clears damp-heat and moves blood; 4) unblocks the intestines.
Indications:	1) For toxic buildup in the blood with heat signs such as rashes and sores, especially those that are very dark in color; 2) for incomplete expression of rashes, chickenpox and measles; 3) applied topically it can be used for damp-heat conditions such as burns, eczema and vaginal itching; 4) for mild cases of constipation.
Contraindications:	Diarrhea due to deficiency of spleen or intestines. It only seems to be effective for measles in the beginning stages and is contraindicated by some for later stages of the disease.
Dose:	3-9g

Other information: This herb is one of the more important anticancer herbs. It expels heat, cools and purifies the blood, resolves rashes, mildly purges and topically resolves damp heat. Animal studies have confirmed its effectiveness against sarcoma-180 (about 30%), leukemia and for the treatment of breast cancer. Topically it can be used in formula to relieve the ulceration of radiation treatments.

Lobeliae chinensis / Ban Bian Lian
Common Name: Chinese lobelia

Family:	Campanulaceae
Part used:	The herb and root (Herba cum Radice)
Energy and flavor:	Neutral and sweet
Organ meridians affected:	Liver, kidney, heart, lung and small intestine
Type of cancer:	Lungs, breast, kidneys, nose, liver and ascites cancer
Actions:	1) Diuretic, reduces edema; 2) detoxifying, and anti-inflammatory; 3) cools the blood and reduces toxicity, being broadly antipathogenic and antifungal.
Indications:	It is used for edema, enteritis, dysentery, eczema, liver cirrhosis, cancer, inflamed sores, abscesses and venomous snakebites.
Contraindications:	Use with caution for individuals with all types of deficiencies.
Dose:	15-30g, and up to 60g
Biochemical constituents:	Lobeline, lobelanine, lobelanidine, isolobelanine, lobelinin, polyfructosan, flavones and saponins.

Other information: It is classified by Li Shi zhen of the Ming Dynasty as acrid, bitter and nonpoisonous, while in Bensky it is described as sweet and neutral. It is interesting that both its flavor and chemistry resembles the North American lobelia inflata. In vivo tests have shown the herb to have inhibitive activity on sarcoma-37 in mice.

Lonicera japonica / Jin Yin Hua
Common Name: Honeysuckle flowers

Family:	Caprifoliaceae
Part used:	The flowers, leaves and vine
Energy and flavor:	Cold and sweet

Lonicera japonica (continued)

Organ meridians affected:	Lung, heart, stomach and large intestine
Type of cancer:	Breast, lungs, various other cancers as well
Actions:	1) Expels heat and fire from toxicity; 2) dispels wind-heat derived from an external pathogen; 3) expels damp-heat from the lower burner.
Indications:	1) For acute infections where there is pain and swelling such as boils, sore throat, conjunctivitis, upper respiratory tract infection and intestinal abscesses; 2) for external wind-heat with symptoms of fever, sore throat, common cold, influenza and headache; 3) for dysentery and acute urinary tract infection. Honeysuckle can be used as a general anti-inflammatory, antibiotic, antiviral, to reduce swellings of the breast, sore and swollen throat and conjunctivitis. It is also good for intestinal abscess.
Contraindications:	This herb should not be used by those with deficiency in the spleen/stomach nor when there are symptoms of coldness and diarrhea. It should be used carefully when there is qi or yin deficiency.
Dose:	6-15g. Large doses (up to 60g) can be used effectively and safely in severe cases.
Biochemical constituents:	Flavones, luteolin, luteolin-7-glucoside, inositol, and saponins.

Other information: Honeysuckle flowers have been found to inhibit ascites carcinoma and exhibit an inhibitory rate of 22.2% on sarcoma-180 in rats. It is commonly used in Chinese formulas especially for the treatment of cancer of the lungs and breast. It is commonly combined with Forsythia blossoms for various inflammatory conditions as well as for cancer.

Lycium barbarum, fructus / Gou Gi Zi
Common Name: Lycii berries

Family:	Solanaceae
Part used:	The berry

Energy and flavor:	Neutral and sweet
Organ meridians affected:	Liver, kidneys and lungs
Types of Cancer:	All cancers, especially good for the liver
Actions:	They tonify both the blood and yin of the liver. Being high in beta-carotene they provide important anticancer fighting nutrients.
Indications:	Consumptive cough, dizziness and blurred vision
Contraindications:	Excess heat and spleen deficiency
Dose:	6-18g
Biochemical constituents:	Betaine, carotene, physalien, thiamin, riboflavin, vitamin C, B-sitosterol and linoleic acid.

Other information: Best of all Lycii berries taste good and can be added to cereals, soups and stews as one would add raisins. In fact the Chinese call them "red raisins." Research has found them to play an important role in DNA protection and therefore useful to prevent cancer.

Magnolia officinalis / Hou Pou
Common Name: Magnolia

Family:	Magnoliaceae
Part used:	The bark (Cortex)
Energy and flavor:	Warm, acrid, bitter and aromatic
Organ meridians affected:	Spleen, lung, stomach and large intestine
Type of cancer:	Cancer of the stomach and esophagus
Actions:	1) Moves rebellious qi downward, dries dampness and relieves food stagnation; 2) transforms phlegm and redirects rebellious qi of the lung.
Indications:	1) For damp conditions with symptoms of nausea, vomiting, abdominal distention, loss of appetite and diarrhea; 2) for cough, wheezing and asthma due to abundant phlegm obstructing the lungs; 3) peach-pit throat, where it feels as if there is something lodged in the throat.
Contraindications:	This herb should not be used by pregnant women or by those with stomach or spleen deficiency.

Magnolia officinalis (continued)

Dose: 3-9g

Biochemical constituents: Magnolol, isomagnolol, essential oil (machilol, eudesmol) and alkaloid (magnocurarine, magnoflorine, salicifoline).

Manis pentadactya-Dactyla / Chuan Shan Jia
Common Name: Pangolin (anteater) scales

Family: Manidae

Part used: The scales (Squama)

Energy and flavor: Cold and salty

Organ meridians affected: Liver and stomach

Type of cancer: Cancer of the breast, cervix and liver

Actions: 1) Disperses congealed blood; 2) promotes menses and lactation; 3) reduces swelling and promotes the discharge of pus from boils, abscesses and carbuncles (can be topically applied); 4) relieves rheumatic pains.

Indications: 1) Delayed or stopped menstruation; 2) arthritic pains; 3) pains from trauma and injuries; 4) promotes the resolution and healing of boils, abscesses and ulcerated sores; 5) stopped lactation.

Contraindications: Use with caution for the treatment of sores caused by deficiency.

Dose: 3-9g

Preparation: Presoak in warm water for 2 hours, then simmer 1 to 3 hours.

Melia Toosendan / Chuan Lian Zi
Common Name: Sichuan chinaberry

Family: Meliaceae

Part used: The fruit

Energy and flavor: Bitter and cold

Organ meridians affected:	Liver and small intestine
Type of cancer:	All kinds but especially abdominal and gastrointestinal cancers.
Actions:	It has broad anti-parasitical, anti-fungal and anti-bacterial properties. It is especially useful to relieve pain associated with the hypochondrium, abdomen and gastrointestinal areas. In this it is particularly effective when combined with corydalis.
Contraindications:	Use with caution or combine if necessary with warming digestive herbs such as saussurea for individuals with cold deficiency and weak digestion.
Dose:	10-15g

Momordica charantia
Common Names: Bitter melon, African pear, Bitter apple, Bitter cucumber, Bitter gourd, Karela and Wild cucumber

Family:	Curcurbitaceae
Part used:	The fruit, leaves and vines
Energy and flavor:	Cool and bitter
Organ meridians affected:	Kidneys, pancreas and spleen
Type of cancer:	All types
Actions:	Cooling, tonic, antidiabetic, abortifacient, alterative, anthelmintic, antiinflammatory, cardiotonic, emmenagogue, laxative, purgative, stomachic and vermifuge.
Indications:	Treats fevers, toxicity, diabetes, worms, bronchitis, anemia, biliousness, gout, HIV infection, hypercholesterolemia, hyperglycemia, jaundice, leprosy, leukemia (leaves and vines), liver problems, malaria, venomous bites and skin ulcers.
Contraindications:	Should not be eaten by pregnant women.
Dose:	9-30g
Biochemical constituents:	Calcium carbohydrates (40%), GABA, iron, magnesium phosphorus, potassium protein (15%) sodium titanium and vitamin C

Momordica charantia (continued)

Other information: Momordica was found to inactivate immunotoxic proteins of human bladder carcinoma cells.[52] Several other studies confirm the anticancer properties of bitter melon. One found that an extract of bitter melon had a 77% inhibition of tumor formation in mice as opposed to untreated mice with tumors that was 33%.[53]

Nidus Vespae / Lu Feng Fang
Common Name: Hornet nest
(It is from the honeycomb of polistes mandarinus)

Family:	Vespidae
Energy and flavors:	Neutral, toxic and sweet
Organ meridians affected:	Lung and stomach
Type of cancer:	Lung, liver and gastrointestinal cancers
Actions:	Clears heat, expels wind, dries damp and relieves pain.
Indications:	Applied topically as an ointment or a wash for a variety of skin ailments including rashes with itch, sores, scabies, carbuncles and wind-damp painful obstruction.
Contraindications:	Those with qi or blood deficiency or those with open sores should not use this herb.
Dose:	6-12g decocted; 1-3g as a powder internally.
Biochemical constituents:	It contains myricin and resin. The volatile oil is toxic.

Other information: It has been found to inhibit both gastric and liver cancers. One method is to burn it to ashes and take it in 6-gram doses twice daily. This can be used for various cancers but especially breast cancer.

Nine times salt (Prepared sodium chloride) / Zi Nao Sha
Common Name: Rock salt

Part used:	Mineral and NaCl
Energy and flavor:	Cold and salty
Organ meridians affected:	Kidneys

Type of cancer:	Used for various types of cancers including esophageal cancer, thyroid and other glandular types of cancers and gastrointestinal tract cancers.
Actions:	Antiinflammatory, astringent, softens and dissolves tumors.
Indications:	Various gastrointestinal complaints including H. pylori and Crohn's disease, periodontal gum disease, cancerous tumors and hard swellings.
Contraindications:	None known
Dose:	1g (1/8th teaspoon) 3 times daily with food

Other information: This is a Korean herbal preparation made by cooking the salt nine times in bamboo with pine in a metal cook stove. In the last firing the salt becomes liquid and hardens again as it cools. Because of this it absorbs all the resins from the bamboo and pine and is considered 'purified.' The salt is so pure that each molecule is approximately 1/100th the size of regular NaCl so that it is able to be absorbed directly in the cell and promote cellular detoxification and healing. It becomes like white metal or platinum and is even able to penetrate the bone marrow and assist in the healing of bone cancer as well as stomach and mouth cancer.

This substance is only available from: Jiang Jing Formulas 4432 156th, S.E., Lynwood, Washington, 98037 USA. (www.Jiangjing.com)

Nymphaea odorata
Common Name: White pond lily, Sweet/fragrant water lily

Family:	Nymphaceae
Part used:	The root
Energy and flavor:	Cool, bitter, astringent and dry
Organ meridians affected:	Liver, kidneys and lungs
Type of cancer:	Uterine and cervical cancer
Actions:	Astringes and dries dampness and clears heat.
Indications:	For damp heat, leucorrhea, spermatorrhea, urinary-genito infections, prostate inflammation, cough, uterine and cervical cancer.
Contraindications:	Do not use if there is dryness and constipation.

Nymphaea odorata (continued)

Dose:	4-8g
Biochemical constituents:	Alkaloids (including nupharine), a phytoestrogen, tannins, gallic and tartaric acids, mucilage, starch, gum, resin, saccharides and ammonia

Other information: Highly recommended by Eli Jones[54] for cancer of the uterus. His formula consists of phytolacca root, nymphaea odorata root and helonias dioca root. Four ounces of the 1:5 tincture of each is mixed with a gallon of syrup. A wineglassful is given three times daily.

Oldenlandiae chrysotrichae / Bai Hua She Shi Cao
Common Name: Oldenlandia

Family:	Rubiaceae
Part used:	The aerial portions
Energy and flavor:	Mild, bitter and non-toxic
Organ meridians affected:	Heart, liver and spleen
Type of cancer:	It is an important anti cancer herb for all cancers but especially gastrointestinal, cervix, breast, rectum and fibrosarcoma.
Actions:	It clears heat, relives dampness, detoxifies, disperses blood and promotes healing.
Indications:	It is used for upper respiratory conditions caused by heat and inflammation, it also treats other infections including tonsillitis, acute appendicitis, urinary tract infections, jaundice and gastrointestinal cancers. Its detoxifying properties make it useful for venomous bites and stings.
Contraindications:	Not to be used by pregnant women.
Dose:	15-30g (up to 60g for treating cancer)
Biochemical constituents:	Corymbosin, argentaffin, diterpenoid acids, B-sitosterol, ursolic acid, stearic acid, oleic acid and linoleic acid

Other information: Interestingly, in vitro, this herb has only weak antibacterial properties, while in vivo, it seems to powerfully stimulate phagocytic activity.

Treating appendicitis experimentally generally lowered the animal's body temperature, significantly reduced leukocyte count, and essentially absorbed inflammation. At a dose of 30 to 60g it is often added to conventional prescriptions for cancer and has exhibited no adverse reaction. It has been shown to inhibit the mitosis process of tumor cells and cause degeneration and necrosis of tumors. Argentaffin surrounds tumors, inhibiting to some degree infiltration and metastasis. Besides gastrointestinal cancers it is also used for leukemia.[55]

For lymphosarcoma, a decoction of equal amounts of oldenlandia and scutellariae barbatae is taken. (*Medicine and Drugs of Fujian, Vol.2, 1976*).

Ophiopogonis Japonici / Mai Men Dong
Common Name: Ophiopogon

Family:	Liliaceae
Part used:	The tuber
Energy and flavor:	Cold, sweet and slightly bitter
Organ meridians affected:	Heart, lung and stomach
Type of cancer:	Lung
Actions:	1) Replenishes yin essence and promotes secretions; 2) lubricates and nourishes the stomach; 3) soothes the lung; 4) nourishes the heart.
Indications:	1) For chronic bronchitis, hemoptysis in pulmonary tuberculosis, restlessness, laryngitis, dry stool caused by heat in the stomach, palpitations, fearfulness and insomnia; 2) irritability due to yin deficiency; 3) constipation and dry mouth.
Contraindications:	Not for those with weak spleen and stomach with coldness and diarrhea.
Dose:	6-12g
Biochemical constituents:	Ophiopogonin, ruscogenin, B-sitosterol and stigmasterol

Ostrea gigas / Mu Li
Common Name: Oyster shell

Family:	Ostreidae
Part used:	The shell
Energy and flavor:	Slightly cold, salty and astringent
Organ meridians affected:	Liver and kidney
Type of cancer:	Stomach, lung, liver and thyroid
Actions:	1) Calms and anchors the spirit; 2) contains fluids; 3) softens and moves lumps.
Indications:	1) For disturbance of shen with symptoms such as headache, insomnia, palpitations and restlessness; 2) for loss of vital fluids such as night sweats, unabating sweating, nocturnal emissions, vaginal discharge and uterine bleeding; 3) for lumps of the neck such as scrofula and goiter.
Contraindications:	Oyster shell should not be used by those who are cold and weak nor by those with high fever without symptoms of sweating.
Dose:	15-30g; it should be cooked for 30 to 45 minutes before the other herbs are added.
Biochemical constituents:	Calcium salts, magnesium, potassium and other minerals.

Panax ginseng / Ren Shen
Common Name: Ginseng

Family:	Araliaceae
Part used:	The root
Energy and flavor:	Warm, sweet and slightly bitter
Organ meridians affected:	Spleen, lung and heart
Type of cancer:	All cancers
Actions:	1) Very strongly tonifies the qi; 2) tonifies the lungs and spleen, helps digestion and assimilation; 3) assists the body in the secretion of fluids and stops thirst and wasting; 4) strengthens the heart and calms the shen.

Indications:	1) For collapse of basal qi with symptoms of very weak and thin pulse, abundant sweating, shallow breathing, extreme fatigue or shock; 2) for deficiency of lung and spleen qi with symptoms of shortness of breath, wheezing, difficulty in breathing, loss of appetite, diarrhea, fatigue and prolapse of the internal organs; 3) for wasting and thirsting disorder or dehydration in the aftermath of febrile diseases; 4) for weakness of the heart caused by either qi or blood deficiency with symptoms of palpitations, insomnia, restlessness and forgetfulness.
Contraindications:	Those with yin deficiency with excess heat signs should not use this herb, nor should it be used when there are acute pathogenic conditions. Finally it is to be avoided when there are symptoms of high blood pressure.
Dose:	3-9g, higher dosages are sometimes used for shock because of blood loss.
Biochemical constituents:	Ginsenosides, essential oil (panacene, panaxynol), saponin, protopanaxadiol, protopanaxatriol and germanium.

Other information: It is considered efficacious for all deficiencies and also promotes the synthesis of immunoglobulin and albumin and the synthesis of DNA and RNA in normal cells. Studies have shown that ginseng is able to turn cancer cells into normal cells and therefore does no harm. It promotes hemoglobin and activates adrenocortical hormones. Its inhibitory effect against cancer is greatly enhanced when combined with astragalus and ganoderma.

Breast cancer: combine approximately 2 to 3g each of ginseng, ligusticum chuanxiong, moutan peony, cinnamon twig, lignum sappan, platycodon, atractylodes, astragalus, saussureae, linderae, magnolia bark, citrus peel (Chen Pi), semen arecae, ledebouriella root, prepared rehmannia, bupleurum, crataegus, poria, angelica sinensis (Dang Gui) and licorice root.

Cancer of the uterus: combine ginseng, poria, magnolia cooked with ginger, citrus peel (Chen Pi), leonurus, sparganii, pinelliae, cortex mori radicis and atractylodes.

Threeg of ginseng, ganoderma and lily bulb can be taken daily to treat the effects of radiation for *cancer of the head and neck.*

Panax pseudoginseng; Notoginseng / Tienchi, San Qi, Tien Qi
Common Name: Tienchi ginseng, Notoginseng, Pseudoginseng, pseudo-ginseng

Family:	Araliaceae
Part used:	The root (Radix)
Energy and flavors:	Warm, sweet and slightly bitter
Organ meridians affected:	Liver and stomach
Type of cancer:	All types including non-solid types such as lymphomas and leukemia
Actions:	1) Stops bleeding and resolves blood stasis; 2) reduces inflammation and associated pain.
Indications:	1) For bleeding either externally caused by injury or internally for bleeding of any kind, it also breaks up stasis that can cause symptoms such as chest pain and menstrual pain; 2) for inflammation and pain caused by injury such as sprained or broken bones as well as joint pain caused by stagnant blood. It increases blood flow to the heart and is effective for coronary heart disease and angina pectoralis. It has antibacterial, anti-fungal and anti-viral properties.
Contraindications:	This herb should not be used by pregnant women and should be used with caution by those with blood deficiency or yin deficiency or without stagnation of blood.
Dose:	1-9g; 1-3g when taken as a powder; can be used topically
Biochemical constituents:	Saponin (arasaponin A,B).

Other information: A strong tea has been found to inhibit over 90% on JTC-26 in vitro. It was also found to inhibit and completely clear sarcoma-180 in mice. For cancer, it has a broad beneficial application for its anticancer properties, ability to promote blood circulation and relieve associated pain of tumors, counteract inflammation, promote healing and tonify the core immune system. Finally, since high blood sugar is commonly associated with cancer, it is effective in helping to lower blood sugar by increasing the uptake of glycogen, making it also useful for the treatment of diabetes.

As with other species in the ginseng family, it is rich in hormone precursor saponins.

Paris polyphylla / Zao Xiu
Common Name: Paris rhizome

Family:	Liliaceae
Part used:	The rhizome
Energy and flavor:	Slightly cold, slightly toxic and bitter
Organ meridians affected:	Heart and liver
Type of cancer:	Several types of cancers, especially lung, liver, breast and brain.
Actions:	It detoxifies and clears inflammation, relieves pain and has antispasmodic properties and relieves convulsions.
Indications:	Sore throat, septicemia, inflammation and acute high fevers.
Contraindications:	Not for a weak or pregnant woman.
Dose:	5-10g. For cancer, higher doses are used ranging from 12 to 100g.
Biochemical constituents:	Pariphyllin, dioscin, diosgenin, saponin and amino acids.

Other information: In vitro tests have found that it inhibits cancer-forming oncocytes.

Patriniae scabiosaefoliae / Bai Jiang Cao
Common Name: Thlaspi, Patrinia

Family:	Valerianaceae
Part used:	Herb and root
Energy and flavor:	Slightly cold, acrid and bitter
Organ meridians affected:	Liver, stomach and large intestine
Type of cancer:	Colorectal cancer
Actions:	It clears heat and toxicity, drains pus, moves blood and reduces inflammation.
Indications:	Inflammation, abscesses and blood stagnation
Contraindications:	None noted

Patriniae scabiosaefoliae (continued)

Dose: 6-15g

Biochemical constituents: It contains an essential oil, saponins, tannins and alkaloids.

Other information: It is very specific for colitis and colo-rectal cancer. Its anticancer properties are demonstrated with its 98.2% inhibitory rate of JTC-26 with no sign of damaging adjacent healthy cells.

Pau d' Arco, Tabebuia heptaphylla, Tabebuia impetiginosa
Common Names: Ipe roxa, Ipes, Lapacho, Lapacho Colorado, Lapacho morado, red lapacho, Taheebo, Amapa, Tecoma and Trumpet bush

---

Family:	Bignoniaceae
Part used:	Inner bark of a deciduous tree
Energy and flavor:	Cold and mildly bitter
Organ meridians affected:	Liver, lungs and blood
Type of cancer:	Various types of cancers including leukemia and lymphomas
Actions:	Moves blood. It has alterative, antifungal, hypotensive, antidiabetic, bitter tonic, digestive, antibacterial (*Helicobacter pylori*) and antitumor properties.
Indications:	Useful for all inflammatory diseases as well as upper respiratory conditions including asthma and bronchitis, skin conditions, colitis, diabetes, liver disorders, jaundice, hepatitis, malaria, fibrocystic disease and Crohn's disease, rheumatic conditions. Unfortunately, its ability to cure cancer has never been substantiated in clinical trials. However, many in both the US and South America have claimed it to be occasionally effective for a wide variety of cancers including solid tumors, non-solid cancers such as leukemia, Hodgkin's and lymphomas. Medically, many have found that pau d' arco tea will significantly reduce the pain associ-

ated with cancer. This, plus the fact that high doses have been associated with slow clotting, indicates that pau d' arco relieves blood stagnation. It is to be assumed that this is the mechanism through which pau d' arco relieves pain associated with different types of cancers. This property alone would attest to the value of pau d' arco in tea or formula at least adjunctively for the treatment of cancer.

Contraindications: It is a cool-natured herb so it should be used with caution by those with severe gastric weakness. Do not take during pregnancy. Normal dosage is well tolerated and has no side effects. However, high doses have been known to cause nausea, vomiting and slow blood clotting.

Dose: *Dried bark:* 3-6g in decoction using three cups of water. One cup is taken three times daily. *Liquid Extract:* 1:1 in 50% alcohol, 15-60 drops up to 5x/day. *Tincture:* 1:5 in 50% alcohol, 1 teaspoon to a tablespoon should be taken up to 4x/day.

Biochemical constituents: Good quality contains from two to seven percent lapachol. Lapachol apparently has shown strong biological activity against cancer.[56] This constituent has been substantiated to have calcium, carbohydrates (70%), cobalt, fats (0.5%), fiber (15%), magnesium, phosphorus, potassium, protein (9%), silicon and vitamin C.

Other information: This tree is found growing in Argentina, Bahamas, Brazil, Central America, India, Mexico and throughout South America. Related species have even been recognized in Africa and Taiwan. The Argentina species is the preferred type. It has a long history of use throughout Latin America as an anticancer agent. In one study, 9 cancer patients with various types of cancers including liver, kidney, breast and prostate were given 250mg of pure lapachol with meals. All 9 patients experienced tumor shrinkage and significant pain reduction. Three had complete remissions of their cancers. None suffered any side effects.[57] One should be careful to get good quality pau d'arco.

Pinellia ternatae / Ban Xia
Common Name: Pinellia

Family: Araceae

Part used: The rhizome (Rhizoma)

Energy and flavor: Warm, acrid and toxic

Organ meridians affected: Lung, spleen and stomach

Type of cancer: Stomach, esophagus, cervix and lungs

Actions: 1) Drains dampness and reduces phlegm; 2) reverses the flow of rebellious qi; 3) reduces hardenings and relieves distention.

Indications: 1) For cough with abundant phlegm especially when associated with dampness in the spleen; 2) for most kinds of rebellious qi especially where there is dampness involved such as vomiting, nausea and morning sickness; 3) for focal distention or the chest or abdomen, lumps, globus hystericus or any stagnation caused by phlegm in the body.

Contraindications: Pregnant women or those with any blood disorders, especially bleeding, should avoid using this herb. Those with heated conditions should use it with caution. This herb should not be used with aconite (Fu Zi).

Dose: 3-12g

Biochemical constituents: Amino acid, choline, fatty acid, b-sitosteril and D-glycoside, 3,4,-diglycosilic, benzaldehyde and l-ephedrine.

Poke root (Phytolacca decandra or P. americana) / Shang Lu
Common Name: Poke

Family: Phytolaccaeae

Part used: The root

Energy and flavors: Cold, bitter and toxic

Organ meridians affected: Spleen and kidney

Type of cancer:	Breast, lungs and lymphatic
Actions:	Diuretic, lymphatic cleanser, resolves lumps, alterative, anodyne, antibiotic, parasiticide, antiinflammatory, antirheumatic, antiscorbutic, antisyphilitic, antitumor, cathartic and emetic.
Indications:	Edema and abdominal distension
Contraindications:	Not for edema caused by qi deficiency.
Dose:	4-9g. No more than five drops of the extract should be taken at a time, since in higher dose poke is toxic.
Biochemical constituents:	It contains saponins, formic acid, tannin, fatty oil, resin and a sugar. Five distinct proteins have been identified with mitogenic (cancer-killing) properties.

Other information: It was official in the USP from 1820-1900 and again in the National Formulary as recent as 1926. Sometimes called "cancer root" the Eclectics used it widely as an alterative or blood and lymphatic purifier for syphilis, arthritic and rheumatic complaints. They also used it for infections of the upper respiratory tract. It has been widely acclaimed as a treatment for chronic skin diseases, lymphatic enlargements and lymphomas. In over 40 years of use, Dr. Eli Jones considered it the most valuable single remedy for the treatment of cancer. He would prescribe only five drops of the tincture every three hours and found it to be especially important for the treatment of cancer of the breast, throat and uterus and especially for patients who were past mid-life.

Because the properties of pokeroot diminish over time, the alcoholic extract should only be made with the fresh, green root, finely chopping it and then blending with vodka. While it is available for use the next day, it is best to allow it to macerate for at least couple of weeks before press-straining it through a cloth.

A practice used in the Appalachian mountains of North America is to apply a poultice of fresh grated pokeroot over a cancerous lesion or tumor. In many cases this has been known to greatly reduce the size of the cancer or eliminate it altogether.

Most herbalists believe that dried pokeroot is practically worthless, at least it is so for topical application.

Poria cocos / Fu Ling
Common Name: Poria, Tuckahoe, China root

Family:	Polyporaceae
Part used:	The fruiting body
Energy and flavor:	Neutral, sweet or no flavor
Organ meridians affected:	Spleen, lung, heart and urinary bladder
Type of cancer:	Various types of solid tumors
Actions:	Diuretic and sedative. It clears dampness, regulates fluid metabolism, assists digestion and calms the spirit.
Indications:	It is used for edema, swollen abdomen, diarrhea, insomnia, palpitations.
Contraindications:	It is contraindicated for someone with frequent urination, spermatorrhea, and prolapse of the uro-genital organs.
Dose:	6-18g
Biochemical constituents:	Tetracyclic triterpenic acid, polysaccharide (pachyman), ergosterol, choline fat, glucose, lipase and protease.

Other information: Poria has been shown to lower blood sugar, which makes it useful for hyperglycemia commonly associated with cancer of various types. As with other medicinal mushrooms, it has been shown to stimulate the immune system and inhibit the proliferation and growth of tumors. One study using a 50% extract demonstrated that it significantly augmented the secretion of interleukins IL-1 beta IL-6 6 h after in vitro cultivation of human peripheral blood monocytes. The augmented effect was dose dependent. Tumor necrosis factor-alpha (TNF-alpha) secretion was also increased as the cells were treated with 0.4 mg/ml or higher doses of Fu-Ling extract.[58] As with many of the other medicinal mushrooms, besides being effective against tumors, Poria also potentiates the positive effects of chemo and radiation therapy while offsetting some of their negative side effects.

Poria umbellata / Zhu Ling
Common Name: Grifola

Family:	Polyporaceae
Part used:	The fruiting body

Energy and flavor:	Slightly cool, sweet and bland
Organ meridians affected:	Spleen, kidney and urinary bladder
Type of cancer:	Various types of solid tumors
Actions:	Drains dampness and clears heat.
Indications:	Used for edema, abdominal distention, vaginal discharge, urinary infections, jaundice, diabetes and diarrhea.
Contraindications:	Use only when there are signs of dampness.
Dose:	6-15g
Biochemical constituents:	Ergosterol, a-hydroxy-tetracosanoic acid, protein, vitamin H and biotin.

Other information: The diuretic action of grifola is stronger than poria cocos or caffeine. Besides its ability to reduce edema, the polysaccharides of grifola has been used on cancer patients since the 1970's with the result of improved appetite, weight gain, mental alertness and varying degrees of improvement of the cancer.[59] Other Chinese clinical studies found that the extract "757" from grifola administered to 50 cases of primary lung cancer as compared to the control exhibited 86.1% improvement as compared to 62.5% of the control. Even more stunning was that the percentage of cases achieving stability after treatment was 70% as opposed to 25% of the control group. It was also found that grifola "757" significantly strengthened the immune system and helped reduce the side effects of chemotherapy.[60]

Prunella vulgaris / Xia Ku Cao
Common Name: Selfheal

Family:	Labiatae
Part used:	The flowering spike
Energy and flavor:	Cold and bitter
Organ meridians affected:	Liver, gallbladder, thyroid, breast and lungs
Type of cancer:	All cancers
Actions:	Clears liver heat, dissolves tumors, nodules and swollen glands and lowers blood pressure.
Indications:	For many inflammatory diseases including conjunctivitis, mastitis, swollen glands and high blood pressure.
Contraindications:	Not for someone with weak digestion.

Prunella vulgaris (continued)

Dose:	6-18g
Biochemical constituents:	Triterpenoidal saponins, vitamins B1, C, K, and carotene. The spike specifically contains delphinidin, cyanidin and ursolic acid.

Other information: This is an important herb in Chinese medicine and has been all but overlooked in Western herbal medicine. Perhaps because the latter does not distinguish the anti-tumor properties of the whole herb. It is used for all solid masses and tumors and as such can be combined with various other herbs in formulas.

Prunus armeniaca / Xing Ren
Common Name: Apricot seed

Family:	Rosaceae
Part used:	Seed (Semen)
Type of cancer:	Lung cancer
Energy and flavor:	Slightly warm, bitter and slightly toxic
Organ meridians affected:	Lung, esophagus and large intestine
Actions:	1) Stops cough and wheezing caused by either heat or cold; 2) lubricates the intestines and aids constipation.
Indications:	1) For cough, asthma and either chronic or acute bronchitis, it is especially good for dry cough; 2) can be used for constipation.
Contraindications:	This herb should be used with caution when there is yin deficiency and with infants. It should not be used when there is diarrhea.
Dose:	3-9g
Biochemical constituents:	The major constituent is amygdalin, which is also known as B17 or laetrile.

Other information: Amygdalin, found in various natural sources including loquat and peach seeds, is also the basis for B17 and laetrile, considered to be a specific cancer preventive nutrient. There is diverse understanding of all of these as having both curative and preventive effects for the treatment of cancer. It is recommended for active cancers that a patient consume 5 Apricot seeds hourly each day for a total of 30 seeds throughout the day.

For prevention 5 kernels are eaten once or twice daily. Chinese research has found the hot water extract of Apricot seeds in vivo to inhibit various types of cancers, inhibiting JTC-26 type cancer from 50% to 70%.

Psoralea corylifolia / Bu Gu Zhi
Common Name: Psoralea

Family:	Leguminosae
Part used:	The fruit (Fructus)
Energy and flavor:	Very warm, acrid and bitter
Organ meridians affected:	Kidney and spleen
Type of cancer:	Various types of cancers
Actions:	1) Tonifies the kidney yang and augments kidney qi; 2) tonifies the spleen yang; 3) restrains leakage of essence (jing) and holds urine; 4) applied topically for psoriasis and vitiligo.
Indications:	1) For deficiency of kidney yang with symptoms of impotence, cold and weak lower back and knees and weakness in the extremities. It is also for kidney unable to grasp the qi of the lung; 2) for deficiency of spleen yang where there is cold diarrhea which is chronic and often "daybreak diarrhea," borborygmus and abdominal pain; 3) for leakage of essence (jing) and urine with symptoms of spermatorrhea, frequent urination, urinary incontinence and enuresis; 4) has recently been used both topically and by injection for psoriasis, vitiligo and alopecia. It tonifies both kidney and spleen yang, restrains leakage of urine, treats coldness with weakness of the lower back and legs. It is also good for deficient spleen syndromes with diarrhea.
Contraindications:	This herb should not be used when there are acute inflammatory symptoms. It also may need to be combined with digestive and carminative herbs, as it may be difficult to digest.
Biochemical constituents:	Furocoumarin (psoralen, angelicin, isop-

Psoralea corylifolia (continued)

soralen), flavonone (bavachinin, bavachin, isobavachin), isobavachalcone, bakuchiol, resin and fatty oil.

Other information: Its value in the treatment of cancer is primarily in its ability to increase an individual's white blood cell count.

Rabdosia rubescens / Dong Ling Cao	
Common Name: Rabdosia	

Part used:	The aerial part of the herb
Energy and flavors:	Not known
Type of cancer:	It has been successfully used for esophageal cancers, breast and prostate cancer, but is probably effective for a wide variety of other cancers as well. It is one of the active anti-cancer herbs in the formula PC SPES, which has undergone successful clinical trials for prostate cancer.
Actions:	It is antibacterial, anti-inflammatory, anti-spasmodic and analgesic. Chinese medicine uses it to treat acute tonsillitis. In Hunan it is widely used to treat esophageal cancer. The mode of action seems to be that DNA synthesis in Ehrlich ascites cells is inhibited by 74% after treatment of oridonin at a concentration of 10 ug/ml.

Experimental data has found that an alcohol-based extract of the herb is highly toxic to HeLa cells. Both oral and parenteral administration of the extract to mice with Ehrlich ascites cells or S-180 sarcoma cells exhibited a marked inhibitory effect.

From 1974 to 1987 Dr. Wang treated 650 cases of moderate to advanced esophageal carcinoma patients using this herb. Of these 40 patients survived over 5 years, 30 over 6 years, 23 over 10 years with a total of 20 patients still living after 18 years of treatment.[61,62] Another study demonstrated the synergistic effect of oridonin and cisplatin on cytotoxicity and DNA cross-link against mouse sarcoma S180 cells in culture.[63]

Dose:
The full standard adult dose for the treatment of cancer is approximately 20 to 25g of the powdered herb, three times daily. A course of treatment is 1 to 1 ½ months. For esophageal cancer it was found that after several doses, the patient was able to swallow food and experienced an appetite improvement.

Biochemical constituents:
It contains several terpenes. The most active is rubescensine B. Other anticancer principles isolated are oridonin and ponicidine. Additionally, being a member of the Labiatae family, it contains essential oils and tannic acid. Rubescensine B has been found to possess anticancer activity against hepatoma cells at a concentration of 4 ug/ml. Additionally, this constituent was found to augment the immunity of animals with cancer. (From the *Pharmacology of Chinese Herbs*, 2nd edition, by Kee Chang Huang).

Other information: Rabdosia rubescens was one of the herbs in the notorious prostate cancer formula by the name of PC-SPES. This formula was found to contain undeclared hormone blockers and was subsequently pulled from the market in February, 2002. Its manufacturer, BotaniLab, closed its doors in June of the same year. Having said this, I have never used BotaniLab's PC-SPES but I secured Rabdosia rubescens directly from China and made my own version – without the drugs, of course. This formula consisted of Rabdosia, Panax pseudo ginseng, Licorice root, Ganoderma lucidum, Scutellaria baicalensis, Dendranthema morifolium and Serenoa repens (Saw Palmetto). This, along with other herbs and formulas including my own Planetary Formula's Saw Palmetto Classic, together with supplementation and the rigorous diet has proven quite successful in returning PSA count to normal and reversing diagnosed Prostate Cancer (see case history in Chapter Eleven).

Realgar / Xiong Huang
Common Name: Arsenic sulfide

Part used: The mineral

Energy and flavors: Hot, bitter, acrid and poisonous

Organ meridians affected: Heart, Liver and stomach.

Type of cancer: It is effective for a wide range of cancers including non-solid cancers such as leukemia. It is best to begin with the lowest possible dose and increase gradually to the recommended dose given below. This substance should not be used without medical supervision.

Actions: 1) Relieves toxicity; 2) kills parasites; 3) relieves itch; 4) heals snakebites and ulcerations ; 5) dries dampness; 6) treats malarial conditions.

Indications: Relieves toxicity, abscesses and sores

Preparations: 1) With borneol and phellodendron it is applied topically for scabies and eczema; 2) with borneol it can be made into an alcoholic tincture and used topically for herpes zoster; 3) as a powder it is mixed with alumen and it can be applied topically to treat nasal polyps; 4) as a powder combined with alumentum trogopteri seu pteromi (Wu Ling Zhi) for poisonous snakebites and other venomous bites and stings.

Contraindications: Internally during pregnancy and for yin and blood deficiency.

Dose: Internally 0.15 to 0.6g in pills or powders. A finely ground powder is applied topically to localized areas. Because its toxicity is absorbed through the skin it should not be applied to a large area.

Biochemical constituents: As2Ss (arsenic disulfide)

Other information: It is anti-toxic and relieves phlegm. It is a recognized protoplasmic toxin and destroys malignant oncocytes. It is violently toxic and is usually not taken internally. Traditionally, for any internal usage it is decocted with mung beans and the dosage and the period of frequency limited to a safe range of no more than one or two weeks at a time. It is widely used in formula with intractable ulcers and cancers externally.

Rehmannia glutinosa (Unprepared) / Sheng Di Huang
Common Name: Rehmannia root, Chinese foxglove

Part used:	The root
Energy and flavor:	Cold, sweet and bitter
Organ meridians affected:	Heart, liver and kidney
Type of cancer:	Cancers associated with dryness, inflammation and yin deficiency
Actions:	1) Antiinflammatory, expels heat by cooling blood; 2) tonifies yin by promoting fluid production; 3) soothes the heart by calming blazing fire; 4) cools and nourishes; 4) arrests cough; 5) tonifies the kidney-adrenals when used in formulas.
Indications:	1) For febrile diseases in the nutritive or blood level with symptoms of high fever, extreme thirst, reckless movement of blood, a red tongue and a rapid pulse; 2) for heat signs associated with yin deficiency with symptoms of low-grade fever, thirst, red tongue body and a thin rapid pulse; 3) for deficiency of heart yin with symptoms of oral sores, insomnia, low-grade fever or irascibility with a red tipped tongue; 4) for chronic diseases where there is yin deficiency and heat such as wasting and thirsting disorders.

Rehmannia glutinosa (Prepared) / Shu Di Huang

Energy and flavor:	Slightly warm and sweet
Organ meridians affected:	Heart, liver and kidney
Type of cancer:	Used as a yin and blood tonic for all types of cancers.
Actions:	1) Tonifies the blood; 2) tonifies the yin of the kidneys.

Rehmannia glutinosa (continued)

Indications: 1) The most commonly used herb for blood deficiency, it can be used for any symptoms associated with that conditions provided the condition does not have dampness in the spleen, as this herb is very damp and can be difficult to digest; 2) for kidney yin deficiency with symptoms of night sweats, chronic low grade fever, dry mouth, tinnitus, premature graying of the hair and wasting and thirsting disorder.

Contraindications: Those with weak digestion yang deficiency and/or stagnation of qi should not use these herbs, especially when there is dampness, as in conditions associated with diarrhea, lack of appetite and/or excess phlegm. Pregnant women should also avoid it.

Dose: 9-30g

Biochemical constituents: Rehmannin, mannitol, sucrose, amino acid, vitamin A, and catalpol.

Other information: The main indication for rehmannia is dryness and wasting. Its contraindication is digestive weakness since an herb that is as heavy and moist as rehmannia is often difficult for a weak stomach to breakdown and assimilate. Too much rehmannia taken over a prolonged period, especially taken by itself without the addition of digestive and carminative herbs can further weaken digestion. Since the single most important strategy in the treatment of cancer is to maintain and optimize digestion, one should use heavy-natured tonics and especially blood and yin tonics such as rehmannia with caution. Nevertheless, because kidney and adrenal deficiency is commonly associated with the after-effects of chemotherapy or with advanced cancer, a small amount of rehmannia may be of great benefit in a carefully balanced formulation.

Rheum palmatum / Da Huang
Common Name: Rhubarb, Chinese rhubarb, Turkey rhubarb

Family: Polygonaceae

Part used: The root

Energy and flavor: Cold and bitter

Organ meridians affected:	Liver, spleen, large intestine, stomach and pericardium
Type of cancer:	Colorectal cancer, uterine and ovarian cancer and granulocytic leukemia
Actions:	1) Drains excess heat and eliminates dampness especially when in the sunlight yang stage; 2) cools the blood and stops bleeding; 3) invigorates blood, breaks up stasis and relieves pain; 4) clears heat and toxins from excess; 5) applied topically for hot sores and blood stasis.
Indications:	1) For damp-heat conditions of excess with symptoms of constipation, high fever, jaundice, painful urination and fullness of the abdomen; 2) for heat in the blood with reckless movement of blood with symptoms of blood in the stool, vomiting of blood or nosebleed; 3) for amenorrhea, dysmenorrhea, sharp pain, pain due to injury and abscesses it can be applied externally or taken internally to break up stasis and relieve pain; 4) for heat at the blood level accompanied by toxic build up with symptoms of fever, jaundice, acute appendicitis, swollen eyes and abscesses; 5) applied topically for burns, abscesses, carbuncles and blood stasis.
Contraindications:	Because of its purging properties, rhubarb is contraindicated for patients with digestive weakness and low energy.
Dose:	3-12g
Biochemical constituents:	Anthraquinones, chrysophanol, tannins, sennidin, rheidine, palmidine, catechin, gallic acid and flavone, many of these have known anticancer properties.

Other information: Turkey rhubarb or Chinese rhubarb is derived from a number of subspecies and have been found to have antitumor activity in the sarcoma 27 of mice. Emodin inhibits the cellular respiration of ascites cancer and emodin inhibits mice melanoma at an effective rate of 76% and anthraquinones have been generally found to inhibit the growth of cancer. A hot water extract of the drug inhibited sarcoma-180 with an effective rate of 48.8%.

Rheum palmatum (continued)

In general, the herb is not used singly but in combinations such as the Essiac formula or with other alterative herbs. Since it has a purging property, the dose is usually individually regulated according to the patient. However, 30g of the dried herb can be decocted in rice wine for uterine cancer. The dose is one to two tablespoons three times daily after meals.

A topical paste for treating breast tumors is to combine 30g each of rhubarb root and licorice root. These are ground to a powder and mixed with rice wine to form a paste. This can then be spread on a cloth or bandage and topically applied daily to dissolve the lesion. The mixture is also taken internally.

Rumex acetosella (Acetosella vulgaris)
Common Name: Sheep sorrel

Family:	Polygonaceae
Part used:	Aerial portions
Energy and flavor:	Cool and sour
Organ meridians affected:	Liver
Type of cancer:	For different types of cancers. It is one of the main ingredients in Essiac tea.
Actions:	Cooling, anti-inflammatory, anti-fever and diuretic
Indications:	Infections, fevers, cancers and tumors
Contraindications:	Generally very safe and mild but its cooling nature may need to be considered for individuals with symptoms of cold deficiency. The leaf is high in oxalic acid and over consumption has been known to cause toxicity.
Dose:	The fresh or dried leaves are used either in a tea or as a food. The leaves can be eaten fresh or parboiled like spinach.
Biochemical constituents:	Adenosine, anthraquinones, emodin, oxalic acid, Chrysophanol, chrysophanic acid, rutin and tannin (root)

Other information: One of the four primary herbs of the famous Essiac formula (the others being burdock, rhubarb and slippery elm), it was tested in Taiwan and there was no activity against mouse leukemia. However, aloe emodin, isolated from sorrel, does show significant antileukemic action. The eclectics found that sorrel was useful for softening and helping to dissolve tumors. However, in general they considered it a weak medicine and later seldom employed it.

The use of Essiac as a treatment for cancer is widespread. While the four herbs in the formula indeed do possess anticancer properties, there has been no evaluation of the many largely anecdotal claims for its efficacy. These claims include reduced tumor growth, quality of life, and prolonged survival. While in vivo antitumor activity has not been revealed in tests, the various herbs in the formula have been found to have antioxidant, antiestrogenic, immunostimulant, antitumor and anticholoretic actions.[64] The popular FlorEssence™ product has been tested and found to have potent antioxidant properties.[65]

I consider Essiac a mild anticancer botanical. This being said, sheep sorrel has a history of use for the treatment of cancer. King's late 19th century *American Dispensatory* mentions the practice of using sheep Sorrel for the treatment of tumors and cancer. The great Eclectic medical doctor, Dr. Scudder, states how a strong tincture of the whole plant in doses ranging from 1 to 30 drops is a remedy where there is a "tendency to degeneration of tissue." He describes its ability to promote the healing of cancer.

Rumex Crispus
Common Name: Yellow dock, Broad leafed dock, Curly dock

Family:	Polygonaceae
Part used:	The root
Energy and flavor:	Cold, bitter and sweetish
Organ meridians affected:	Liver and colon
Type of cancer:	Leukemia, liver and colo-rectal
Actions:	Clears heat, clears damp heat, detoxifies, mild laxative, cholagogue and blood tonic.
Indications:	Used for anemia, skin diseases, herpes simplex, acne and liver congestion.
Contraindications:	Not for pregnant women and use with caution for people with internal coldness. There are a few reported acute cases of fatal oxalate poisoning from the ingestion of Yellow dock root.
Dose:	3-6g, of the tincture 10 to 30 drops for each dose.

Rumex Crispus (continued)

Biochemical constituents: Anthraquinone glycosides, rhein, emodin, rumicin, chrysarobin, tannins and oxalates

Other information: In China, rumex root has been used for acute leukemia at a dose of 30-60g taken in two doses daily. Considering its well-known benefit in Western herbal medicine for anemia, this sounds like it might be an effective use for this herb. The anthraquinones, rhein and emodin are known to have antitumor properties.

Salvia milthiorrhiza / Dan Shen
Common Name: Chinese red sage root

Family: Labiatae

Part used: The root

Energy and flavor: Slightly cold and bitter

Organ meridians affected: Heart and liver

Type of cancer: For a wide variety of cancers including thyroid, thymus, abdomen, breast, esophageal, liver and reproductive organs.

Actions: Moves blood, promotes circulation, eliminates blood stagnation, anti-inflammatory, sedative and tranquilizer.

Indications: Coronary heart disease, angina, palpitations, menstrual irregularity, irritability, ulcers and carbuncles.

Contraindications: Not for individuals with loose bowels with no signs of blood stagnation.

Dose: 3-15g

Biochemical constituents: Tanshinone, tanshinol, salviol and vitamin E

Other information: At least one study has indicated that salvia enhanced the power of chemotherapy by facilitating mutations of the p53 gene for the treatment of colorectal cancer.[66,66] These and other studies have also indicated that salvia miltiorrhiza increases apoptosis (cancer cell death) in patients.[68] It has been suggested that the antineoplastic properties of red sage root is in its ability to inhibit the respiration and glucolysis of cancer cells.

Sanguinarea canadensis
Common Name: Bloodroot

Family:	Papaveraceae
Part used:	The rhizome
Energy and flavor:	Hot, dry, spicy and bitter
Organ meridians affected:	Lungs and liver
Type of cancer:	Lungs and liver
Actions:	Expectorant, antiinflammatory, antifungal, escharotic, antibiotic, antiseptic, blood coagulant, cathartic, diaphoretic, emetic and emmenagogue
Indications:	It is used for cold phlegm in the lungs, and also for sinus congestion, asthma (sub-acute or chronic), bronchitis, common cold, edema, influenza, skin eruptions, swollen glands and tumors. Sanguinarine is used as a dentifrice against plaque.
Contraindications:	It is toxic in higher dosages and should not be taken by pregnant or lactating women. It should not be taken internally for more than three or four days at a time. Do not take with heparin and other anticoagulants, which are opposed by berberine.
Dose:	10 to 30 drops of the tincture. Externally it is combined with zinc chloride to make a famous escharotic paste.
Biochemical constituents:	Various alkaloids including berberine, sanguinarine, protopine, chelerythrine, resin, sanguinaric acid, citric and malic acids and starch.

Other information: Jones recommends it for colo-rectal cancer, one eighth of a grain once every three hours.

Sargassii pallidum / Hai Zao
Common Name: Sargassum, Seaweed

Family:	Sargassum
Part used:	The aerial portion (Herba)
Energy and flavor:	Cold, bitter and salty
Organ meridians affected:	Lung, kidney, liver, spleen and stomach
Type of cancer:	Thyroid, liver, lung and stomach
Actions:	1) Clears heat and reduces hardenings associated with phlegm-fire; 2) encourages urination and lessens edema; 3) expels phlegm from the lungs; 4) softens goiter, swollen and hard lymph glands and other hardened lumps and nodules.
Indications:	1) For phlegm-fire with symptoms of goiter, scrofula and tuberculosis of the lymph nodes; 2) this herb can be used in combination with other herbs for edema; 3) for phlegm in the lungs due to chronic bronchitis or other similar chronic conditions.
Contraindications:	This herb should not be used by those with symptoms of coldness due to spleen and stomach deficiency.
Dose:	6-15g
Biochemical constituents:	Alginic acid, mannitol, glucose, mucilage, potassium and iodine

Other information: Commonly combined with laminaria (kelp), it has very similar properties. It is useful for softening, dissolving and inhibiting a wide variety of cancers. Being nutritive, both of these herbs are especially effective in softening and dissolving tumors when combined with other herbs for specific cancers.

Saussurea, Aucklandiae lappae / Mu Xiang
Common Name: Saussurea, Costus root, Saussurea lappa

Family:	Compositae
Part used:	The root (Radix)
Energy and flavor:	Warm, acrid and bitter

Organ meridians affected:	Spleen, liver, lung, gallbladder, large intestine and stomach
Type of cancer:	Cancer of the esophagus and stomach
Actions:	1) Relieves qi stagnation of digestion in the spleen, stomach and intestines; 2) relieves qi stagnation of the liver and gallbladder; 3) strengthens the spleen and is used with tonifying herbs to prevent their potential cloying effects.
Indications:	1) For digestive stagnation with symptoms of pain and distention in the abdominal region, nausea, loss of appetite and vomiting; 2) for stagnant qi of the liver and gallbladder with symptoms of flank pain and abdominal distention; 3) typically used with tonifying herbs to prevent the potential cloying effect they can have on the spleen.
Contraindications:	Those with yin and blood deficiency should not use this herb.
Dose:	3-9g
Biochemical constituents:	Essential oil (should not be boiled), stigmasterol, betulin and saussurine

---

Schisandra chinensis / Wu Wei Zi
Common Name: Schisandra berries, Five flavored fruit

Family:	Magnoliaceae
Part used:	The berries
Energy and flavor:	Warm and sour
Organ meridians affected:	Lung, heart and kidney
Type of cancer:	Used as a tonic for all cancers to counteract wasting, nervousness, insomnia and for lung cancer.
Actions:	1) Tonifies the kidneys and preserves the essence; 2) astringes the lung qi and stops coughing; 3) retains bodily fluids and encourages their production; 4) tonifies the heart and calms the spirit (shen).
Indications:	1) For kidney deficiency causing leakage of essence with symptoms such as exces-

sive sweating and night sweats, nocturnal emissions, vaginal discharge, urinary incontinence and daybreak diarrhea; 2) for lung qi and kidney deficiency leading to chronic cough, especially dry cough, wheezing and asthma; 3) for spontaneous sweating, seminal emissions, night sweats, wasting and thirsting disorder and frequent urination; 4) for deficiency of heart blood and yin with symptoms such as palpitations, forgetfulness, insomnia and irritability.

Dose: 2-9g

Contraindications: Those with internal heat should not use this herb nor should it be used by those with an externally contracted disease.

Biochemical constituents: Essential oil (sesquicarene, B-bisabolene, B-chamigrene, A-ylangene), citric acid, malic acid, tartaric acid, sugars, resin, schizandrin, pseudo-y-schizandrin, deoxyschizandrin, schizandrol, stigmasterol and vitamins C and E

Other information: It maintains the normal function of the liver.

Scolopendra Subspinipes / Wu Gong
Common Name: Centipede

Family: Scolopendridae

Energy and flavors: Warm, pungent and toxic

Organ meridians affected: Liver

Type of cancer: Liver and brain

Actions: 1) Antispasmodic, subdues internal wind; 2) clears toxins; 3) opens the channels and stops pain.

Indications: 1) For spasms, tetany, convulsions and epilepsy; 2) treats venomous bites and stings, clears toxins and reduces swollen glands; 3) treats stubborn migraine headaches and rheumatic pains.

Contraindications: This is a toxic substance and the dosage should be conservative. It is contraindicated during pregnancy.

Dose: 1-3g or 0.6 to 0.9g as a powder

Biochemical constituents: (235)-hydroxylysine, taurine and histamine-like substance

Other information: Just as some cultures consume roasted grasshoppers as a food, the Chinese roast scorpions and treat them as a healthful delicacy and recommend consuming 10 each month to protect one from all diseases.

Scrophularia nodosa et species / Xuan Shen species
Common Name: Figwort, Heal all, Carpenter's square

Family: Scrophulariae

Part used: The root and herb

Energy and flavor: Cool, bitter, slightly spicy and dry

Organ meridians affected: Kidneys, liver, large intestines and lymph

Type of cancer: Breast, lungs, glands, lymphoma and other cancers

Actions: Clears heat and dampness, detoxifies and emmenagogue.

Indications: Used for liver congestion, chronic constipation, edema, treats damp eczema, swollen glands, reduces lymph congestion and reduces and softens tumors. It is also used for marked evidence of cachexia, glandular diseases, glandular inflammations of the mammary glands, testicles, etc, difficult menstruation and helping to expel the placenta after childbirth. It also has a beneficial effect for many heart conditions, including palpitations. Externally it is effective for burns, injuries, sprains, swellings, fungal infections and impetigo.

Contraindications: It should not be used during pregnancy, lactation, diabetes, or with ventricular tachycardia. Large doses are poisonous. The use of any cardioactives can potentiate herbs with cardiac glycosides. It can also interfere with

Scrophularia nodosa et species (continued)

antidiabetic drugs.

Dose: Of the tincture take from 5 to 30 drops three or four times daily. Of the whole herb use 6-9g daily.

Biochemical constituents: Harpagophytum, iridoid glycosides, cardioactive glycosides, saponins (diosmin, hesperidin), flavonoids (including aucubin), alkaloid, organic acids, and pectin

Other information: Different scrophularia are known to possess potent antiinflammatory properties that make it useful for different stages of cancer.[69] Jones describes this as one of the most valuable remedies for advanced stages of cancer. It is especially indicated when there is metastasis of lumps to the neck and axilla. It is the principle ingredient in his compound syrup of scrophularia.

Scutellariae barbatae / Ban Zhi Lian
Common Name: Barbat skullcap

Family: Labiatae

Part used: The whole plant

Energy and flavor: Cold, acrid and bitter

Organ meridians affected: Liver, lung and stomach

Type of cancer: Lung, breast and various types of cancers

Actions: It is antitoxic, cools the blood and removes blood stagnation.

Indications: It is particularly effective for various liver diseases such as hepatitis and cirrhosis.

Contraindications: Not for use during pregnancy

Dose: 15-30g

Biochemical constituents: Portual, betacyanin, betanin and betanidin

Other information: Various pharmacological studies have thus far revealed that this herb has a strong inhibitive action on JTC-26 (over 90% rate) with only a slight inhibition of normal cells. It has proven anticancer action, it is antibacterial, inhibiting to granular leukemia with an inhibition rate of over 75%. Animal studies have shown it to be inhibitive on sarcoma-180, Ehrlich's ascites carcinoma and cerebroma-B22 in rats. It is widely used in

Chinese anti-cancer herb formulas. 30g of S. barbatae is twice decocted in water morning and evening for esophageal cancer. The same amount is prepared with an equal amount of solani lyrati and taken once daily. It is commonly combined with oldenlandia and many other anticancer herbs. The fresh juice is the most effective.

Serenoa Serrulata
Common Name: Saw palmetto, Sabal, Serenoa

Family:	Palmaceae, Aracaceae
Part used:	The fruit
Energy and flavor:	Warm, pungent, acrid and sweet
Organ meridians affected:	Kidney, spleen and liver
Type of cancer:	Prostate
Actions:	Nutritive yin tonic, diuretic, expectorant, roborant, sedative, endocrine and anabolic agent and aphrodisiac.
Indications:	Wasting diseases, underweight, upper respiratory conditions, prostate hyperplasia, urinary tract infections, impotence and frigidity. According to Donny Yance, since it has anti-androgenic and estrogenic properties, it is also useful for women who have an excess of androgenic hormones with symptoms of hirsutism, infertility, acne, amenorrhea, polycystic ovaries, debility and deficiency. Traditionally the Eclectics claimed that it helped to stimulate breast growth.
Contraindications:	Gastrointestinal inflammation, esophageal reflux, lactation and pregnancy.
Dose:	3-12g three times daily
Biochemical constituents:	Essential oil, fatty acids, carotene, polysaccharides, tannin, sitosterol, invert sugar and estrogenic substance

Other information: Because of its anabolic, antiandrogenic and estrogenic properties, saw palmetto would be especially useful for prostate cancer. Dihydrotestosterone (DHT) is believed to be the primary cause of prostate hyperplasia that can lead to prostate cancer. Saw palmetto inhibits the conversion of DHT and helps to break down and eliminate the excess testosterone.

Serenoa Serrulata (continued)

It is an adjunctive herb for prostate cancer and should be combined with other anticancer herbs such as andrographis, isatis, barberry and pipsissewa for treating prostate cancer.

Silybum marianum (Carduus marianus)
Common Name: Milk thistle, Silymarin

Family:	Compositae
Part used:	The seeds
Energy and flavor:	Cool, bitter, mildly sweet and dry
Organ meridians affected:	Liver and spleen-pancreas
Type of cancer:	Liver, kidneys, reproductive organs, skin and other cancers
Actions:	Hepatoprotective, bitter tonic, demulcent and antidepressant
Indications:	Used for various acute and chronic liver conditions including hepatitis A, B and C as well as liver cirrhosis. It also helps the cardiovascular system by lowering blood lipids.
Contraindications:	None noted
Dose:	At least 420 ml daily
Biochemical constituents:	Flavonol, silymarin, flavonoid, bitter amines, tannin and polyacetylenes

Other information: There is some very good research attesting to the broad anticarcinogenic effects of silymarin. There is one astounding case of a spontaneous regression of hepatocellular carcinoma of a 52-year-old man who happened to be taking silymarin.[70] Silymarin has also been shown to have antiproliferative and apoptotic effects in skin cancer.[71] In vitro studies have shown that silibinin from silymarin seeds is able to inhibit the prostate-specific antigen involved with prostate cancer.[72] Another in vitro study investigating the effects of flavonoids found in silymarin among other natural substances the ability to exert an antioxidant protective effect on the DNA, thus helping normalize cell growth.[73] More than one study has demonstrated the kidney-protective effects of silibinin against cisplatin-induced nephrotoxicity without compromising the intended beneficial effects of these potent chemotherapeutic agents.[74,75] From all of this evidence it seems that anyone who is dealing with cancer, treatment prevention or possibly recurrence should include milk thistle seeds as a regular part of their supplement program.

Silymarin seasoning: One practical and possibly tasty way to do this was offered by herbalist Ed Smith who describes how to make milk thistle seed gomasio. This is somewhat modified by myself to include another potent anticancer botanical, kelp. Combine equal parts toasted silymarin seeds, Kelp or Nori seaweed, natural sea or rock salt or the Nine Times salt described elsewhere in this book. Use only 1/7th to 1/10th salt or make it to taste. Grind together and use as a regular seasoning on food.

Solanum nigrum / Long Kui
Common Name: Black nightshade

Family:	Solanaceae
Part used:	The aerial portions
Organ meridians affected:	Liver and lungs
Type of cancer:	Lungs, breast and liver
Energies and Flavors:	Cool, bitter and mildly toxic
Actions:	Anti-inflammatory, demulcent, analgesic, antitussive, antiasthmatic, antibacterial, antivenin, antidiabetic, hypotensive, antineoplastic and mildly toxic
Indications:	Used for inflammations, to relieve pain, inhibit coughs, quell asthma, diabetes, lower blood pressure and treat malignancies.
Biochemical constituents:	Glycoalkaloids solanine, solasonine and solamargine. It also has small amounts of atropine and saponins. The alkaloids are highest in the unripe fruit. Solanine extracted from the unripe fruit of S. nigrum provided a 40 to 50% inhibition rate of transplanted animal tumors

Other information: Chinese medicine has found this herb to be effective against Ehrlich's ascites carcinoma, lymphatic leukemia-615, sarcoma-180 and sarcoma-37 in rats. Further research has found that it inhibits cancer cells of the stomach and finally in vitro with methylene-blue test tube experiments, on leukemia cancer cells. It is widely used for various cancers by the Chinese including cancer of the lungs, liver and cervix.

It is most effective when fresh and combined with astringent herbs including agrimony and sanguisorba, which limits its demulcent properties. When it is decocted for at least 45 minutes to one hour, its mild toxicity is greatly reduced.

Solanum nigrum (continued)

The approximate daily dose is 150g of the fresh herb and 30 to 60g of the freshly dried herb double decocted in 800ml of water. This is then slowly reduced to 300 ml of water and taken orally in three doses three times each day. Do this for 15 days and stop or change the formulation for a week or two and repeat as needed.

Solanum nigrum is regarded as one of the more important of Chinese anticancer herbs and is commonly found throughout various countries of the west including Europe and North America. **Nightshades** (Solani nigri, Solani lyrati), which are not to be confused with another member of the Solanaceae family that is closely related but toxic, Belladonna (Atropa belladonna), both S. nigri and S. lyrati are classified in Chinese Medicine as cold with lubricating functions. They are among the more important Chinese anticancer herbs also found growing throughout various countries of the West including Europe and North America. Pharmacologically they have been found to be effective for inhibiting Ehrlich's ascites, carcinoma, lymphatic leukemia-615 and sarcoma-37. Dosages range from 30 to 60g daily of the dried herb, more if it is used fresh. Western herbalists tend to shy away from the use of these plants because of reported toxicity. While the Chinese classify them as slightly toxic, decocting them over a prolonged period of 45 minutes to an hour mitigates their toxicity (something evidently never realized over the centuries of use by Western herbalists and the Eclectics).

The herbs are commonly combined in formula with agrimony and burnet (Sanguisorba), astringents with anti-cancer properties that serve to counterbalance the demulcent properties of the two benign nightshades.

Black nightshade is a very ancient remedy in the history of western herbalism. It was commonly employed topically in the form of a poultice or the expressed juice for a wide variety of inflammatory diseases. Caesalpinus also states that it was used internally for inflammations of the stomach, intestines and urinary tract. Infusions of even so much as 1 grain of the leaf taken at bedtime could have a profound effect that would include vomiting, sweating, purging and significant increase of urinary output. Its slight narcotic effect, which was inconsistent, might result in a state of giddiness possibly with strong evacuative effects from any or all of the eliminative systems. There are stories of children eating the raw berries and falling into a stupor. One of these, Eberle[77], mentions its use for foul, painful and chronic ulcers and pains in particular parts of the body. He also corroborates the Chinese use both for the treatment and attendant pain of cancer when he indicates its use for "scorbutic eruptions, and ulcers of a cancerous nature." In fact, there are at least ten biochemical constituents in black nightshade that have individually demonstrated anticancer properties. These include ascorbic acid, beta-carotene, beta-sitosterol, artemicide, citric acid, solamargine, solasodine, tannin and quercetin. These have variously showed positive activity for a variety of cancers including but not necessarily exclusively breast cancer, lung cancer, prostate cancer, lymphomas and skin cancers.

Sophora flavescentis / Ku Shen
Common name: Sophora

Family:	Leguminosae
Part used:	The root
Energy and flavor:	Cold and bitter
Organ meridians affected:	Heart, liver, stomach, large and small intestine and urinary bladder
Type of cancer:	Cervix, stomach, liver, respiratory tract, urinary and reproductive system
Actions:	1) Expels damp-heat; 2) scatters wind and relieves itching; 3) promotes urination and expels heat; 4) kills parasites; 5) applied externally for damp-heat.
Indications:	1) For damp-heat with symptoms of vaginal discharge, jaundice, dysentery and carbuncles; 2) for wind itching with symptoms of damp-heat sores, vaginitis, eczema and genital itching; 3) for damp-heat conditions of the urinary bladder and small intestine with symptoms of acute urinary tract infection, dysentery and edema associated with damp-heat; 4) for external application to damp-heat sores.
Other Indications:	It is used for jaundice, acute dysentery, leucorrhea, vaginitis, eczema, ringworm and acute urinary tract infections.
Contraindications:	Those with weakness and coldness in the spleen and stomach should not use this herb.
Dose:	3-12g
Biochemical constituents:	It contains various alkaloids including matrine, oxymatrine, sophocarpine and flavones.

Other information: The alkaloids have been found to have various percentages of inhibitory rates on various cancers. It is particularly effective for tumors of the chest, abdomen and cervix.

Sophora subprostrata / Shan Dou Gen
Common Name: Pigeon pea, Subprostrate sophora

Family:	Leguminosae
Energy and flavor:	Cold and bitter
Organ meridians affected:	Heart, lung, throat, large intestine, leukemia and lymphoma
Type of cancers:	Lungs, breast, gastrointestinal, large intestine, cervix, pancreas and urinary bladder
Actions:	It is antiinflammatory, detoxifying and one of the more important anticancer herbs.
Indications:	It is used for gingivitis, sore throat and cancer of the respiratory tract (lung and throat), digestive, urinary and reproductive systems. It is also used for leukemia. It increases the reticuloendothelium and increases white blood cells.
Dose:	6-9g
Biochemical constituents:	It contains alkaloid (matrine, oxymatrine, anagyrine, methylcytisine) flavonoid (sophoranone, sophoradin, sophoranochromene, sophoradochromene, genistein, pterocarpine, maackian, trifolirhizin) and caffeic acid.

Other information: It has been found to inhibit cervical tumors in mice, sarcoma-190, dehydrogenase in patients with acute lymphocytic leukemia and acute granulocytic leukemia. It has minimal adverse effects and will not reduce white blood cells.

Sparganium stoloniferium; Scirpus martimus / San Leng
Common Name: Bur reed tuber, Sparganium, Scirpus

Families:	Sparganium – Sparganiaciae; Scirpus – Cyperaceae
Energy and flavor:	Neutral to cold, pungent and bitter
Organ meridians affected:	Liver and spleen
Type of cancers:	Various cancers, especially liver cancer and cancer of the gastrointestinal and genitourinary organs

Actions:	Removes blood stagnation, moves blood and qi and relieves pain.
Indications:	For irregular menstruation, abdominal pains, abdominal distention, indigestion and tumor pain.
Contraindications:	Not for pregnant women or those with symptoms of excess menstruation.
Dose:	3-9g

Other information: It has been found to inhibit the growth of tumors and is particularly effective for treating abdominal cancers. It is, however, useful for other cancers and especially in helping to relieve the pain of tumors.

For stomach cancer decoct ten pounds of the dried herb. The tea is then strained, boiled and slowly reduced to thick syrup. Add 60% vegetable glycerin. Take 4 tablespoons three times daily.

Stillingia Root, Stillingia sylvatica, Stillingia ligustina, Stillingia treculeana
Common Name: Queen's delight, Queen's root, Silver leaf, Stillingia, Yaw root

Family:	Euphorbiaceae
Part used:	The root
Organ meridians affected:	Liver, lungs and bladder
Type of cancer:	Various types of cancers
Actions:	Alterative, anti-inflammatory, diuretic, laxative (large doses), astringent, cathartic (large doses), cholagogue, diaphoretic, diuretic (small doses), emetic, expectorant, flea repellant, laxative (small doses), sialagogue and spasmolytic
Indications:	It is used for various skin diseases, inflammations, bronchitis, cancer, constipation, dermatitis, eczema, fever, hemorrhoids, hepatitis, laryngismus stridulus, laryngitis, liver congestion, painful menstruation, scrofula, skin disorders, skin rash, sore throat and syphilis.
Contraindications:	Lactation and during pregnancy. Overdose can cause vertigo, burning sensation of the

Stillingia Root (continued)

mouth, throat and gastrointestinal tract, diarrhea, nausea, vomiting, dysuria, pruritus, skin eruptions, cough, depression, fatigue and perspiration. When stored for more than 2 years, stillingia seems to lose all potency. Fresh stillingia is a skin irritant, and the powder is a sternutatory (causes sneezing). Large doses can irritate mucous membranes. Leaves and stems are toxic to sheep due to the HCN content.

Dose: 3x/day

Dried Root: 1-6g or by decoction. *Liquid Extract:* 1:1 in 25 % alcohol, dose 0.5-2 ml. *Tincture:* 1:5 in 45 % alcohol, dose 1-4 ml. *Tincture, Dried Root:* 1:5 in 50 % alcohol; dose: 10-30 drops. *Tincture, Fresh Root:* 1:2 in 50% alcohol; dose: 10-30 drops

Biochemical constituents: Diterpene esters of the daphnane and tigliane type, including prostatin and gnidilatin, fixed oil, volatile oil and resins

Other information: Stillingia has a respected history of use in various North American preparations along with red clover for the treatment of cancer.

Strychnos Nux-vomica / Ma Qian Zi
Common Name: Nux-vomica, Strychnine; Semen strychni

Family: Loganiaceae

Part used: The seeds

Energy and flavor: Cold, bitter and poisonous

Organ meridians affected: Liver and spleen

Type of cancers: For a wide variety of cancers including lungs, breast, nasopharyngeal, uterine, colorectal and leukemia.

Actions: It clears the channels, subsides infection, assuages pain and promotes the circulation of qi and blood.

Indications: It is used for various types of pains and swellings from trauma. It is also used for rheumatic conditions, hemiplegia, spasms, facial paralysis, lymph tuberculosis and carcinoma. Topically it can be powdered and applied for carbuncle, furuncle and scabies.

Contraindications:	*Strychnine, the primary constituent, is very toxic with 5-10 mg causing poisoning and 30 mg death. Thus, it should be used with great caution internally and certainly not during pregnancy or for very weak individuals.* Processing will greatly reduce its toxicity. The procedure to detoxify it is to boil it first, strip off the shell, cut into slices and stir-fry or roast with sesame oil.
Dose:	0.3 to 0.9g per day. An appropriate amount is powdered and applied topically for external application. It is also safe and effective to use in homeopathic dilution up to 30X.
Biochemical constituents:	It contains pseudobrucine, strychnos alkaloids, pseudo-strychnine, strychnine, brucine, romicine, B-colubrine, fatty oil, protein and chlorogenic oil

Other information: It is used both in the East and West to stimulate nerve conduction, to relieve tension and spasm and increases gastric secretion to aid digestion. It also relieves chronic bronchitis and cough with phlegm. When used for a long time, it increases the function of antihistamine. In overdose, it causes tetanic convulsion and paralytic breath. The central nerve system has a strong affinity for it, and a long-term administration may result in poisoning. It is also both antiviral against influenza virus and antifungal. It has been found to inhibit sarcoma-180 and leukemia cells.

For cancer of the digestive tract: Process 30g of semen strychni by boiling them in water, removing the shell, cutting them into slices, roasting with sesame oil and grinding into powder. Combine with 9g of licorice powder and make into pills by mixing a little rice flour or slippery elm powder as a binder and adding a small amount of water. This is then rolled into small pills and taken in dosage of 0.3 to 0.6g each time with boiled water or tea. Because this is a highly toxic herb, only qualified medical practitioners should use it. However, it is also available in homeopathic dose and many of the western Eclectics freely and safely used it in 30X potency.

It is especially important but generally beneficial to have a periodic break from all long-term herbal prescriptions, especially those that contain strong toxic herbs. This formula can be used six days a week with a one-day interval.

Taraxacum officinalis / Pu Gong Yin
Common Name: Dandelion

Family:	Compositae
Part used:	The whole plant
Energy and flavors:	Cool, bitter and sweet
Organ meridians affected:	Liver and stomach
Type of cancer:	Breast, liver, lungs and pancreas
Actions:	Clears heat and toxicity
Indications:	It is used for abscesses, boils and carbuncles and for inflammation of the breasts. It also will increase lactation.
Contraindications:	Overdose can cause mild diarrhea.
Dose:	10-30g
Biochemical constituents:	Taraxasterol, choline, inulin and pectin

Other information: It is specifically indicated for breast abscess and mammitis as well as other cancers. Research has demonstrated that the hot-water extract inhibits sarcoma-180 with an effective rate of 43.5% while the alcoholic extract has no effect. A polyose constituent is responsible for its anticarcinogenic and immune strengthening properties.

Because dandelion activates liver function, it helps the liver neutralize estrogen, which can activate certain cancer cells. For breast abscess and breast cancer angioma, rub the white milk of fresh dandelion root on the lesions 5 to 10 times daily. Dandelion and flos lonicera (honeysuckle flowers) have complementing and synergistic effects for the treatment of breast cancer.

For breast cancer:

Dandelion herb	9g
Red clover blossoms	15g
Angelica sinensis (Dang Gui)	15g
Trichosanthes root	9g
Boswellia resin	3g
Guggul (Myrrh extract)	3g
Licorice	6g
Orange or Tangerine leaves	10 leaves

Terminalia chebula / He Zi
Common Name: Myrobalan fruit, Terminalia, Chebula, Haridra

Family:	Combretaceae
Part used:	Dried ripe fruit, green fruit, leaf or kernel
Energy and flavor:	Neutral, bitter, sour and astringent
Organ meridians affected:	Lung, stomach and large intestine
Type of cancer:	Stomach, esophagus and large intestine
Actions:	Astringent, anti-dysenteric and laxative
Indications:	Stops diarrhea treats dysentery, stops chronic cough, wheezing and various conditions of the throat including loss of voice.
Contraindications:	Not for external conditions such as colds, flus and fevers.
Dose:	3-9g
Biochemical constituents:	It contains a high amount of tannic substances (approximately 23.6-37.36%) in addition to shikimic acid, quinic acid, fructose, amino acids and sennoside A in the fruit. When the tannin is removed from the fruit, it first has a laxative effect and then an astringent property.

Other information: Pharmacological studies have demonstrated that both the alcoholic and hot water extract works on JTC-26 with an inhibiting rate of 100%. In vivo, studies have shown that the hot water extract inhibits sarcoma-180 in mice with a rate of 20.9% and the alcohol extract with 7.6%. Additionally, it seems to inhibit Ehrlich's ascites carcinoma in mice and fusocellular (spindle cell) sarcoma.

The fruit of a myrobalan tree, which also grows in India and Tibet, is widely used and revered and used in ancient formulas such as Triphala.

This is one of the four ingredients in the Japanese-Kanpo anticancer formula called WTTC. The formula consists of 10g each of Fructus chebula, Caulis wisteria, and Fructus trapae bispinosae and semen coicis. Double blind clinical studies using the formula for gastrointestinal and other cancers were conducted in 1959. It was found to inhibit the regeneration of cancer cells by repressing their division and slowing the division and multiplication.

Thea Sinensis
Common Name: Green tea

Family:	Theaceae
Part used:	Young leaves and leaf buds
Energy and flavor:	Cool, mildly bitter and astringent
Organ meridians affected:	Liver
Type of cancer:	All types
Actions:	Stimulant, diuretic and astringent
Indications:	Useful for diarrhea, fatigue and as an antioxidant.
Contraindications:	Not to be used in excess for individuals with frequent urination or night urination.
Dose:	1 to 4 cups daily
Biochemical constituents:	Caffeine, tannins of which the main one is epigallocatechin, flavonoids including quercitin and kaempferol

Other information: Researchers of Purdue University found that the EGCG compound of Green tea inhibits an enzyme required for cancer cell growth and selectively kills cultured cancer cells with no ill effect on healthy cells.[77] The amount required to achieve high enough concentration was about four cups of Green tea per day.

Because black tea is oxidized, it does not have the same cancer fighting properties of green tea.

Thuja occidentalis
Common Name: Thuja, White cedar, Arbor vitae

Family:	Cupressaceae
Part used:	Leaves and tops
Energy and flavor:	Warm, spicy and astringent
Organ meridians affected:	Lungs, liver and colon
Type of cancer:	Various types of cancers
Actions:	It is expectorant, stimulant, lymphatic cleanser, emmenagogue and anthelmintic.
Indications:	It expels and clears phlegm, treats cystitis and amenorrhea, detoxifies the lymphatic system

and treats warts. Thuja is indicated for all abnormal growths. Externally the tincture is applied to treat fungus and warts. Internally the homeopathic preparation, or a small dose taken for 4 days every two weeks in three cycles will stimulate the disappearance of warts. It is also considered an antidote to conditions caused as a result of vaccinations.

Contraindications: Thuja should absolutely be avoided during pregnancy. Thujone is toxic in large doses and should be taken internally only occasionally. The exception, in terms of the practice of the Eclectics, is that it be taken in frequent small doses for the treatment of cancer.

Dose: From one to ten drops every two or three waking hours for malignancy. For non-malignant growths one only needs to take a drop two or three times a day for four days. The excrescences will fall off, especially if it is also applied externally. One can use either the 1:1 fluid extract or the 1:5 tincture. Good results can also be obtained with homeopathic 30X dosage.

Biochemical constituents: Volatile oil containing thujone as the major component, it also contains isothujone, borneol, bornyl acetate, l-fenchone, limonin, sabinene, camphor, thujone and others, flavonoids, mucilage and tannins.

Other information: It has shown in vitro antiviral properties and stimulates phagocytosis. [78, 79] Eli Jones injected twenty to sixty drops into the rectum for colon cancer and also, as he calls it, the cauliflower variety of uterine cancer.[80] It is recommended both internally and externally, however it can be applied for all growths, cancers, swollen glands and breast cancer and for attendant pains associated with cancer. Ellingwood describes the practice of numerous Eclectic physicians of the late 19th and early 20th centuries who found that by keeping Thuja applied externally to cancers and taken internally it "is claimed to exercise an abortive influence over incipient cancer, and to retard the progress of more advanced cases. In extreme cases it will remove the fetor, retard the growth, and materially prolong the life of the patient." [81] The eclectics claimed good results by injecting Thuja directly into the tumor. This is not recommended unless a qualified practitioner does it, especially to assure that the extract is of injectibles quality.

Tinospora cordifolia (T. sinensis) / Kuan Jin Teng
Common Name: Guduchi

Family:	Menispermaceae
Part used:	The stem and vine
Energy and flavor:	Very cold and bitter
Organ meridians affected:	Liver
Type of cancer:	Liver cancer
Actions:	It detoxifies, clears heat and dampness, and has antispasmodic properties.
Indications:	It detoxifies the blood. The vine relaxes the tendons and resolves swelling from arthritis, injury or trauma.
Contraindications:	Not to be used during pregnancy or immediately after childbirth.
Dose:	Of the root, 6-9g; of the vine, 15-30g
Biochemical constituents:	Palmatine, flavonoid glycoside, amino acid and saccharides

Other information: Tinospora cordifolia is a widely used detoxifying herb in the system of Ayurvedic medicine. One study showed that it had powerful antioxidant properties suggesting its value in the prevention and treatment of different types of cancer.[82] The root can be ground to a paste and mixed with wine and applied topically for lipomas and angiomas.[83]

Trapae bispinosae, fructus / Chi Shih
Common Name: Water caltrop, water chestnut and water truffle

Family:	Trapaceae
Part used:	The stalk, leaf and stem are used
Energy and flavor:	Mild, sweet, and non-toxic
Organ meridians affected:	Regulates the middle warmer to supplement the viscera.
Type of cancer:	Mostly gastrointestinal cancers
Actions:	Relieves thirst, reduces fever, diuretic and nutritional
Indications:	Used for fevers, thirst, sunstroke, nocturnal

emission, leucorrhea, numbness, skin diseases and alcoholism.

Contraindications: Not for individuals with weak digestion.

Dose: 9-30g

Biochemical constituents: It contains ergostatetraen, B-sitosterol and large quantities of starch.

Other information: Water chestnuts can be eaten as a food. The seeds are eaten raw or cooked. They can be reduced to flour to make porridge but lack sufficient starch to make bread.

It is cultivated in the lakes of China and Asia. It has been shown to be effective for cancer of the liver, AH-13 in mice, and it inhibits mice sarcoma-180 with an effective rate of 60%. It is effective for gastrointestinal cancers, cancer of the esophagus, breast, uterus, cervix, ovaries and other types of cancers. It is widely used for all types of cancers both in China and Japan. For cancers that seem curable decoct 30 grains of the fresh or dried fruit daily into a strong decoction. Take four times daily. It can be used both internally and externally as well as used as a douche for cervical cancer.

Interestingly King's *American Dispensatory* describes how a close European relative of this plant, trapa natans, is one of a number of manganivorous plants that have a special ability to take up manganese. Manganese in turn has the following uses: it acts as a purgative, treats ascites, hepatic conditions, skin conditions and when combined with iodide of iron in a syrup it is recommended for the use of swollen glands, cancer, glandular enlargements and anemia.

Trichosanthes kirilowii / Tian Hua Fen
Common Name: Trichosanthes

Family: Cucurbitaceae

Part used: The root

Energy and flavor: Cold, bitter, slightly sweet and sour

Organ meridians affected: Lungs and stomach

Type of cancer: Lungs, breast and gastrointestinal

Actions: Anti-inflammatory, demulcent, anti-mucus yet moistens dryness of the lungs and abortifacient. It clears lung heat and evil phlegm, detoxifies and clears pus. It is considered one of the most powerful of all antibacterial herbs.

Trichosanthes kirilowii (continued)

Indications:	Cough with thick sputum or blood-streaked sputum, breast abscess, hot toxic carbuncles and sores
Contraindications:	Do not use during pregnancy. It can be toxic and even fatal in higher dosages because of its ability to impair hepatic and renal function. It is also contraindicated for weak digestion. This means that its use for cancer patients should probably include digestives as part of the formula.
Dose:	9-15g
Biochemical constituents:	Saponins, a peculiar glucoprotein comprised of citruline, arginine, glutamic acid, aspartic acid and lesser amounts of serine, glycine, threonine and alanine

Other information: Its anti-cancer properties are due to a number of potent alkaloids and saponins. The latter may serve as important hormone precursors that by occupying the hormone receptor sites can regulate the over utilization of hormones such as estrogen and testosterone that can especially provoke the growth and proliferation of breast, ovarian and male prostate cancer. Chinese research has found that the glucoprotein it contains causes necrosis to trophocytes and interferes with the respiration and anaerobic glycolysis of cancer cells.

One formula for breast cancer:

Trichosanthes root	30g
Oyster shell	30g
Prunella spike	30g
Dandelion root	30g
Kelp	12g
Scrophularia	4g
Centipede powder	2g
Scorpion powder	2g

Boil the broken oyster shell alone for 30 minutes before adding the other ingredients. Then add everything except the last two ingredients and continue to simmer in a covered container for an additional 30 minutes. Mix the powdered centipede and scorpion in gelatin capsules. Divide everything equally in two doses, which are taken A.M. and P.M. daily.

For esophageal cancer:

Trichosanthes root	15g
Burdock root	60g
Codonopsis root	15g
Scrophularia root	12g
Ophiopogonis root	12g
Asparagus root	9g
Peach seed	9g

Because the formula calls for the use of iron, the above herbs should be boiled in an iron kettle or pot. Otherwise, 30g of hematite is crushed and preboiled for 30 minutes before adding the remaining herbs for another 30 minutes decoction. The entire preparation should be reduced to two cups that are taken A.M. and P.M. daily.

Formula for lung cancer:

Trichosanthes root	15g
Burdock root	60g
Fritillary bulbs	30g
Lonicera blossoms	30g
Violet leaves and flowers	30g
Red clover blossoms	30g

Simmer trichosanthes and burdock root in 4 cups of water for 30 minutes; add the remaining herbs and enough water to completely cover all the ingredients. Simmer on low heat for 20 minutes more and strain. Reduce to two or three cups, which are taken throughout the day.

For nasopharyngeal cancer: Immerse 10g of sliced trichosanthes and 10g of hydrastis in 25 ml of 75% ethanol; after a day add 25 ml of distilled water and after an additonal three days add 50 ml more of distilled water. Let stand another day and press strain the ingredients. To the reserved liquor add 20 ml of vegetable glycerin. Drops of this are applied into the nose 3 to 6 times daily. Accompany this with an internal prescription consisting of the powder of 3 centipedes, 3g of squama manitis (Anteater scales), 3g of Cockroach, 3g of lumbricus and 3g of tienchi ginseng. Divide this formula into three equal doses. Mix in gelatin capsules and take three times daily.

	Trifolium pratense **Common Name: Red Clover**

Family:	Leguminaceae
Part used:	The flowers with a few of the accompanying leaves
Energy and flavors:	Cool, sweet and bitter
Organ meridians affected:	Lungs and liver
Type of cancer:	All types but especially the lungs and breast
Actions:	Detoxifies, moves blood and removes stagnation and has nutritive properties.
Indications:	Toxicity, infections, inflammations and coughs
Contraindications:	Not for those who are taking other blood thinning agents.
Dose:	9-15g
Biochemical constituents:	Isoflavones, flavonoids, coumarins, resins, minerals and vitamins

Other information: A key ingredient of the Hoxsey formula and the proprietary Jason Winters tea. Red Clover blossoms were used by the Eclectics as an alterative, blood purifier and a treatment for coughs and other acute upper respiratory complaints. It was the key ingredient of their trifolium compound, considered the basis of the later Hoxsey formula. Parke Davis produced it in 1890 as Syrup Trifolium, which like the Hoxsey formula contained potassium iodide but no licorice. In 1898, it was also listed in King's *American Dispensatory*, the Bible of Eclectic physicians. This all-purpose alterative, which at that time also contained Podophyllum (may apple) root, an herb known to be toxic in certain dosage but also to possess definite anti-cancer properties was used for a wide range of conditions including syphilis, scrofula, rheumatism and glandular and skin conditions including cancer and tumors.

Red clover blossoms are high in beta-carotene and vitamin E, which is one reason why the dried purplish-red blossoms should be predominately used. Like soy, red clover is high in isoflavones that possess estrogen-like actions.

Coumarin, one of the primary active constituents of both red clover and dang gui, stimulates phagocytosis and significantly inhibits metastasis. Coumarins also mildly thin the blood and thereby help to remove stagnation and improve circulation generally.

Breast cancer: a strong decoction of a half-ounce each of red clover blossoms and dandelion root can be simmered in an ounce of water. Three cups should be taken daily.

For all cancers: a gentle treatment for all cancers is a combination of equal parts red clover blossoms, Violet leaves and blossoms, burdock and Yellow dock roots. Simmer at least two ounces of the combination in a quart of water for 20 minutes and drink three to four cups daily.

Tulipa edulis, Pseudobulbus / Shan Ci Gu
Cremastra variabilis
(Sometimes a toxic plant, iphigenia indica, is mistaken for this herb.)
Common Name: Tulip bulb

Family:	Liliaceae
Part used:	The bulb
Energy and flavor:	Cold, sweet and slightly toxic
Organ meridians affected:	Liver and stomach
Type of cancer:	It is used for a wide variety of cancers, especially breast and esophageal cancers.
Actions:	Clears heat and toxicity, dissolves nodules such as swollen glands and tumors and clears heat and various types of inflammations.
Indications:	It is used for sores, ulcers, carbuncles, boils, toxic swelling and swollen glands.
Contraindications:	Use with caution internally on weak patients.
Dose:	3-9g in decoctions
Biochemical constituents:	Glucomannan, colchicine and alkaloids

Other information: The anticancer property is probably based on the ability of colchicine to inhibit the dehydrogenase of the cells of acute lymphocytic and acute granulocytic leukemia. Colchicine is very toxic and its onset tends to be slow, over 3 to 6 hours after ingestion. Symptoms of toxicity include nausea, vomiting, diarrhea, weakness and in advanced stages, respiratory failure. It can also cause blood disorders such as granulocytopenia.[84]

Uncaria Tomentosa
Common Name: Cat's claw, Una de gato

Family:	Rubiaceae
Part used:	The inner bark
Energy and flavor:	Cold and bitter
Organ meridians affected:	Liver and lungs
Type of cancer:	Cancers of various types
Actions:	Clears heat, antimicrobial, antiviral, anti-hypertensive, antirheumatic, contraceptive, cytostatic, immune tonic, astringent, stimulates the immune system and promotes wound healing.
Indications:	It is used for a variety of ailments, including various types of inflammatory conditions, rheumatism, gastric ulcers, tumors, dysentery, arthritis, asthma, diabetes, cancer and tumors, viral infections, menstrual disorders, AIDS, gonorrhea, convalescence and general debility.
Contraindications:	No serious side effects have as yet been reported. However, in Europe, health care providers avoid combining this herb with hormonal drugs, insulin or vaccines. Do not take this product if you are pregnant or breast-feeding. Cat's claw may have platelet blocking constituents that would warrant using it with caution if one is using other medications, such as and including aspirin, which thin the blood.
Dose:	This product can be taken as a tincture (1-2 ml) up to 2 times per day, as a capsule (350-500 mg) once or twice per day, or as tea (1 gram of root bark per cup of boiling water), and drunk 1-3 times each day. It can be combined with other herbs or therapies for cancer.
Biochemical constituents:	Oxindole-alkaloids, N-oxide, rhyncophylline, N-oxide, carboline alkaloid, hirustine N-oxide triterpenes, polyphenols, phytosterols (stigmasterol and campsterol). Some studies

have identified the alkaloid isoteropodine as the primary constituent.

Other information: Only the aerial parts of cat's claw are harvested for medicine and it regrows itself from the root in about 4 years so there should not be significant ecological concerns for the use of this potent herb.

The activity of an extract of the bark both in vitro and in vivo has shown positive antimutagenic effects.[85,86] Research by Wagner and Kreutzamp identified the active constituents as a group of alkaloids with immune stimulating activity. Further research by Dr. Felipe Melgarejo, again with the extracts of the bark or stem confirmed the herb to have both antiinflammatory as well as anti-cancer and antitumor activity.[87]

There are actually several species of South American plants that are popularly called cat's claw. For this reason, one should find a reputable supply specifically of *uncaria tomentosa*.

Verbena hastate
Common Name: Blue vervaine

Family:	Verbenaceae
Part used:	The whole herb
Energy and flavor:	Cold and bitter
Organ meridians affected:	Liver and stomach
Types of Cancer:	Cervical, liver and ascites
Actions:	Antiinflammatory, blood moving, cholagogue, diuretic and anthelmintic (removes parasites)
Indications:	Liver congestion, hepatitis, cirrhosis, ascites and menstrual irregularities
Contraindications:	Not for pregnant women or those with a cold deficient constitution unless it is combined with other herbs to counterbalance it.
Dose:	15–30g
Biochemical constituents:	Iridoids, verbenallin, verbenine, essential oil, tannin and mucilage

Viola odorata
Common Name: Violet

Family:	Violaceae
Part used:	The leaves and flowers. The Chinese use the whole plant.
Energy and flavor:	Cool, sweet and mildly bitter
Organ meridians affected:	Lungs, stomach and liver
Type of cancer:	Especially for cancers of the breast, lungs and gastrointestinal organs
Actions:	Demulcent, expectorant, alterative, antipyretic, antiseptic, vulnerary and antispasmodic
Indications:	It is used both internally and topically for various types of inflammations of bacterial or viral origin. It is also used to lubricate dryness of the lungs and in syrup for the relief of coughs.
Contraindications:	None noted
Dose:	One ounce of the aerial portion of the plant steeped in three cups of boiling water. Consume a cupful three times daily.
Biochemical constituents:	Phenolic mucilage glycosides, saponins, flavonoids, carotenoids and vitamin C

Other information: Violet leaves are well known throughout the history of Western herbal medicine as a treatment for cancer. The Chinese use it as an herb to soften and dissolve tumors and hardened nodules. The steamed leaves make a delicious potherb.

Viscum album
Common Name: European mistletoe, Birdlime, Iscador

Family:	Loranthaceae
Part used:	Foliage, including the stem and branches
Energy and flavor:	Neutral and bitter
Organ meridians affected:	Liver, kidneys and heart
Type of cancer:	All cancers
Actions:	Calms the spirit, antispasmodic, antihyper-

	tensive, replenishes kidney and liver energy and antirheumatic.
Indications:	For insomnia, nervousness, hypertension, coronary heart disease, arthritis and rheumatic complaints, epilepsy, chorea, asthma, migraine headaches, skin conditions and hypoglycemia.
Contraindications:	Not for pregnant women. Large doses in animals have been known to cause vomiting and death.
Dose:	2.5g infused in cold water for 10 to 12 hours, taken up to two times daily. Blood pressure should be regu`larly monitored.
Biochemical constituents:	Quercetin, avicularin, arabinose, oleanolic acid, B-amyrin, mesoinositol, lupeol, b-sitosterol, myristic acid and viscum flavones.

Other information: There are several species of mistletoe. Chinese mistletoe (Loranthes parasiticus), specifically grows on mulberry leaves and is widely used for back pain, arthritis and rheumatic complaints. American mistletoe (viscum flavescens), found growing on juniper and oak trees, is regarded as toxic and has opposite properties to the European mistletoe in that it tends to raise rather than lower blood pressure in some individuals. They all share the ability to relieve spasmodic tension. All Mistletoes have strong emmenagogue and uterus contracting properties so that they should not be used during pregnancy. However, small amounts are useful for reducing bleeding and promoting clotting.[88]

Rudolf Steiner (1864-1925), the scientifically-oriented German mystic first suggested the use of European mistletoe for cancer in the 1920's. Since then it has been used as a mainstay herb by Anthroposophical medical doctors[1] in the form of Iscador. Since then there has been literally thousands of reported case studies substantiating its benefit for the treatment of different types of cancers.[89] Only European mistletoe should be used since this is what all of the studies are based upon.[90]

In Europe there is a long history of traditional use of mistletoe found growing on oak trees dating back to the druids. Culpepper mentions that it "mollifies knots, tumors and imposthumes, ripens and discusses them, and draws forth thick as well as thin humours from the remote parts of the body, digesting and separating them, being mixed with resin and wax, mollifies the hardness of the spleen, and helps old ulcers and sores, mixed with sanderic

---

[1] A system of herbal medicine based on Steiner's teachings.

Viscum album (continued)

and orpiment, it helps to draw off foul nails, and if quick lime and wine lees be added thereto, it works the stronger." He then goes on to mention its traditional use for epilepsy, palsy and vertigo.

Because it is parasitic, it is expected that there would be a difference between Mistletoes that grow on different trees. Anthroposophical medicine uses different types of mistletoe based on the type of cancer, the trees from which it is harvested and methods of preparation, since different forms of Iscador are prepared with added homeopathic metals. Only qualified practitioners should administer Iscador, especially since one of the usual modes of application is through injection.

There are numerous studies, both positive and inconclusive, that substantiate the possible benefit of mistletoe and Iscador for the treatment of various cancers. Two publications based on Anthroposophical medicine strongly support the value of Iscador, properly administered by a trained practitioner. They found that more breast cancer patients were alive after 10 years compared to those who did not receive Iscador; people who had a combination of surgery and Iscador had an 83% survival rate after 5 years as compared to 69% for those who only received radiation. About 50% of bladder papillomas become malignant after 3 years, with Iscador only 3 out of 14 did; 75% of bronchial patients given Iscador were alive after 4 years as compared to only 35% of those without Iscador; 80% of skin patients treated with Iscador were alive after 3 years as compared to 35% of those without it. Iscador seemed to also extend the survival rate of patients with various other types of cancers including cancers of the lung, breast, gastrointestinal, ovaries and cervix.

One of the questions that should be asked here, however, is to what extent a substance such as Iscador plays in increasing survival statistics as opposed to patients whose lives may have been shortened as a result of damaging chemotherapy and radiation. I have personally met many patients who choose to receive no medical intervention for their cancers and lived on far beyond what is normally expected.

In any case, recent studies have confirmed the ability of mistletoe to stimulate the production of cancer killing Natural Killer (NK) cells, which may account for a large percentage of the benefit from the use of European mistletoe and Iscador.[91]

Iscador is available to qualified health practitioners in liquid form from Biological Homeopathic Industries (BH) 11600 Cochite, SE P.O. Box 11280, Albuquerque, NM 87123; Tel: (505) 293-3843, Fax: (505) 275-1672. One may also contact the Physician's Association for Anthroposophical Medicine, 7953 California Ave., Fair Oaks, CA 95628, Tel: (916) 967-8250, Fax: (916) 966-5314, or check for sources on the Internet.

Withania somnifera
Common Name: Ashwagandha

Family:	Solanaceae
Part used:	The root
Energy and flavor:	Neutral, bitter and acrid
Organ meridians affected:	Lungs and kidneys
Type of cancer:	All types
Actions:	Tonic, antirheumatic, aphrodisiac, sedative, astringent, anodyne, antifungal, antihypertensive, antiinflammatory and immunostimulant.
Indications:	Joint and nerve pains, low energy, insomnia, weakness of the back and knees, impotence, infertility, wasting diseases and diseases of aging.
Contraindications:	Do not use during pregnancy.
Dose:	3-12g or 3g of the powder boiled in warm milk for a tonic. The powder can be taken mixed with ghee (clarified butter) and honey.
Biochemical constituents:	Bitter alkaloid, warfarin, somniferine, and beta-sitosterol

Other information: There is considerable evidence that withania somnifera taken in conjunction with radiation therapy enhances the effect of radiotherapy and significantly decreases adverse reactions. In one study on mice, an extract of withania increased the total WBC count of mice and reduced the leucopenia induced by a sub lethal dose of gamma radiation. It also increased bone marrow cellularity and normalized the ration of erythrocytes and polychromatic erythrocytes in mice after the radiation exposure. [92,93]

Besides its use in integrative treatment with radiation and chemotherapy, withania has demonstrated a significant inhibitory effect in mice against sarcoma 180.[94]

* * *

Various Cancer Formulas

Thyroid cancer:

Fifty grams each of the following: sparganii. aurantii, curcumae, angelicae sinensis, salviae miltiorrhizae, paeoniae alba, citri reticulatae, sinapis albae, prepared squama manitis; 100g each of thallus laminariae seu eckloniae, sargassum, spica prunellae; twenty fiveg of flos carthami; one hundred and fiftyg of rhizoma zedoariae, herba taraxaci and concha ostreae. Grind all the herbs into a fine powder, put into 00 sized capsules and take 6 three times daily.

Lung cancer:

Black nightshade	30g
Lonicera	30g
Forsythia	30g
Scutellaria	30g
Houttuyniae	30g
Scrophularia root	30g
Trichosanthes root	30g
Codonopsis	9g
Agrimonia	9g
Sanguisorba	9g

Simmer in enough water to cover on a low flame for one hour. Strain and reduce to 3 cups. Take three cups daily.

For all cancers:

Oldenlandiae diffusae	250g
Scolopendra (centipede)	30g
Nidus vespae	30g
Herba taraxaci	30g
Rx isatis	30g
Scorpion	30g
Periostracum serpentis	30g

Pound into a fine powder, blend with honey and make into pills (each about 6g) for oral administration morning and evening. (*Herbal Handbook*)

Esophageal cancer:

Lithospermi	30g
Scutellariae barbatae	30g
Oldenlandiae	30g
Dioscoreae (Shan Yao)	15g
Corium stomachichum galli (chicken gizzard skins)	9g

Adenophorae	9g
Poria	6g
Codonopsis	6g
Pinelliae	6g
Citri reticulatae	6g
Saussureae	9g
Rice sprouts	30g
Barley sprouts	30g
Spicy prunellae	30g
Jujube dates	5 pieces

Ulceration caused by radiation:

Lithospermi	60g
Angelica (Dang Gui)	60g
Angelica dahuricae	15g
Calomelas	12g
Sanguis draconis	12g
Licorice	26g
Bee's wax	60g
Sesame oil	500g

Heat the sesame oil, add the finely powdered herbs and simmer for a few minutes, melt the bee's wax into the mixture and blend in the powdered calomelas.

Bone cancer:

Astragalus	30g
Hawthorn berries	30g
Poria mushroom	30g
Coix	30g
Oldenlandia herb	30g
Angelica sinensis (Dang Gui)	10g
Mume plum	10g
Trichosanthes root	10g

Brain cancer:

Rhz. paris	30g
Rx. Clematidis	30g
Fr. Chaenomelis	9g
Rx. Notoginseng powder	3g

Make into a decoction and take twice daily.

Chemotherapy, supporting the immune system:

Astragalus root	30g
Ganoderma mushroom	30g
Codonopsis	30g
Licorice	10g
Ginger	10g

Simmer in 6 cups of water down to 3. Take one cup three times daily. Ideally begin using this formula a week before beginning chemotherapy and radiation and continue through the course of treatment and after completion.

Thyroid cancer:

Prunella spike	20g
Polygonum multiflorum stems	20g
Oyster shell	30g
Kelp	30g
Dioscorea villosa	9g
Turmeric root	15g
Acorus graminei	15g
American ginseng	15g
Bupleurum root	10g
Zedoariae	10g

Simmer in 4 cups of water, slowly down to two and take one cup A.M. and P.M. This is contraindicated for those who suffer from chronically low energy.

Thyroid cyst:

Spica prunellae	60g
Rx. Salvia milthiorrhiza	24g
Pericarpium trichosanthes	24g

Thallus laminariae seu eckloniae	24g
Sargassum	24g
Rhz. Cyperus	24g
Cormus iphigeniae	24g
Rx bupleurum	15g
Rx Paeoniae lactiflorae	18g

This is decocted and taken in two doses daily. In addition take 60g each of Spica prunellae and 60g of pork simmered and taken every other day.

Colon and appendix cancer:

Herba Patriniae Scabiosaefoliae	30g
Flos Lonicerae	30g
Semen coicis	30g
Herba violae yedoensis	30g
Herba scutellariae barbatae	15g
Rhz. Zedoariae	9g
Rhz. sparganii	9g

For various cancers:

Fructus trapae bispinosae	60g
Coix	30g
Herba tetragoniae	30g
Caulis wisteriae sinensis	9g

Take one dose daily. This is from the *Journal of Jiangsu*, Vol 1. 1962. It is claimed by Chang Minyi to have a miraculous effect.

Cancer of the stomach, nasopharynx, lung and cervix:

Make a decoction of 30g each of duchesnea, scutellaria barbata, Trapae bispinosae and Sophora. Take 3 cups daily.

Strategies for Creating
an Effective Herbal Treatment

Herbs

According to the internal organs and bodily area involved:

Lungs – Black nightshade, Mullein, Herba solani lyrati, Fructificatio lasiopherae seu calvatae

Spleen-pancreas – Radix sophorae

Liver – Calculus bovis, Radix sophorae, Herba solani lyrati

Urinary system – Chapparal, coix, cleavers, houttuyniae, leonurus, lindera

Stomach – Radix sophorae, Radix paridis, Herba oldenlandiae, Herba solani lyrati

Large intestine – Rhubarb, coix, coptis, goldenseal, lonicera, partriniae

Esophagus – Rhizoma balamcandae, Radix sophorae, Herba scutellariae barbatae, Rhizoma paradis, Fructificatio lasiopherae seu calvatae

Nasopharyngeal – Fructus xanthii, Rhizoma paradis

Brain – Rhizoma paridis

Lymphoma – Rhizoma paridis

Pharyngeal – Fructificatio lasiopherae seu calvatae

Tongue – Fructificatio lasiopherae seu calvatae

Various cancers – Herba scutellariae barbatae, flos lonicera, spica prunella

Salves and Poultices

A powder for external application on *cancerous lesions:*

Arsenicum	3g
Coptis	3g
Phellodendron	3g
Agrimony ashes	20g
Slippery elm powder	50g

Add enough water to bind it together. Separate into small one-inch diameter balls and roast in the oven until it appears burnt. Grind into a powder and sprinkle the powder topically over cancerous lesions. To aid its adherence, it can be moistened with a little water. This can be used for any open cancerous lesion such as breast cancer, anal fistula, over infested lymph nodes, cervical cancer, etc. One should be cautioned against any accidental ingesting of this powder.

For skin cancer:

Hirudo	30g
Rhubarb root	5g
Indigo	3g

Grind to a fine powder and mix decoction in heated sesame oil, dissolve bee's wax to form the consistency of an ointment and apply topically.

For malignant lymphoma:

Laminaria	30g
Sargassum	30g
Arisaematis	90g
Pinellia	90g
Moschus	6g
Borneol	6g
Carthami, flos	60g
Concha ostreae	60g
Halitum	18g

Grind to a powder and mix with a decoction of 250g of rhz. Bletillae for external application to the lesion. (From *Rhymed Discourse on External Therapy*.)

Breast cancer:

Make a powder of 30g each of rhubarb and licorice. Decoct in wine to form a paste. Apply topically. Also take a spoonful several times daily by mouth.

Endnotes

[1] Minyi, Chang, *Anticancer Medicinal Herbs*, Hunan Science and Technology Publishing House (1992)

[2] *Guangdong Traditional Chinese Medicine*, (Vol. 3, 1960)

[3] Minyi, Chang, ibid.

[4] Minyi, Chang, ibid.

[5] Ahn, B.Z.; Yoon, Y.D.; Lee, Y.H.; Kim, B.H.; Sok, D.E., "Inhibitory effect of bupleuri radix saponins on adhesion of some solid tumor cells and relation to hemolytic action:

screening of 232 herbal drugs for anti-cell adhesion." College of Pharmacy, Chungnam National University, Taejon, Korea. Source: Planta Med, 64(3):220-4 1998 Apr., College of Pharmacy, Chungnam National University, Taejon, Korea. Source: Planta Med, 64(3): 220-4 1998 Apr

[6] Nakano, Y.; Matsunaga, H.; Saita, T.; Mori, M.; Katano, M.; Okabe, H., "Antiproliferative constituents in Umbelliferae plants II. Screening for polyacetylenes in some Umbelliferae plants, and isolation of panaxynol and falcarindiol from the root of Heracleum moellendorffii." Faculty of Hospital Pharmacy, Saga Medical School, Nabeshima, Japan. Source: Biol Pharm Bull, 21(3):257-61 1998 Mar

[7] Chakraborty, A., et al. "Anticarcinogenic Promoting Activities of Herbal Extracts Used in Tropical Ethnomedicine," Poster Presentation, 48th Annual Meeting of the International Congress of the Society of Medicinal Plant Research, P2A/17, Sept. 5, 2000

[8] Zollner, T.M. et al. "Induction of NK-like Activity in T cells by Il-s/anti-cd3 is linked to expression of a new antitumor receptor with specificity for acetylated manose." Anticancer Research 13:4 (1993). 923-930 (Cited from Goldberg, et al. An Alternative Medicine Definitive Guide to Cancer, 1997, pub. Future Medicine Publishing, Inc.)

[9] Pienta, K.J. et al, "Inhibition of Spontaneous Metastasis in a Rat Prostate Model by Oral Administration of Modified Citrus Pectin." Journal of the National Cancer Institute 87: 5 (1995), 348-353

[10] Crowell, P.L.; Gould, M.N., "Chemoprevention and therapy of cancer by d-limonene." Crit Rev Oncog 1994;5(1):1-22

[11] Xu, R.H.; Peng, X.E.; Chen, G.Z.; Chen, G.L., "Effects of cordyceps sinensis on natural activity and colony formation of B16 melanoma." Chin Med J (Engl) 1992 Feb;105(2): 97-101 (ISSN: 0366-6999) Institute of Combined Traditional Chinese and Western Medicine, Hunan Medical University, Changsha.

[12] Nakamura, K.; Yamaguchi, Y.; Kagota, S.; Kwon, Y.M.; Shinozuka, K.; Kunitomo, M., "Inhibitory effect of Cordyceps sinensis on spontaneous liver metastasis of Lewis Lung carcinoma and B16 melanoma cells in syngeneic mice." Jpn J Pharmacol 1999 Mar;79(3): 335-41 (ISSN: 0021-5198), Department of Pharmacology, Faculty of Pharmaceutical Sciences, Mukogawa Women's University, Nishinomiya, Japan.

[13] Yang et al, 1993. "A new biological response modifier-PSP. From Mushroom Biology and Mushroom Products." S.T. Chang et al (eds.) Hong Kong: The Chinese University Press, 247-259.

[14] Ebina, T. 1987a. "Antitumor effect of PSK. Interferon inducing activity and intratumoral administration." Gon to Kagaku Ryoho 14:1841-1846. From CA 107:108960. Also 1987b (2) Effector mechanism of antimetastic effect in the "double grafted tumor system." CA 107:108961f. – From Hobbs, Christopher, Medicinal Mushrooms 1995, Botanica Press.

[15] Zhou, Jin-Xu, et al. "Antitumor effect of PSP of coriolus versicolor and its mechanics."

[16] Verma, S.P.; Salamone, E.; Goldin, B., Department of Community Health. Tufts University School of Medicine, Boston, Massachusetts 02111, USA., Biochem Biophys Res Commun, 233(3):692-6 1997 Apr 28

[17] Singh, S.V.; Hu, X.; Srivastava, S.K.; Singh, M.; Xia, H.; Orchard, J.L.; Zaren, H.A., "Mechanism of inhibition of benzo[a]pyrene-induced forestomach cancer in mice by dietary curcumin." Cancer Research Laboratory, Mercy Cancer Institute, Pittsburgh, PA 15219, USA. Source Carcinogenesis, 19(8):1357-60 1998 Aug

[18] Krishnaswamy, K., "Indian functional foods: role in prevention of cancer." National Institute of Nutrition, Hyderabad, India. Nutr Rev, 54(11 Pt 2):S127-31, 1996 Nov

[19] Beal and E. Reinhard, Natural Products as Medicinal Agents, Hippokrates, 1981

[20] Yance, Donny, *Herbal Medicine, Healing & Cancer*, 1999, pub by Keats

[21] Lersch, C.; Zeuner, M.; Bauer, A.; Siemens, M.; Hart, R.; Drescher, M.; Fink, U.; Dancygier, H.; Classen, M., "Nonspecific immunostimulation with low doses of cyclophosphamide (LDCY), thymostimulin, and Echinacea purpurea extracts (echinacin) in patients with far advanced colorectal cancers: preliminary results." Kliniken und Polikliniken der Technischen, University at Munchen, Germany.

[22] Chubarev, V.N., Rubtsova, E.R., Filatova, I.V., Krendal,' F.P., Davydova, O.N., [Immunotropic effect of a tincture of the tissue culture biomass of Ginseng cells and of an Eleutherococcus extract in mice]. Farmakol Toksikol 1989 Mar-Apr;52(2):55-9

[23] Ronichevskaia, G.M., "The effect of large doses of extracts of Ginseng and Eleutherococcus extracts on the occurrence of spontaneous tumors in hybrid mice," Vopr Onkol 1967;13(3):67-71 J Pharm Sci 1984 Feb;73(2):270-2

[24] Bespalov, V.G.; Aleksandrov, V.A.; Iaremenko, K.V.; Davydov, V.V.; Lazareva, N.L.; Limarenko, AIu; Slepian, L.I.; Petrov, A.S.; Troian, [The inhibiting effect of phytoadaptogenic preparations from bioGinseng, Eleutherococcus senticosus and Rhaponticum carthamoides on the development of nervous system tumors in rats induced by N-nitrosoethylurea] Vopr Onkol 1992;38(9):1073-80

[25] Hacke, B.; Medon, P.J., "Cytotoxic effects of Eleutherococcus senticosus aqueous extracts in combination with N6-(delta 2-isopentenyl)-adenosine and 1-beta-D-arabinofuranosylcytosine against L1210 leukemia cells." J Pharm Sci (United States), Feb 1984, 73(2) p270-2

[26] Willard, T., 1990. *Reishi Mushroom. Herb of Spiritual Potency and Medical Wonder*, Issaquah: Sylvan Press.

[27] Wang, S.Y. et al, 1994. "The role of Ganoderma Lucidum in immunopotentiation: effect on cytokine release from human macrophages and T-lymphocytes." From Program and Abstracts of the '94 International Symposium on Ganoderma Research. Beijing: Beijing University.

[28] Wang, S.Y.; Hsu, M.L.; Hsu, H.C.; Tzeng, C.H.; Lee, S.S.; Shiao, M.S.; Ho, C.K.; Department of Medical Research, Veterans General Hospital-Taipei, Taiwan, Republic of China. *Int J Cancer*, 70(6):699-705 1997 Mar 17

[29] Wang, G. et al. 1993. "Antitumor active polysaccharides from the Chinese mushroom Songshan Lingzhi, the fruiting body of Ganoderma tsugae." *Bioscience, Biotechnology and Biochemistry* 57:894-900

[30] Chang and But, 1986; Kasahara & Hikino, 1987.

[31] Ha, S.W.; Yi, C.J.; Cho, C.K.; Cho, M.J.; Shin, K.H.; Park, C.I., "Enhancement of radiation effect by Ginkgo biloba extract in C3H mouse fibrosarcoma." *Radiother Oncol* 1996 Nov;41(2):163-7 Laboratory of Radiation Biology, Seoul National University Medical College, South Korea.

[32] Fukaya, H., "Experimental studies of the protective effect of ginkgo biloba extract (GBE) on cisplatin-induced toxicity in rats." Nippon Jibiinkoka Gakkai Kaiho 1999 Jul;102(7):907-917 Department of Otolaryngology, Fukushima Medical University School of Medicine.

[33] Kubo, K.; Nanba, H., "Anti-hyperliposis effect of Maitake fruit body (Grifola frondosa) I." Department of Microbial Chemistry, Kobe Pharmaceutical University, Japan. Source, *Biol Pharm Bull*, 20(7):781-5 1997 Jul

[34] Mori, K., et al. 1987. "Antitumor activities of edible mushrooms by oral administration." From Wuest, P.J., et al. (eds.) *Cultivating Edible Fungi*, Amsterdam: Elsevier: 1-6.

[35] Hobbs

[36] Miller, D. 1994. Current protocol submitted to the N.I.H. Scientific Director Cancer Treatment Research Foundation, Arlington Heights, IL. (Cited from Hobbs)

[37] Zhu et al, 1994 (cited from Hobbs)

[38] Nanba, H., 1993, "Antitumor activity of orally administered "D-fraction" from Maitake mushroom (Grifola frondosa)"; J. Naturopathic Med. 4:10-15

[39] Nanba, H. 1994b. "Activity of Maitake D-fraction to prevent cancer growth and metastasis." J. Naturopathic Med.

[40] Nanba, H. et al. 1994c, Biol. and Pharm. Bull. "Antidiabetic activity present in the fruit body of Grifola frondosa (Maitake) I." 1106-1110

[41] Nanba, H. 1993, ibid

[42] Jones, Eli, Cancer, Its Causes, Symptoms & Treatment, B. Jain pub.

[43] Ying, J. et al. 1987. "Icones of Medicinal Fungi From China." Translated by X.Yuehan, Beijing: Science Press (Cited from Hobbs, Christopher Medicinal Mushrooms, Botanica Press, 1995).

[44] Hartwell, J.L. 1971. Plants used against cancer. Lloydia 34:386-96 (Cited from Hobbs, Medicinal Mushrooms, Botanica Press 1995).

[45] Larionov, L.F., 1965. Cancer Chemotherapy, Translated from the Russian by A. Crozy. New York: Pergamon Press. As quoted by Heinerman, J. The Treatment of Cancer with Herbs. Orem, Biworld pub., (Cited from Hobbs, Medicinal Mushrooms, Botanica Press 1995).

[46] Hobbs, Christopher Medicinal Mushrooms, Botanica Press, 1995

[47] Piaskowski, S. 1957. "Preliminary studies on the preparation and application of preparations from black birch touchwood in human cases of malignant tumors." Sylwan 101:5-11.

[48] Chang Minyi, AntiCancer Medicinal Herbs, publ by Hunan Science and Technology Publishing House, 1992.

[49] Kurashige, S.; Akuzawa, Y.; Endo, F., "Effects of Lentinus edodes, Grifola frondosa and Pleurotus ostreatus administration on cancer outbreak, and activities of macrophages and lymphocytes in mice treated with a carcinogen, N-butyl-N-butanolnitrosoamine." Department of Laboratory Sciences, Gunma University School of Health Sciences, Japan. Immunopharmacol Immunotoxicol, 19(2):175-83 1997 May

[50] Liu, M.; Li, J.; Kong, F.; Lin, J.; Gao, Y., "Induction of immunomodulating cytokines by a new polysaccharide-peptide complex from culture mycelia of Lentinus edodes." Research Center for Eco-Environmental Sciences, Chinese Academy of Sciences, Beijing. lmq@bltd.com.bta.net.cn Immunopharmacology, 40(3):187-98, 1998 Nov

[51] Lau, B.H.; Ruckle, H.C.; Botolazzo, T.; Lui, P.D., "Chinese medicinal herbs inhibit growth of murine renal cell carcinoma." Cancer Biother 1994 Summer;9(2):153-61

[52] Battelli, M.G. et al. "Toxicity of ribosome-inactivating proteins-containing immunotoxins to a human bladder carcinoma cell line." Int J Cancer 1996 Feb 8;65(4): 485-90 Department of Experimental Pathology, University of Bologna, Italy.

[53] Jilka, C.; Strifler, B.; Fortner, G.W.; Hays, E.F.; Takemoto, D.J., "In vivo antitumor activity of the bitter melon (Momordica charantia)." Cancer Res 1983 Nov;43 (11):5151-5

[54] Jones, Eli, Cancer, Its Causes, Symptoms & Treatment, B. Jain pub.

[55] Yeung, Him Che, Handbook of Chinese Herbs Vol 1, 1996, pub by the Institute of Chinese Medicine, 602 San Gabriel Blvd., Rosemead, CA 91770 (818)280-8811

[56] Rao, K.V., "Quinone Natural Products, Streptonigrin (NSC-45383) and Lapachol (NSC 11905) Structure-activity relationships." Cancer Chemotherapy Reports (part2)

4:4 (1974) 11:17. Also Rao K.V. et al. "Recognition and Evaluation of Lapachol as an Antitumor Agent." Cancer Research 28 (1968), 1952-1954.

[57] Santana, C.F. et al. "Preliminary Observations with the Use of Lapachol in Human Patients Bearing Malignant Neoplasms." Revista de Instituto de Antibioticos 20 (1980/1981), 61-68. Cited in: Werbach, M.R., and M.T. Murray, Botanical Influences on Illness (Tarzana, CA: Thirk Line Press, 1994), cited in An Alternative Medicine Definitive Guide to Cancer pub by Future Medicine Publishing Inc., Tiburon, Ca. 1997

[58] Yu SJ; Tseng J, "Fu-Ling, a Chinese herbal drug, modulates cytokine secretion by human peripheral blood monocytes." Department of Biology, National Taiwan Normal University, Taipei, Int J Immunopharmacol, 18(1):37-44 1996 Jan

[59] Zhu, D. 1987. "Recent advances on the active components in Chinese medicines." Abstracts of Chinese Medicines. 1:251-286 (cited from Hobbs)

[60] Chang & But 1987, World Scientific vol 2, pg 1106

[61] Wang, R.L., Tumor Department, First Affiliated Hospital of Henan Medical University, Zhengzhou.

[62] Chung Hua Chung Liu Tsa Chih 1993 Jul;15(4):300-2, Related Articles, Books, LinkOut [A report of 40 cases of esophageal carcinoma surviving for more than 5 years after treatment with drugs].

[63] Gao, Z.G., Ye, Q.X., Zhang, T.M., "Synergistic effect of oridonin and cisplatin on cytotoxicity and DNA cross-link against mouse sarcoma S180 cells in culture." Department of Pharmacology, He-nan Institute of Medical Sciences, Zhengzhou, China.

[64] Tamayo, C., M.A. Richardson, S. Diamond, I. Skoda. "The Chemistry and Biological Activity of Herbs Used in Flor-Essence™ Herbal Tonic and Essiac™." Phytotherapy Research 2000;14:1-14.

[65] Richardson, Mary Ann, DrPH, et al, "Flor-Essence Herbal Tonic Use in North America: A Profile of General Consumers and Cancer Patients," HerbalGram, 50, 2000

[66] Zheng, M.; Wang, H.; Zhang, H.; Ou, Q.; Shen, B.; Li, N.; Yu, B., "The influence of the p53 gene on the in vitro chemosensitivity of colorectal cancer cells." Department of Surgery, Rui Jin Hospital, Shanghai Second Medical University, P.R. China., J Cancer Res Clin Oncol, 125(6):357-60 1999

[67] Bulletin of Pharmaceutics, Vol.7 1980

[68] Zhang, G.G.; Ye, R.G.; Kong, Q.Y., "Effects of radix Salivae miltiorrhizae on proliferation, apoptosis and c-myc protein expression of fibroblast in culture of kidney with lupus nephritis," Department of Surgery, Rui Jin Hospital, Shanghai Second Medical University, P.R. China. Source Chung Kuo Chung Hsi I Chieh Ho Tsa Chih, 125(6):473-5 1997 Aug

[69] Fernandez, M.A.; Saenz, M.T.; Garcia, M.D., "Anti-inflammatory activity in rats and mice of phenolic acids isolated from Scrophularia frutescens." J Pharm Pharmacol 1998 Oct;50(10):1183-6

[70] Grossmann, M.; Hoermann, R.; Weiss, M.; Jauch, K.W.; Oertel, H.; Staebler, A.; Mann, K.; Engelhardt, D., "Spontaneous regression of hepatocellular carcinoma." Am J Gastroenterol 1995 Sep;90(9):1500-3 (ISSN: 0002-9270)

[71] Zi Xi, et al. "Modulation of Mitogen-Activated Protein Kinase Activation and Cell Cycle Regulators by the Potent Skin Cancer Preventive Agent Silymarin." Biochem Biophys Res Commun 1999 Sep 24;263(2):528-536

[72] Proc Natl Acad Sci U S A 1999 Jun 22;96(13):7490-5 (ISSN: 0027-8424) Zi X; Agarwal R, "Silibinin decreases prostate-specific antigen with cell growth inhibition via G1 arrest, leading to differentiation of prostate carcinoma cells: implications for prostate cancer intervention." Center for Cancer Causation and Prevention, AMC Cancer Research

Center, 1600 Pierce Street, Denver, CO 80214, USA.

[73] Duthie, S.J.; Johnson, W.; Dobson, V.L., "The effect of dietary flavonoids on DNA damage (strand breaks and oxidised pyrimdines) and growth in human cells". *Mutat Res* 1997 Apr 24;390(1-2):141-51

[74] Bokemeyer, C.; Fels, L.M.; Dunn, T.; Voigt, W.; Gaedeke, J.; Schmoll, H.J.; Stolte, H.; Lentzen, H., "Silibinin protects against cisplatin-induced nephrotoxicity without compromising cisplatin or ifosfamide anti-tumour activity." *Br J Cancer* 1996 Dec;74(12): 2036-41

[75] G. Scambia et al., "Antiprotective Effect of Silybin on Gynaecological Malignancies: synergism with Cisplatin and Doxorubicin," *European Journal of Cancer* 32A (5): 877-82 (1996.

[76] John Eberle, M.D., *A Treatise of the Materia Medica and Therapeutics,* 1830.

[77] Morre, Dorothy and James, presented at the 38th annual meeting of the American Society for Cell Biology in San Francisco. 1998

[78] Vomel, T. Arzneim, forsch, 35 II (9), 1437, (1985)

[79] Beuscher, N. and Kopanski, L. *Planta Med.* 14, 376, (1986)

[80] Ellingwood, Finley, M.D., *American Materia Medica, Therapeutics and Pharmacognosy.* 1898

[81] Ellinwood ibid.

[82] Mathew, S.; Kuttan, G., "Antioxidant activity of Tinospora cordifolia and its usefulness in the amelioration of cyclophosphamide induced toxicity." *J Exp Clin Cancer Res* 1997 Dec;16(4):407-11

[83] Dictionary of Traditional Chinese Medicinal Herbs (cited from Chang Minyi)

[84] Bensky, Gamble, *Chinese Herbal Medicine Materia Medica, Revised Edition,* 1993, Eastland Press

[85] Rizzi, R., Re, F., Bianchi, A., et al. "Mutagenic and antimutagenic activities of uncaria tomentosa and its extracts." *Journal of Ethnopharmacology,* 1993;38:63-77.

[86] Duke, J.A., *Handbook of Medicinal Herbs,* Boca Raton, FL, CRC Press. 1992.

[87] Blumenthal, M., "Una de Gato (Cat's Claw): Rainforest herb gets scientific and industry attention." Whole Foods (Herb Clip). 1995:62-5.

[88] Moore, Michael, *Medicinal Plants of the Mountain West,* 1978, Museum of New Mexico Press. Pg 107-109

[89] Keine, H. "Clinical Studies on Mistletoe Therapy for Cancerous diseases: A Review." Therapeutikon 3:6 (1989). 347-350 (citation from Goldberg, et al. *An Alternative Medicine Definitive Guide to Cancer,* 1997, pub. Future Medicine Publishing, Inc.)

[90] Office of Technology Assessment. Unconventional Cancer Treatments (Washington DC: US government Printing Office, 1990), 83. Iscador with copper is used for primary tumors of the liver, gallbladder, stomach and kidneys; Iscador with mercury is used to treat tumors of the intestines and lymphatic system; Iscador with silver is used to treat cancers of the breast and urogenital tract; and Iscador without any added metals is used to treat most other cancers. This report notes the marked difference between European Mistletoe and the American species. (Cited from Goldberg, et al. *An Alternative Medicine Definitive Guide to Cancer,* 1997, pub. Future Medicine Publishing, Inc.)

[91] Schink, M., "Mistletoe therapy for human cancer: the role of the natural killer cells." Verein Filderklinik e.V., Research Department, Filderstadt, Germany. Anticancer Drugs, 8 Suppl 1():S47-51 1997 Apr

[92] Kuttan, G., "Use of Withania somnifera Dunal as an adjuvant during radiation

therapy." *Indian J Exp Biol* 1996 Sep;34(9):854-6   Amala Cancer Research Centre, Amala Nagar, Thrissur, India.

[93] Devi, P.U., "Withania somnifera Dunal (Ashwagandha): potential plant source of a promising drug for cancer chemotherapy and radiosensitization." *Indian J Exp Biol* 1996 Oct;34(10):927-32 Department of Radiobiology, Kasturba Medical College, Manipal, India.

[94] Devi, P.U.; Sharada, A.C.; Solomon, F.E.; Kamath, M.S., "In vivo growth inhibitory effect of Withania somnifera (Ashwagandha) on a transplantable mouse tumor, Sarcoma 180." *Indian J Exp Biol* 1992 Mar;30(3):169-72   Department of Radiobiology, Kasturba Medical College, Manipal, India.

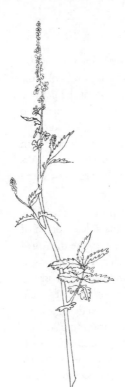

CHAPTER SEVEN

TREATING SPECIFIC CANCERS ACCORDING TO THE SIX METHODS

The following represents an herbal and supplement approach to the treatment of a few of the more common and representative types of cancers. Many formulas may be more appropriate to a specific patient than those presented here. These are primarily offered as examples using the principles and herbs described in this book. By so doing, it is possible to create the most powerful integrated herbal and supplement program for cancer patients.

These are not intended as an alternative to qualified medical care. However, in the absence of such care or in the event that what is being offered is deemed unsuitable by the patient, they certainly can be tried.

In creating an herbal treatment program for cancer there are some general principles that should be considered.

1. *Root and Branch:* First one should distinguish between the root and branch of the disease. The root is the underlying weakness that allows the disease to flourish while the branch is the acute manifestations. Generally in treating the root one emphasizes the use of blood and qi tonics, while treating the branch involves using a higher dose of those herbs that clear

toxic heat and have anticancer properties.

2. *Energetic basis of treatment:* One should prescribe herbs as much as possible according to the energetic principles of excess-deficiency and cold-hot-cool-warm properties and natures based on the symptoms of the patient. Even though cancer itself is regarded as a condition of stagnant heat and dampness, other systems of the body may be dry, cold and/or deficient so that herbs that treat dryness may involve deficiency of blood or yin hormonal reserves or hypo-functioning internal organs. The best results will be obtained if one learns to prescribe herbs according to these more wholistic indications.

3. *Excess-deficiency:* Cancer is regarded as an extreme condition of toxicity. This is not necessarily the fault of the patient but it is a description of the disease. Such an extreme toxic condition requires extreme measures of treatment, which is one reason that treatments such as chemotherapy, radiation and surgery are used. Similarly one will find the use of strong detoxifying herbs that may include nux vomica seeds (the source of strychnine), nightshade family of plants, apricot and peach seeds that have cyanide-type compounds (also called laetrile), animal substances such as scorpions, centipedes, silkworms, lumbricus, wasp nests and poisonous substances such as arsenic used in Chinese herbal medicine. Western herbs such as chelidonium, carnivora, and sanguinaria are also strong herbs with toxic potential. Therefore one will generally include along with these mildly toxic substances, herbs such as ganoderma, astragalus, jujube date, licorice and codonopsis to protect the "righteous qi," or the normal processes of the body.

In this way, one must regard the use of radiation and chemotherapy drugs as strong cancer killing compounds. One of the cutting edges of contemporary cancer medicine is like herbal medicine where the creation of a "chemotherapy cocktail," consisting of several chemotherapy drugs, is combined together like an herbal formula. As with the combination of anticancer herbs, combining several chemotherapy drugs, each one in smaller amounts, works synergistically better together than the use of only one or two. Following this with herbs or drugs that support those processes of the body that may be injured by the strong drugs will give the body more strength to have a stronger energetic response.

4. *Strengthening the body's reserves:* One should also pay attention to the use of herbs according to the energetic and organ-symptom sign understanding. Generally one uses herbs that strengthen the spleen-stomach, thereby promoting digestion and elimination and helping the entire body. Similarly because chronic diseases such as cancer tend to weaken the internal reserves implied by the concept of kidney energy, one would also use herbs to tonify the kidneys according to TCM theory. This may include herbs

such as ginseng, codonopsis, astragalus, ganoderma, atractylodes for the qi of the spleen and stomach and herbs such as prepared asparagus root, angelica sinensis, prepared Rehmannia, peony and lycii berries to tonify blood and herbs such as prepared rehmannia again, ligustrum berries, asparagus root, to nourish kidney yin which are the hormonal reserves of the body. It is with the use of such herbs and formulas such as Six Gentlemen Combination (Liu Junza Tang), Ginseng and Astragalus (Bu Zhong Yi Qi Tang) and Rehmannia Six pills (Liu Wei Wan) that patients undergoing conventional treatment are able to function much better than those who do not take these.

5. *Conventional medicine and herbal therapy:* In general, when one is undergoing chemotherapy or radiation, one would consider diminishing the dosage by approximately one third of those herbs that remove toxic heat while leaving a higher dose of herbs that supplement Zheng Qi and stimulate blood circulation. This is because the primary effect of chemotherapy is already focused on detoxification, which is the role that herbs that remove toxic heat would be doing. As for radiation, again the greater emphasis is on the supplement Zheng Qi, maintaining what is normal while the effects of radiation are focused on attacking the cancer. Herbs that stimulate blood and qi, on the other hand, are among the most important class for the treatment of cancer because they not only prevent metastasis by keeping the blood more viscous, thus inhibiting the ability of cancer cells to adhere to distant sites of the body, but they also have been shown to enhance the effects of both chemo and radiation therapy.

Some of the main problems attendant to undergoing chemotherapy are as follows:

6) *Digestive disorders* including loss of taste, anorexia, nausea, diarrhea and abdominal distension. Loss of taste as well as nausea and vomiting are usually caused by cold deficiency of the spleen and stomach. Because digestion is so seriously impaired, further intake of supplements can be difficult and of little value. Instead, until digestion and appetite is restored one should focus on using those herbs and supplements that will benefit digestion. This of course would include digestive enzymes, bromelain, etc. as well as one or two herbal formulas that are focused on treating specific digestive disorders. For these conditions, one would create formulas incorporating herbs with carminatives, spleen qi tonic and herbs that relieve food stagnation. Many of these are available as patents in liquid or pill form and can be easily added to the regime.
    Carminative herbs for loss of taste and appetite are cardamon, tangerine peel, cloves, and anise seed. Chinese patent formula: Shu Gan

Wan, Bao He Wan, Ping Wei San, Planetary's Digestive Comfort.

Nausea and vomiting of hot or acid fluid is a hot condition and one would use citrus peel, poria mushroom, ophiopogon, coptis, goldenseal, Oregon grape, tangerine peel or dandelion root. Nausea and vomiting of clear fluid is a cold condition and one would use ginger fried pinellia, tangerine peel, poria mushroom, honey-fried licorice, cloves, ginger and jujube dates.

A powder can be made for either hot or cold type nausea and vomiting and this can be taken with warm water.

An Ayurvedic formula that is useful for this is called *Draksha* and contains a large number of herbs in fermented grape liquor. This is one of the best digestive tonics and all cancer patients would benefit from taking one or two tablespoons of Draksha 10 or 15 minutes before eating. It is commonly available from Indian importers throughout the country (see resources at the end of the book). Planetary Formulas has Digestive Grape Bitters that can be similarly used before meals.

Foods and substances that relieve food stagnation include acidophilus, digestive enzymes, Massa Fermentata and hawthorn berries. These can be taken separately before meals or combined in a formula with the above ingredients.

7) *Low white or red blood cell count* following chemo or radiation therapies – a wide number of herbs is effective to counteract this tendency. Some Chinese herbs and substances to consider include ganoderma, astragalus, panax ginseng and panax quinquefolium, lycii berries, angelica sinensis, placenta, cordyceps, maitake mushroom, schizandra berries, jujube dates, pseudoginseng (tienchi), donkey skin hide gelatin. Western herbs would include comfrey root, slippery elm bark, elecampane root and aralia root. Other substances on the market include colostrum, various mushroom products such as Planetary's Reishi Mushroom Supreme, or Maitake Mushroom, Beta Glucan (also derived from mushrooms), folic acid and B12. I especially recommend injectables of tonic herbs such as ginseng, dang gui, astragalus, B12 and/or folic acid. These are made even more efficacious when they are injected into certain well known acupuncture points such as Stomach 36 on the lateral and upper side of the tibia 3 inches distal to the top of the knee and Conception vessel 6 with is on the medial anterior line one and one half inches below the navel. I recommend that cancer patients solicit their doctors to administer B12 injections after chemo or radiation therapy. I have seen these be very helpful in regaining their strength.

In the case of surgery, one would use herbs that promote healing and stimulate blood circulation. Comfrey root is ideal for this and can be used with benefit along with irish moss for two weeks to a month after surgery to promote healing. In my experience, the toxicity of comfrey root is far exaggerated and it remains one of the best Western herbs to take for a limited period, ideally of no more than two weeks at a time, to promote healing. Yarrow leaves and blossoms and agrimony herb are also useful to stop bleeding while promoting circulation and healing. One of the most beneficial Chinese herbs is tienchi ginseng (ginseng pseudo-ginseng), which tonifies the blood Qi as well as promotes circulation while stopping bleeding and it is ideal to use after surgery. As in most cases, a formula is generally safer and better to use than a single herb. One can boil an ounce each of crushed tienchi ginseng roots, comfrey root and irish moss (*chondrus crispus*) for 30 to 40 minutes in a quart and a half of water, covered. Then add an ounce each of yarrow leaves and blossoms and agrimony leaves with 4 or 5 slices of fresh ginger to steep the hot tea until cool. This is then strained and all the herbs can be boiled a second time in half as much water for 20 or 30 minutes. Combine the two and cook down to a pint. Add a half pint of blackstrap molasses and a half pint of honey to make syrup. Keep refrigerated. Administer 2 or 3 tablespoons three times daily.

The most important categories for creating an individualized cancer formula are the first three:

1) **Immune tonic herbs** that supplement Shang Qi or normal processes of the body,

2) **Anticancer herbs** that clear toxic heat, and

3) **Blood moving herbs.** Herbs in the remaining three categories are usually given as indicated according to each patient's needs.

I have broadened the category of herbs that clear phlegm to include removing dampness. Generally phlegm denoting a thicker substance is regarded as a stage of advanced dampness and the mushrooms, poria, grifola, shiitake and indeed all mushrooms have the ability to relieve dampness and are especially beneficial in the treatment of cancer. The two primary herbs for removing phlegm are pinellia and the somewhat stronger acting arisaema. These have specific applications for phlegm especially involving the respiratory system.

Herbs that relieve qi stagnation are:

1) Bupleurum and verbena hastata that clear the liver and help regulate hormones

2) Herbs such as saussurea and lindera that help to relieve pain

3) Herbs such as magnolia bark, cardamon, and Massa fermentata that help to promote digestion.

Furthermore, the combination of herbs that relieve qi stagnation together with herbs that promote blood circulation are often combined because they tend to have a synergistic effect with each other and pain often involves both qi and blood stagnation. The combination of corydalis, a strong blood-moving herb together with melia for qi stagnation is often used because these two herbs work synergistically to relieve various pains especially of gastrointestinal origin. Even if it only means adding herbs that promote digestion and assimilation such as Massa fermentata and cardamon, or the use of citrus peel, herbs that relieve qi stagnation have a wide application for most types of cancer.

Herbs that soften and dissolve the mass mostly include various seaweeds, which apart from their known anticancer properties, also tend to soften and dissolve hard masses. Personally I have found this latter property to be slight with the exception of certain types of goiters. Other herbs used in this way including prunella and violet leaves together with the various seaweeds, are useful if for nothing else than the fact that they all have effective anticancer properties generally.

Finally, a seventh category that I think is useful for obvious reasons are **herbs that calm and settle the spirit.** I usually give these in a separate formula but certain of them, especially oyster shell and skullcap, have other properties that are useful for the treatment of cancer. The herb zizyphus spinosa is an important herb for treating nervousness, insomnia and exerting a generally calming effect.

Herbal Formulas According to the Six Methods

Breast Cancer

Supplement Zheng Qi (maintain normal and support the immune system)	Astragalus – 30g Codonopsis – 9g Dang Gui Angelica – 9g
Remove toxic heat	Taraxacum (dandelion) – 15g Trichosanthes root – 9g Solanum nigri and/or lyratum – 30g Lithospermum – 12g
Stimulate blood circulation	Persica seed – 9g Corydalis – 9g
Clear phlegm and/or dampness	Fritillaria bulb – 9g Poria – 9g Coix – 9g

Relieve qi stagnation	Bupleurum – 9g Cyperus – 9g Chenpi citrus – 3g
Soften and dissolve the mass	Violet (whole herb) – 30g Prunella spike – 30g

Cook the entire amount for 40 minutes with enough water so that the water is approximately 2 inches above the settled herbs. Strain and save the resultant tea. Then add more water to the reserved herbs and cool 20 minutes. Strain and discard the herbs. Combine the first and second teas and slowly reduce down to 2 cups. These are taken morning and early evening.

Alternatively, if these herbs are supplied as a dried extract, the daily dose is one tablespoon twice a day with a tea of dandelion root, burdock root, red clover tea and violet leaf.

Topical application (combine the following):

Faeces Trogopterorum	30g
Sulphur	30g
Strychnine	30g
Donkey skin gelatin	30g
Realgar	30g
Ginger	30g

Grind all herbs to a fine powder. Slowly add a small amount of hot water while mixing to form a paste. Spread about ¼ inch thick on a cloth and apply directly over the tumorous area. Reapply daily.

Supplemental Planetary Herbal Formulas:

Red Clover Cleanser	Two tablets 3 times daily
Soy Isoflavones	Two tablets 3 times daily
Triphala	Two tablets 3 times daily
Bupleurum Liver Cleanse	Two tablets 3 times daily
Reishi Mushroom supreme	Two tablets 3 times daily
Easy Sleep	Four tablets taken before retiring in the evening.

Apricot seeds:

Buy one pound and keep refrigerated. Take 5 seeds hourly for a total of 30 seeds daily.

Frozen blueberries:

Consume at least a quarter package daily frozen and thawed. They contain ellagic acid and have powerful antioxidant properties against cancer.

In addition, the following nutritional supplements should be taken daily:

Nutritional supplements:

Calcium D-glucarate (CDG): Four 500 mg capsules twice daily; this is used to detoxify estrogen.

Quercetin: 1 to 3g to be taken with vitamin C and bromelain in two or three divided doses. Inhibits cancer growth, assists conventional western therapies, especially good for genetically driven cancers because it inhibits the tumor-suppressing gene P53.

Omega 3 Fatty acids: 12g of Eskimo oil tablets daily. It inhibits the spread of cancer.

Inosital Hexaphosphate (IP6): 10 capsules twice daily. Regulates normal cellular functions, prevents genetic mutations of cells, increases natural killer cells.

Folic acid and B12: 800 mcg. Protects and inhibits cancer growth.

Mixed Carotenoid supplement: 100,000 IU's

Vitamin D: 400 IU's daily

Vitamin A: 25,000 IU's daily

Bromelain: 4000 mg daily

Vitamin C: 2000 mgs daily

CoQ10: 400 mlg daily. Antioxidant and detoxifying agent.

Selenium: 700 mcg daily. Free radical, used to make glutathione, inhibits cancer growth.

Zinc: 20 mlgs. Immune system stimulant, promotes healing. Should not be taken along with cisplatin or carboplatin chemotherapeutic drugs.

Chlorella: 1 to 2 teaspoons two or more times daily. Dense and nutrient rich in vitamins, minerals and easily assimilable protein, it supports the immune system of patients undergoing chemo and radiation therapy, increases phagocytes, T-cells and cancer killing B cells.

Kelp and other seaweeds: Take several commercially available seaweed tablets two or three times daily. It contains important cancer fighting nutrients including calcium, potassium, many other minerals and iodine.

Daily regime:

Coffee enema once or twice daily.

Epsom salt bath twice a week.

Prostate Cancer

Supplement Zheng Qi (maintain normal and support the immune system)	Ganoderma lucidum (reishi or ling zhi) Astragalus – 30g Milk thistle, Silymarin – 30g (freshly crushed seeds) Saw Palmetto – 9g
Remove Toxic Heat	Rabdosia rubescens – 9g Andrographis – 15g Scutellaria baicalensis – 15g Chrysanthemum morifolium – 9g
Stimulate Blood circulation	Panax pseudo ginseng (Tienchi or Sanqi) – 9g
Clear Phlegm and/or Dampness	Poria – 9g Coix – 9g
Relieve Qi stagnation	Bupleurum – 9g Green citrus peel – 3g
Soften and Dissolve the Mass	Prunella spike – 30g

Cook the entire amount as previously described for 40 minutes with enough water so the water is approximately 2 inches above the settled herbs. Strain and save the resultant tea. Then add more water to the reserved herbs and cool 20 minutes. Strain and discard the herbs. Combine the first and second teas and slowly reduce down to 2 cups. These are taken morning and early evening.

Alternatively, if these herbs are supplied as a dried extract, the daily dose is one or two tablespoonful twice a day with a tea of dandelion root, burdock root, red clover tea, sarsaparilla and a quarter part chaparral.

Additional herbal supplements:

Planetary Formulas

Saw Palmetto Classic – Three tablets 3 times daily.

Bupleurum Liver cleanse – Two tablets 2 times daily.

Triphala – Two tablets 3 times daily.

Diurite – Two tablets 3 times daily.

Reishi Mushroom Supreme – Two tablets 3 times daily.

Easy Sleep – Four tablets one half hour before retiring in the evening.

Apricot seeds:

Buy one pound and keep refrigerated. Take 5 seeds hourly for a total of 30 seeds daily.

Frozen blueberries:

Consume at least a quarter package daily frozen and thawed. They contain ellagic acid and have powerful antioxidant properties against cancer.

Nutritional supplements:

Inosital Hexaphosphate (IP6): 10 capsules twice daily. Regulates normal cellular functions, prevents genetic mutations of cells, increases natural killer cells.

Folic acid and B12: 800 mcg. Protects and inhibits cancer growth.

Mixed Carotenoid supplement: 100,000 IU's daily. Powerful antioxidant, especially good for prostate cancer.

Vitamin C: 2000 mgs daily – powerful antioxidant

Vitamin E: 1000 IU's daily – powerful antioxidant

Vitamin D: 400 IU's daily – powerful antioxidant

Vitamin A: 25,000 IU's daily – Taken with Vitamin D as an antioxidant.

Selenium: 700 mcg daily. Free radical, used to make glutathione, inhibits cancer growth.

Zinc: 30 mlg daily. Used for prostate cancer. (Do not take if you are given cisplatin or carboplatin).

Pycnogenol: 50 mlg daily from combined grape seed and pine bark. Powerful antioxidant and preventive for prostate cancer.

Quercetin: 1 to 3g to be taken with vitamin C and bromelain in two or three divided doses. Inhibits cancer growth, assists conventional western therapies, especially good for genetically driven cancers because it inhibits the tumor-suppressing gene P53.

Omega 3 Fatty acids: 12g of Eskimo oil tablets daily. It inhibits the spread of cancer.

Modified Citrus Pectin (MCP): 1 tablespoon mixed with water, vegetable juice or a green drink, three times daily between meals. Especially good for prostate cancer, prevents metastasis.

Chlorella: 1 to 2 teaspoons two or more times daily. Dense and nutrient rich in vitamins, minerals and easily assimilable protein, it supports the immune system of patients undergoing chemo and radiation therapy, increases phagocytes, T-cells and cancer killing B cells.

Kelp and other seaweeds: Take several commercially available seaweed tablets two or three times daily. It contains important cancer fighting nutrients including calcium potassium, many other minerals and iodine.

Daily regime:

Coffee enema once or twice daily.
Epsom salt bath twice a week.

Lung Cancer

Supplement Zheng Qi (maintain normal and support the immune system)	Ganoderma lucidum (reishi or ling zhi) Astragalus – 30g Codonopsis – 30g Asparagus root – 9g Apricot seeds – 9g Schizandra – 9g
Remove Toxic Heat	Lonicera – 10g Scutellaria barbata – 15g Solanum Nigra – 15g (or solanum lyratum) Houttuynia herb – 15g Trichosanthes root – 15g
Stimulate Blood circulation	Panax pseudo ginseng (Tienchi or Sanqi) – 10g
Clear Phlegm and/or Dampness	Pinellia – 9g Poria – 9g
Relieve Qi stagnation	Bupleurum – 9g Chenpi citrus – 3g
Soften and Dissolve the Mass	Lilium brownii – 9g Oyster shell – 15g Prunella spike – 30g Violet leaves – 30g

Cook the entire amount as previously described for 40 minutes with enough water so that the water is approximately 2 inches above the settled herbs. Strain and save the resultant tea. Then add more water to the reserved herbs and cool 20 minutes. Strain and discard the herbs. Combine the first and second teas and slowly reduce down to 2 cups. These are taken morning and early evening.

Alternatively, if these herbs are supplied as a dried extract, the daily dose is one or two tablespoonsful twice a day with a tea of dandelion root, burdock root, red clover tea, sarsaparilla and a quarter part chaparral.

Additional Planetary Herbal supplements:

Triphala – Two tablets 3 times daily
Bupleurum Liver Cleanse – Two tablets 3 times daily

Apricot seeds:

Buy one pound and keep refrigerated. Take 5 seeds hourly for a total of 30 seeds daily.

Nutritional supplements:

Inosital Hexaphosphate (IP6): 10 capsules twice daily. Regulates normal cellular functions, prevents genetic mutations of cells, increases natural killer cells.

Folic acid and B12: 800 mcg. Protects and inhibits cancer growth.

Mixed Carotenoid supplement: 100,000 IU's daily. Powerful antioxidant against cancer.

Vitamin C: 2000 mgs daily – powerful antioxidant

Vitamin E: 1000 IU's daily – powerful antioxidant

Vitamin D: 400 IU's daily – powerful antioxidant

Vitamin A: 25,000 IU's daily – taken with Vitamin D as an antioxidant.

Vitamin K: 300 mcg once daily – inhibits lung cancer.

Selenium: 700 mcg daily. Free radical. Used to make glutathione, inhibits cancer growth.

Zinc: 20 mlgs. Immune system stimulant, promotes healing. Should not be taken along with cisplatin or carboplatin chemotherapeutic drugs.

N-Acetyl Cysteine: 2000 mg daily. Powerful free radical, glutathione precursor, inhibits cancer growth.

Quercetin: 1 to 3g to be taken with vitamin C and bromelain in two or three divided doses. Inhibits cancer growth, assists conventional western therapies, especially good for genetically driven cancers because it inhibits the tumor-suppressing gene P53.

Omega 3 Fatty acids: 12g of Eskimo oil tablets daily. It inhibits the spread of cancer.

Chlorella: 1 to 2 teaspoons two or more times daily. Dense and nutrient rich in vitamins, minerals and easily assimilable protein, it supports the immune system of patients undergoing chemo and radiation therapy, increases phagocytes, T-cells and cancer killing B cells.

Kelp and other seaweeds: Take several commercially available seaweed tablets two or three times daily. They contain important cancer fighting nutrients including calcium, potassium, many other minerals and iodine.

Daily regime:

Coffee enema once or twice daily.
Epsom salt bath twice a week.

Liver Cancer

Supplement Zheng Qi by restoring normal health and supporting the immune system	Dioscorea – 9g Codonopsis – 9g
Remove toxic heat	Oregon Grape root – 9g Dandelion – 9g Scutellaria barbata – 9g
Stimulate blood circulation	Angelica dang gui – 9g
Clear phlegm	Magnolia bark – 9g
Relieve qi stagnation	Citrus Immaturus aurantii (Chih shih or zhi shi) – 9g Bupleurum – 9g
Soften and dissolve the mass	Prunella – 15g

Other herbs to consider:

For constipation add 9g of rhubarb root.

For pain add 9g each of corydalis and melia.

For jaundice add capillaris and gardenia, 15g each.

For swollen abdomen add 3g fresh ginger and 9g of pinellia.

For yin deficiency add 20g each of adenophora and trichosanthes root.

Cook the entire amount for 40 minutes with enough water so that the water is approximately 2 inches above the settled herbs. Strain and save the resultant tea. Then add more water to the reserved herbs and cool 20 minutes. Strain and discard the herbs. Combine the first and second teas and slowly reduce down to 2 cups. These are taken morning and early evening.

Alternatively, if these herbs are supplied as a dried extract, the daily dose is one or two tablespoonsful twice a day with a tea of dandelion root, burdock root, red clover tea, sarsaparilla and a quarter part chaparral.

Additional Planetary Herbal supplements:

Triphala – Two tablets 3 times daily
Bupleurum Liver Cleanse – Two tablets 3 times daily

Apricot seeds:

Buy one pound and keep refrigerated. Take 5 seeds hourly for a total of 30 seeds daily.

Nutritional supplements:

Inosital Hexaphosphate (IP6): 10 capsules twice daily. Regulates normal cellular functions, prevents genetic mutations of cells, increases natural killer cells.

Folic acid and B12: 800 mcg. Protects and inhibits cancer growth.

Mixed Carotenoid supplement: 100,000 IU's daily. A powerful antioxidant against cancer.

Vitamin C: 2000 mgs daily – powerful antioxidant

Vitamin E: 1000 IU's daily – powerful antioxidant

Vitamin D: 400 IU's daily – powerful antioxidant

Vitamin A: 25,000 IU's daily. Taken with Vitamin D as an antioxidant.

Vitamin K: 300 mcg once daily. Inhibits lung cancer.

Selenium: 700 mcg daily. Free radical, used to make glutathione, inhibits cancer growth.

Zinc: 20 mlgs. Immune system stimulant, promotes healing. Should not be taken along with cisplatin or carboplatin chemotherapeutic drugs.

Lactobacillus Acidophilus: Take indicated dose twice daily with whey protein before meals – helps digestion, assimilation and elimination and promotes general intestinal health.

Wobenzyme: 2-4 tablets three or four times' daily a half hour before meals. It can be taken with the acidophilus for convenience. – Maintains digestion and assimilation, activates the immune system and inhibits metastasis.

Lipoic acid: 400 mg Activates the immune system by stimulating T-cells, prevents oncogene activation and helps regenerate glutathione.

N-Acetyl Cysteine: 2000 mg daily. Powerful free radical, glutathione precursor, inhibits cancer growth.

Quercetin: 1 to 3g to be taken with vitamin C and bromelain in two or three divided doses. Inhibits cancer growth, assists conventional western therapies, especially good for genetically driven cancers because it inhibits the tumor-suppressing gene P53.

Omega 3 Fatty acids: 12g of Eskimo oil tablets daily. It inhibits the spread of cancer.

Chlorella: 1 to 2 teaspoons two or more times daily. Dense and nutrient rich in vitamins, minerals and easily assimilable protein, it supports the immune system of patients undergoing chemo and radiation therapy, increases phagocytes, T-cells and cancer killing B cells.

Kelp and other seaweeds: Take several commercially available seaweed tablets two or three times daily. It contains important cancer fighting nutrients including calcium potassium, many other minerals and iodine.

Daily regime:

Coffee enema once or twice daily.
Epsom salt bath twice a week.

Large Intestine Cancer

Most cancers of the large intestine occur in the recto-sigmoid section. Because it is a small distance from the rectum, diagnosis is easily performed by direct inspection. Any unusual signs of bleeding from the rectum should warrant a medical examination.

Following is one of several possible formulas one can create using the principle of the Six methods for treating large intestine cancer. This formula is similar to many that have actually been used in China with some success.

Supplement Zheng Qi by restoring normal health and supporting the immune system.	Codonopsis – 15g Coix – 30g
Remove toxic heat	Oldenlandia – 15g Scutellaria barbata – 15g Solanum nigrum or S. lyratum – 15g
Stimulate blood circulation	Angelica dang gui – 9g Corydalis – 9g Melia – 9g Persica – 9g
Clear phlegm and dampness	Magnolia bark – 9g

Relieve qi stagnation	Citrus Immaturus aurantii (Chih shih or zhi shi) – 9g
Soften and dissolve the mass	Laminaria kelp – 9g Sargassum seaweed – 9g

Other herbs to consider:

For constipation add 9g rhubarb.

For dry stool add 15g hemp seed (crushed) or flax seed.

For blood in the stool add Nelumbinis rhizoma (charred), unprepared rehmannia 9g, artemisia vulgaris ashes or the ash of human hair 12g.

Cook the entire amount for 40 minutes with enough water so that the water is approximately 2 inches above the settled herbs. Strain and save the resultant tea. Then add more water to the reserved herbs and cool 20 minutes. Strain and discard the herbs. Combine the first and second teas and slowly reduce down to 2 cups. These are taken morning and early evening.

Alternatively, if these herbs are supplied as a dried extract, the daily dose is one or two tablespoonsful twice a day with a tea of dandelion root, burdock root, red clover tea, sarsaparilla and a quarter part chaparral.

Planetary Herbal Formulas:

Triphala – Two tablets 3 times daily
Bupleurum Liver Cleanse – Two tablets 3 times daily

Peach seeds:

Buy one pound and keep refrigerated. Take 5 seeds hourly for a total of 30 seeds daily.

Nutritional supplements:

Inosital Hexaphosphate (IP6): 10 capsules twice daily. Regulates normal cellular functions, prevents genetic mutations of cells and increases natural killer cells.

Folic acid and B12: 800 mcg. Protects and inhibits cancer growth.

Mixed Carotenoid supplement: 100,000 IU's daily. Powerful antioxidant against cancer.

Vitamin C: 2000 mgs daily – powerful antioxidant

Vitamin E: 1000 IU's daily – powerful antioxidant

Vitamin D: 400 IU's daily – powerful antioxidant

Vitamin A: 25,000 IU's daily. Taken with Vitamin D as an antioxidant.

Vitamin K: 300 mcg once daily – inhibits lung cancer.

Selenium: 700 mcg daily. Free radical, used to make glutathione, inhibits cancer growth.

Zinc: 20 mlgs. Immune system stimulant, promotes healing. Should not be taken along with cisplatin or carboplatin chemotherapeutic drugs.

Lactobacillus Acidophilus: Take indicated dose twice daily with whey protein before meals – helps digestion, assimilation and elimination and promotes general intestinal health.

Wobenzyme: 2-4 tablets three or four times daily a half hour before meals. It can be taken with the acidophilus for convenience. It maintains digestion and assimilation, activates the immune system and inhibits metastasis.

Lipoic acid: 400 mg. Activates the immune system by stimulating T-cells, prevents oncogene activation and helps regenerate glutathione.

N-Acetyl Cysteine: 2000 mg daily. Powerful free radical, glutathione precursor, inhibits cancer growth.

Quercetin: 1 to 3g to be taken with vitamin C and bromelain in two or three divided doses. Inhibits cancer growth, assists conventional western therapies, especially good for genetically driven cancers because it inhibits the tumor-suppressing gene P53.

Omega 3 Fatty acids: 12g of Eskimo oil tablets daily. It inhibits the spread of cancer.

Chlorella: 1 to 2 teaspoons two or more times daily. Dense and nutrient rich in vitamins, minerals and easily assimilable protein, it supports the immune system of patients undergoing chemo and radiation therapy, increases phagocytes, T-cells and cancer killing B cells.

Kelp and other seaweeds: Take several commercially available seaweed tablets 2 or 3 times daily. It contains important cancer fighting nutrients including calcium, potassium, many other minerals and iodine.

Daily regime:

Coffee enema once or twice daily.
Epsom salt bath twice a week.

Skin Cancer

There are three main common types of skin cancer. Squamous cell carcinoma (also known as flat epithelial cell cancer, coarse cell or cuticular cancers) appears as a crusty or scale-like growth often in the form of a cauliflower or nipple. Basal cell carcinoma is the most common and usually forms on the face, nose or eyelids. The tumor may form a thick lump, which can appear encrusted or flat. While metastasis is rare, as it enlarges it will tend to ulcerate. The third and most deadly cancer is melanoma. The reason is that if it enters the lymphatics and blood vessels, it tends to metastasize readily to distant areas of the body.

For cancer of the skin, the use of escharotic salves offers several advantages. According to Mohs these are:

1) unprecedented reliability

2) conservatism

3) low operative risk

4) excellent healing, and

5) can be used on patients for which the cancers are too widely extended or are too complicated to cure.[1]

For both squamous and basal cell application confined directly to the affected area is sufficient. For melanomas the cancerous cells may undetectably occupy areas slightly more distant from the primary site. This plus the fact that melanomas tend to penetrate vascular walls and travel under the skin to adjacent lymph nodes, a somewhat larger area may be treated ranging at least two inches around the periphery of the primary site. It is recommended that all melanomas be evaluated by an oncologist who may choose to do an adjacent lymph node biopsy to determine if it has invaded other areas. After excision of a skin cancer with any method the Amas test may be especially useful since its major virtue is in detecting cancer antibodies before actual tumors arise.

For internal treatment of skin cancers, the major methods that are emphasized are to first of all remove toxic heat, stimulate blood circulation, and finally to supplement the Zheng Qi or immune system.

One **Chinese formula** used is called Salvia Root and Pyrola combination (Lian hsieh szu wu tang ho tzu yin chu shih tang). It consists of the following herbs, combined and decocted and taken orally twice a day:

Salvia Milthiorrhiza root	15g
Pyrola	15g
Pteris multifida	15g
Red peony	12g
Scutellaria baicalensis	12g
Unprocessed rehmannia	12g
Lonicera	12g
Coix	30g

---

[1] Mohs, Frederic E., M.D., *Chemosurgery*, p 160-161, Charles Thomas, publisher, 1978

Moutan peony	9g
Ligusticum	6g
Carthamus	4.5g
Licorice	3g

Western herbs would be a combination of the following:

Yellow dock	Oregon Grape
Boneset	Chaparral
Dandelion	Motherwort
Calendula	Angelica archangelica
Licorice	

Nutritional supplements:

Folic acid and B12: 800 mcg. Protects and inhibits cancer growth.

Mixed Carotenoid supplement: 100,000 IU's daily. Powerful antioxidant against cancer.

Vitamin C: 2000 mgs daily – powerful antioxidant

Vitamin E: 1000 IU's daily – powerful antioxidant

Vitamin D: 400 IU's daily – powerful antioxidant

Vitamin A: 25,000 IU's daily – taken with Vitamin D as an antioxidant.

Vitamin K: 300 mcg once daily – inhibits lung cancer.

Selenium: 700 mcg daily. Free radical, used to make glutathione, inhibits cancer growth.

Zinc: 20 mlg daily. Antioxidant mineral that is useful for the prevention and treatment of cancer. Prevents DNA damage.

N-Acetyl Cysteine: 2000 mg daily – powerful free radical, glutathione precursor, inhibits cancer growth.

Quercetin: 1 to 3g to be taken with vitamin C and bromelain in two or three divided doses. It inhibits cancer growth and assists conventional western therapies. It is especially good for genetically driven cancers because it inhibits the tumor-suppressing gene P53.

Omega 3 Fatty acids: 12g of Eskimo oil tablets daily. Inhibits the spread of cancer.

Chlorella: 1 to 2 teaspoons two or more times daily. Dense and nutrient rich in vitamins, minerals and easily assimilable protein, it supports the immune system of patients undergoing chemo and radiation therapy, increases phagocytes, T-cells and cancer-killing B cells.

Kelp and other seaweeds: Take several commercially available seaweed tablets two or three times daily. It contains important cancer fighting nutrients including calcium, potassium, many other minerals and iodine.

Planetary Herbal Formulas:

Bupleurum Liver Cleanse

Yellow Dock Skin Cleanse

Triphala

Take two tablets of each two or three times daily with a tea of equal parts sarsaparilla, yellow dock root, burdock root, and dandelion root.

This should be followed strictly for at least three months, then it can be modified according to convenience and need.

Non-Solid Cancers

Leukemia

Supplement Zheng Qi by restoring normal health and supporting the immune system.	Asparagus cochinensis – 9g Cordyceps sinensis – 9g Astragalus – 15g Ginseng – 9g Rehmannia (prepared) – 9g
Remove toxic heat	Lithospermum – 9g Isatis – 4g Andrographis – 9g Oldenlandia – 15g Scutellaria barbata – 9g
Stimulate blood circulation	Angelica Sinensis – 9g Paeonia alba – 9g Salvia miltiorrhiza – 9g Panax pseudoginseng (Tienchi) – 9g
Clear phlegm	N/A
Relieve qi stagnation	N/A
Soften and dissolve the mass	N/A

Nutritional supplements:

Folic acid and B12: 800 mcg. Protects and inhibits cancer growth.

Mixed Carotenoid supplement: 100,000 IU's daily. Powerful antioxidant against cancer.

Vitamin C: 2000 mgs daily – powerful antioxidant

Vitamin E: 1000 IU's daily – powerful antioxidant

Vitamin D: 400 IU's daily – powerful antioxidant

Vitamin A: 25,000 IU's daily. Taken with Vitamin D as an antioxidant.

Vitamin K: 300 mcg once daily – inhibits lung cancer.

Selenium: 700 mcg daily. It is a free radical, used to make glutathione and inhibits cancer growth.

Zinc: 20 mlg daily. Antioxidant mineral useful for the prevention and treatment of cancer. Prevents DNA damage.

N-Acetyl Cysteine: 2000 mg daily. Powerful free radical, glutathione precursor, inhibits cancer growth.

Lipoic Acid: 600 mg daily. Antioxidant, glutathione precursor, detoxifies the blood and liver.

Glutathione: 2500 mg daily. Powerful antioxidant, repairs DNA, stimulates immune system.

Quercetin: 1 to 3g to be taken with vitamin C and bromelain in two or three divided doses. Inhibits cancer growth, assists conventional western therapies, especially good for genetically driven cancers because it inhibits the tumor-suppressing gene P53.

Omega 3 Fatty acids: 12g of Eskimo oil tablets daily. It inhibits the spread of cancer.

Hydrazine Sulfate: It is effective against cachexia, increases the appetite, decreases pain, lessens anorexia, inhibits tumor growth and enhances the cytotoxic effects of chemotherapeutic drugs. See the section on supplements for specific protocol.

Chlorella: 1 to 2 teaspoons two or more times daily. Dense and nutrient rich in vitamins, minerals and easily assimilable protein, it supports the immune system of patients undergoing chemo and radiation therapy, increases phagocytes, T-cells and cancer killing B cells.

Kelp and other seaweeds: Take several commercially available seaweed tablets two or three times daily. It contains important cancer fighting nutrients including calcium, potassium, many other minerals and iodine.

Planetary Herbal Formulas:

>Reishi Mushroom Supreme
>
>Women's Treasure
>
>Yellow Dock Skin Cleanse
>
>Triphala

Take two tablets of each two or three times daily with a tea of equal parts violet leaves, yellow dock root, burdock root, and dandelion root. This should be followed strictly for at least three months, then it can be modified according to convenience and need.

Hodgkin's Lymphoma

Supplement Zheng Qi by restoring normal health and supporting the immune system.	Atractylodes – 9g Cordyceps sinensis – 9g Astragalus – 15g Ginseng – 9g Scrophularia – 9g
Remove toxic heat	Oldenlandia – 30g Lithospermum – 9g Andrographis – 9g
Stimulate blood circulation	Turmeric – 9g Carthamus – 9g Salvia miltiorrhiza – 9g Panax pseudoginseng (Tienchi) – 9g
Clear phlegm	Trichosanthes root – 9g Fritillary – 6g
Relieve qi stagnation	Saussurea – 6g Cardamon – 6g Bupleurum – 9g Chenpi Citrus – 6g Corium stomachichum galli (chicken gizzard skins) – 9g
Soften and dissolve the mass	Oyster shell – 30g Prunella – 15g

Nutritional supplements:

Folic acid and B12: 800 mcg. Protects and inhibits cancer growth.

Mixed Carotenoid supplement: 100,000 IU's daily. Powerful antioxidant against cancer.

Vitamin C: 2000 mgs daily – powerful antioxidant

Vitamin E: 1000 IU's daily – powerful antioxidant

Vitamin D: 400 IU's daily – powerful antioxidant

Vitamin A: 25,000 IU's daily. Taken with Vitamin D as an antioxidant.

Vitamin K: 300 mcg once daily – inhibits lung cancer.

Selenium: 700 mcg daily. Free radical, used to make glutathione, inhibits cancer growth.

Zinc: 20 mlg daily. Antioxidant mineral useful for the prevention and treatment of cancer. Prevents DNA damage.

N-Acetyl Cysteine: 2000 mg daily. Powerful free radical, glutathione precursor, inhibits cancer growth.

Lipoic Acid: 600 mg daily. Antioxidant, glutathione precursor, detoxifies the blood and liver.

Glutathione: 2500 mg daily. Powerful antioxidant, repairs DNA, stimulates immune system.

Quercetin: 1 to 3g to be taken with vitamin C and bromelain in two or three divided doses. Inhibits cancer growth, assists conventional western therapies, especially good for genetically driven cancers because it inhibits the tumor-suppressing gene P53.

Omega 3 Fatty acids: 12g of Eskimo oil tablets daily. It inhibits the spread of cancer.

Hydrazine Sulfate: It is effective against cachexia, increases the appetite, decreases pain, lessens anorexia, inhibits tumor growth and enhanced the cytotoxic effects of chemotherapeutic drugs. See the section on supplements for specific protocol.

Chlorella: 1 to 2 teaspoons two or more times daily. Dense and nutrient rich in vitamins, minerals and easily assimilable protein, it supports the immune system of patients undergoing chemo and radiation therapy, increases phagocytes, T-cells and cancer killing B cells.

Kelp and other seaweeds: Take several commercially available seaweed tablets two or three times daily. It contains important cancer fighting nutrients including calcium, potassium, many other minerals and iodine.

Planetary Herbal Formulas:

  Reishi Mushroom Supreme

  Bupleurum Liver Cleanse

  Complete Pau D'Arco

  Guggul

  Take two tablets of each two or three times daily with a tea of equal parts violet leaves, cleavers herb, yellow dock root, burdock root, and dandelion root.

  This should be followed strictly for at least three months, then it can be modified according to convenience and need.

Part Three

OTHER IMPORTANT CANCER TREATMENTS

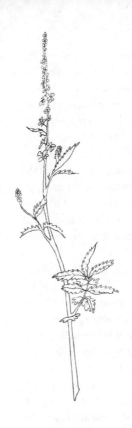

DIET & CANCER

"Let your food be your medicine and your medicine your food"

Hippocrates

Diet is the first line for both the treatment and prevention of cancer. This is especially true in herbal therapy since herbs are ingested and used by the body like 'special foods.' One may not be able to cure all diseases with dietary adjustment but it is safe to say that if a disease can't be cured with diet, it probably can't be cured or controlled through any other natural means. Nutritionist Patrick Quillin corroborates this when he states, "Proper nutrition could prevent from 50-90% of all cancer.[1,2] Our food and water supply contains thousands of carcinogens that can both initiate as well as promote the development of cancer. These include over three thousand additives used to color, flavor, preserve and extend the shelf life of foods as well as various herbicides, pesticides and fertilizers that are routinely used on crops. These eventually find their way into our water supply and affect

---

[1] Quillin, Patrick., *Healing Nutrients*, Random House, NY, 1987
[2] Quillin, Patrick. and Noreen Quillin, "Beating Cancer With Nutrition," *Nutrition Times Press*, 1994

all life that are exposed to these pollutants. Humans who consume milk, poultry, eggs and the flesh of animals reared with antibiotics to prevent disease contribute to our antibiotic resistance. The same is true with the use of growth hormones that are fed to animals to speed their growth and increase their bulk for market. When humans consume these products they have been known to form what is known as 'xeno-hormones,' creating hormonal imbalances and increasing cancer risk. While individuals might question the degree of carcinogenic impact of any one of these influences, taken as a whole they represent a substantial burden on the body's ability to counteract their debilitating effects on our health. Notwithstanding this, chemical additives in food have been linked to a wide variety of health problems including various autoimmune diseases, hyperactivity, allergies, hormone imbalances, birth defects, arthritis and cancer.

When we read or hear of spokespersons and researchers defending the use of one or another of these additives and pollutants, we are often persuaded by their academic credentials to ignore the direct or indirect connection with the various industries that control their purse strings. The influence and control of industry and organized medicine can be either blatant or subtly insinuated. Through the funding by agribusiness, chemical and manufacturing companies of academic research or a university science department chair may tend to slant research in favor of the company's financial interests rather than purely objective findings. Individuals who do independent research and arrive at data and information that supports the need for pure, organic air, food and water, such as the late noble prize winning physicist, Linus Pauling, are often ostracized and made the object of criticism and ridicule by their peers.

Even those with genetic predisposition towards cancer can prevent its occurrence through proper nutrition and balanced lifestyle. To emphasize genetics as the cause of cancer is too often a ruse disguising other economic and politically knotty concerns such as the regulation of food, water and air quality. An example is the abuse of smoking tobacco as the major cause of lung cancer, still the world's leading form of cancer. For decades many held the unpopular view of tobacco as being a primary cause of lung cancer while tobacco industry defendants ranging from hired medical researchers, medical doctors and representatives of the AMA publicly proclaimed its safety.

Genetic Engineering

In fact there is no question that the major causes for the dramatic increase of cancer are lifestyle, environmental degradation and food and water quality. In regards to the latter, genetically engineered foods loom as an even further threat. With little or no regard for its long-term impact based on the interconnectedness of life on this planet, genetic industries pursue a relentless course of genetically altered food primarily for the purpose of short-term profitability.

What is the carrot held out through genetically engineering our food? Though the genetically engineered carrot may bear superficial resemblance to one that is non-genetically manipulated, it is possible to splice the genes into a carrot's DNA not only from other plants but insects, fish and mammals veritably creating 'frankenfoods,' so named after Mary Shelley's 19th century manmade monster. There may be many worthwhile uses for genetic engineering but moral, ethical and environmental issues arise when it is done solely for the purpose of increasing resistance to plant diseases, insects and other pests or to allow them to grow in different climates or adverse circumstances solely to increase profitability. In all of this there are serious concerns of possible "genetic fallout" if and when any of these freak foods work their way into the food chain. However it may look or taste, a genetically engineered carrot is very different from a non-genetic organically grown carrot and as things stand at this time and as stated, we lack sufficient long-term evaluation of the impact of genetically engineered foods both on our own bodies as well as on all life on the earth.

Instead of achieving strength and integrity by fostering long-term organic agricultural practices, the effect of genetically engineered food defies nature's laws far beyond any previously known attempts at hybridization. Of course, what is not known is the impact this will have on the evolution of increasing strains of virulent bacteria and other pathogens including the proliferation of super-weeds. As it stands, genetic engineering is being pursued by agribusiness to increase crop resistance to diseases and increase yields. All of this in lieu of putting into place appropriate practices of organic farming and animal husbandry.

Because of the pollution of the gene pool, it is not difficult to imagine how the general consumption of genetically engineered foods will increase the risk of cancer and other degenerative diseases as a result of further weakening of the immune system.

Cancer is first and foremost a disease directly or indirectly affecting all of nature. The negative impact of destroying forests, burning fossil fuels and various toxic chemicals discharged into the environment is already associated with the increase of cancer not only of humans but also nearby wildlife in various areas around the world. The awareness of this continues to fuel the widespread interest and phenomenal growth of the ecology movement, the organic natural food industry and the interest in more natural treatments of disease.

Genetic engineering, which already extends to the manipulation of the gender of the newborn will undoubtedly include the manipulation and control of various personality traits in humans and other creatures. All of this poses not only an ecological but a moral dilemma as well. It is difficult to imagine the outcome and the grave responsibility involved as we superimpose our will upon the process of natural selection. Such knowledge and control, if used at all, should not be made subservient to the purpose of short-term gain or profit without sufficient long-term evaluation of its impact on all life.

The Importance of Organic Foods

Fresh organic foods have always and will always be best for the general health of people as well as in the prevention and treatment of cancer. Our bodies are simply not equipped to efficiently utilize or adequately discharge refined foods lacking in naturally associated nutrients, or the residues from various unnatural additives such as artificial food coloring or preservatives. The use of irradiated foods have been shown to cause DNA damage, especially in small children, while at the same time the use of microwave cooking further compromises the molecular structure of foods and places additional burdens on the already compromised immune system of cancer patients.

Studies corroborate that the increase of a wide variety of cancers is associated with the increased use of pesticides and herbicides in agriculture. Specifically, pesticides that interfere with the reproductive cycle of insects have similar adverse effects on humans at even very low concentrations. Studies comparing organically grown food with the same food grown with chemical fertilizers have demonstrated organic food to have as much as a 50% nutritional increase.

Diet Strategies for Cancer Patients and for General Health and Well Being

Foods to Eliminate

The basis of a healthy diet begins with eating healthy food. The goal is to eliminate as much as possible those foods that injure or sabotage our health and maximize those that will optimize it.

There are many foods that should be either limited or altogether eliminated as part of the prevention and treatment of cancer. These include the following:

The Three Whites – white sugar, white flour and refined salt: the common denominator for all of these is that they have been subjected to a process where vital components necessary for their utilization by the body have been removed. The result is not simply that they are lacking in nutritional value but that in order for them to be utilized at all, they actually draw upon vital bodily reserves.

Considering that as much as 20% of calories in a typical American diet are derived from refined sugar, it is no surprise that glucose intolerance ranging from both hypoglycemia to hyperglycemia is rampant. The increase of blood glucose results in the increase of insulin from the pancreas, which in turn reduces the sex-binding hormone globulin. The increase of hormone levels increases the risk factors for hormone dependent cancers including breast cancer, prostate cancer and other reproductive cancers. In essence, refined sugar increases the growth of cancer and tumors while low blood-glucose levels tend to slow tumor growth.

Substituting naturally derived sweeteners in unrefined sugar such as with the use of sucanat, fruit, maple syrup, agave plant syrup and barley or rice syrup offer better alternatives because they are broken down and utilized by the system more slowly and thus lessen the tendency of abnormal insulin spikes. Even these, however, should be limited when treating cancer patients.

White flour is made from grains whose fiber has been removed. The reasons, if any, are aesthetic since fiber depleted flour tends to have a lighter, whiter texture and appearance. Fiber has been found to offer significant benefits for digestion and elimination and the lack of it has been associated with the occurrence of a variety of cancers including colon and breast cancer.

Refined salt is almost pure sodium chloride. As a result, it is lacking in the naturally occurring trace minerals that are found in unrefined sea salt and rock salt. The various trace minerals are important catalysts for numerous vital functions throughout the body. It is their presence in unrefined salt that imparts the naturally darker colored appearance based on the particular concentration of minerals.

One disadvantage of sea salt is that it also contains chlorine, a moderately toxic and volatile element. To purify sea salt simply place it in an open pan and heat it to the point where you smell the volatilized chlorine. It is then purified and the sea salt can be cooled and stored for use.

Other foods that put a stress on the body's repair systems include coffee and alcohol. Coffee is a stimulant that uses reserves of energy from the adrenal glands to give one a temporary sense of energy. This, of course, impairs the innate recuperative energy necessary for coping with cancer. Furthermore, being a diuretic, the habitual use of coffee contributes to the potential for a number of deficiencies as well as hypertension and other cardiovascular diseases. Finally, coffee has been associated with increased risk of prostate cancer.

Other substances that rob our system of vital nutrients include alcohol and recreational drug abuse. All of these negatively affect our immune system and should be avoided as part of a cancer prevention and treatment program.

Macronutrients Guideline for Cancer Patients

Protein & Cancer

Protein is comprised of amino acids (amine meaning nitrogen containing) with both enzymes and many hormones being proteins. Protein is so essential to the body that the only bodily constituents that do not contain protein are urine and bile. While carbohydrates and lipids are burned as fuel, the main function of protein is as the foundation of the body. About 20 to 30 pounds of an adult's weight is protein with half again of that being found in the muscles. From this it is reasonable to assume that about 20 to 30% of one's diet should consist of protein from various sources. While protein can be converted to fuel if necessary, being a structural constituent, an insufficient amount over a period of time will causes conditions and diseases associated with chronic protein deficiency. Protein deficiency is associated either with individuals with a thin, emaciated appearance or a 'fat and flabby' edemic appearance.

Why is protein an important consideration in cancer? One of the main reasons is that at least in one important sense, cancer represents flawed protein metabolism and this almost always shows up as cachexia or protein malabsorption in advanced stages. In fact this is so much of a problem that anywhere from 40 to 80% of oncologists believe that the primary cause of death in cancer patients is cachexia or protein malabsorption associated with severe weight loss in the final stages. Because protein is the only nitrogen-containing nutrient, tumors cause a corresponding negative nitrogen imbalance favorable to the growth and proliferation of cancer by altering the metabolism of protein to make the amino acids available for the growth of tumors.

Animal sources of protein are considered first class proteins because they are more readily absorbed while vegetable sources are second-class proteins because they are slower to breakdown and convert into vital constituents. At first it may seem advantageous to partake of animal protein sources, however, the saturated fats found in dairy, pork, beef and other types of red meat, negatively effect the composition and liquidity of macrophage membranes thus impairing their ability to destroy tumor cells. Animals fed on high polyunsaturated fats show a decrease in the cytotoxic ability of macrophages. This is also seen with the use of unsaturated fats from certain fish, flaxseed oil and commercial omega 3 fatty acid supplements, making these variously desirable additions to the anticancer diet.

Some Traditional Chinese practitioners regard chicken, and by implication other poultry, as being contraindicated for cancer patients. Dr. Miriam Lee, one of the most reknowned acupuncturists of Northern California, described a chicken as a "dirty" animal and while not harmful for people with normal health, for patients fighting cancer she said it was contraindicated. Interestingly, there may be some corroboration with the findings of Virginia Livingston-Wheeler of the Livingston Foundation Medical Center in San Diego, who identified a bacterium she named Progenitor cryptocides, which she classified as a member of the mycobacterium family, order actinomycetales. According to her, this ubiquitous microorganism in humans and animals (especially chickens) becomes pathogenic only when the immune response is inadequate. Ignorant of any Chinese opinions on the contraindications of the use of chicken for cancer patients, Virginia Wheeler theorized that P. cryptocides was at least one of the causes of cancer, an opinion that I personally cannot corroborate. She consequently developed a treatment designed to stimulate the patient's immune system to produce antibodies against P. cryptocides.[1,2] It was a multifaceted approach that incorporated various nutritional supplements, vaccines, antibiotics, anti-parasite medicine, megavitamins, and other nutritional supplements, digestive enzymes, and enemas; and a vegetarian whole-foods diet that allows dairy products only after the patient has recovered.

For these reasons, a primarily vegetarian diet is emphasized for most cancers. Vegetable sources of protein including beans and legumes, especially soy, should be emphasized because they have powerful nutritional value but also supply cancer-fighting isoflavones. Fish, especially the fattier fish such as salmon, are another valuable supplement because of their Essential Fatty acid content. Whey protein is also useful because it contains small mounts of antioxidants, glutathione and L-cysteine. Whey also contains lactoferrin and lactalbumin, which increase the conversion rate of L-cysteine to glutathione.[3]

The Question of Dairy

In India, when one is weak and deficient, they are given boiled warm milk mixed with ginger, honey and other spices. Wholesome milk is similarly given in Middle and Northern European, Russia and Balkan countries as well. Contrast this with the fact that at the same time milk and other dairy products are regarded as primary allergens in Western industrial countries. Perhaps the difference is in the quality of the milk resulting from the manner in which cows are handled. As any nursing mother knows how improper diet and stress can adversely affect her milk causing sickness and colic in nursing children, so also the adverse treatment of cows cause toxins and stress hormones to be present in their milk and consequently adversely affect its quality. Perhaps it is more important that we emphasize the use of the milk

---

[3] *Dr. Gaynor's Cancer Prevention Program*, by Mitchell L. Gaynor M.D. and Jerry Hickey pub. By Kensington, 1999, p. 47.

from free grazing, gently handled 'contented cows.'

The question of whether milk should be pasteurized or not begs the real issue of milk quality. In fact, milk is best served scalded and warm. It has a long protein chain that when cold is difficult to assimilate properly. Therefore, many milk allergies are not seen when the milk is first scalded and then taken warm as opposed to the use of cold milk. As with pasteurization, scalding milk over the stove will also destroy most harmful pathogens. The difference is that pasteurization is usually flash heated at the lowest possible temperature, while bringing milk to a boil over the stove is a more prolonged cooking process resulting in a breakdown of the long chain fatty acids that tend to cause allergic reactions. In many countries this process is similarly achieved through the use of fermented dairy in the form of yogurt which greatly assists in its assimilation and utilization.

Next to human milk, by far the best quality milk for most people is raw goat's milk. The fat content of goat's milk, unlike that of the cow, is closest to human breast milk. As such it is a good alternative to cow's milk for infants who are unable to be breast-fed. Japanese macrobiotics does not recommend milk in any form other than human breast milk for infants. Besides a basic cultural difference, one reason may be that Japan is a densely populated country with hardly the type of space required for cattle grazing.

Carbohydrates and Cancer

Carbohydrates are a way that plants store energy. When animals eat plants, they must convert their carbohydrates to glucose through the hormone insulin. Excess glucose is stored in the liver as glycogen.

There are two broad forms of carbohydrates, simple and complex. Simple carbohydrates are the monosacharides in the form of sugar, which give certain foods their characteristic sweet flavor. These include glucose, fructose and galactose. When two monosacharides join together, a disaccharide is formed. Sucrose from white sugar is the most well known, however there is also lactose from milk which enhances calcium uptake and maltose from germinating grains. The problem with simple carbohydrates are that they have the potential of being too rapidly absorbed putting a severe burden on the overtaxed adrenals and pancreas. Ultimately this compromises the integrity of the immune system but it also increases the replication of cancer cells. If one must use sweeteners, the most preferable are those that breakdown more slowly which include sugar from fruit, called fructose, honey, maple syrup and barley or rice malt syrup.

Polysaccharides are complex carbohydrates found in food in the form of starch, dextrin, cellulose and glycogen. Each type of plant produces its own type of starch with most of them being broken down and converted to sugar more slowly before entering the bloodstream. The overall effect of this is that it tends to be less of an overload on the body's innate resources. In fact many polysaccharides actually have tonic properties that are useful for strengthening the immune system. These are found in many of the tonic herbs such as ginseng, codonopsis and astragalus, for instance.

Dry roasting grains or toasting bread converts complex carbohydrates into dextrin's, which are partially broken down starches. Glycogen is a form of glucose that is stored in the liver and muscles. In most people, there is usually enough to fuel the body for about half a day. Individuals with hypoglycemia lack sufficient glycogen stores and must therefore eat small meals more frequently to maintain blood sugar ratios.

When eaten, muscle meat has very little glycogen because when the animal is slaughtered the glycogen that normally present is converted to the more toxic lactic acid. This is one reason for the tradition of bleeding an animal and/or soaking meat in cool water to leach out as much of the blood as possible.

From the above we may better understand why cancer patients should primarily limit themselves to a high complex carbohydrate diet based on the use of whole grains (if they can be digested or partially refined grains for those with weak digestion) and a variety of vegetables. If one experiences a sweet craving it should be indulged in only after eating a diet with the proper balance of protein and complex carbohydrates.

The Oxygen Connection

Cancer does not exist in the presence of life-giving oxygen. In 1966, Professor Otto Warburg, a man who received two Nobel prizes in 1931 and 1944 for his work on cellular energetics, stated "... the prime cause of cancer is the replacement of the respiration of oxygen in normal body cells by a fermentation of sugar." This further provides many important clues for the treatment of cancer that supports the idea of limiting or altogether eliminating the use of sugar that literally serves to feed and speed the replication of cancer cells and the excessive use of cooked red meat and saturated fats that slow and inhibit aerobic activity in the intestines.

Healthy metabolism requires oxygen in the mitochondria of the cells to generate heat necessary for the conversion of food to energy. A diet high in saturated fat gradually makes the mitochondria less permeable and thus reduces its aerobic, oxygenating, metabolic capacity. Cancer and tumors live in an anaerobic (oxygen-less) environment. Instead of utilizing nutrients from external sources, they derive their life energy as a result of the breakdown of the stored protein and muscle. This in turn is converted into a type of sugar through a process of dark (anaerobic) fermentation.

Fiber

Cellulose is the most abundant form of carbohydrate and is found in all whole fruits, grains and vegetables. Since the human body lacks the enzyme to breakdown cellulose, it enters the colon as fiber without being digested. There it serves an important function by helping to absorb and retain water in the colon for proper elimination.

Fiber can be divided into two main categories: soluble and insoluble. Soluble fiber found in pectin, gums and mucilage's such as psyllium, algae, flax seed, etc. is easily fermented by friendly intestinal bacteria. This in turn has a number of beneficial effects, creating short-chain fatty acids that go to the liver and help to reduce cholesterol and assist in the breakdown of glucose and fats.

Insoluble fiber is not broken down but has a local 'broom-like' effect on the intestinal walls as they stimulate peristalsis and increase the frequency of bowel movements. The use of insoluble fiber is associated with a decreased risk of intestinal cancer, decreased constipation and a reduction of blood pressure.

Lipids, Fats & Oils for Cancer

Ever speculate why we crave fats? Fats are the most concentrated form of energy, providing nine calories for every gram burned. This is more than double that of carbohydrates. Furthermore, an adequate amount of fat is necessary for insulation and warmth. Fat also saves the B vitamin, thiamin, that is required for metabolizing carbohydrates. When an adequate amount of fat is available, the body will not have to resort to burning protein for fuel. Fats also help in the transportation of fat-soluble vitamins A, D, E, and K. They help to maintain more balanced blood sugar levels by slowing the rate at which food, especially carbohydrates, leave the stomach. Thus they decrease appetite and give one a feeling of satiety. Fats also make foods more palatable and delicious. Finally, last but not least they are the building blocks of bodily hormones.

An excess of fat, especially saturated fat, consists of a fatty acid that is replete with hydrogen atoms. This makes for a denser type of fat that increases cholesterol production and blood cholesterol levels. Butter is a natural fat high in saturated fatty acids. Lightly heating butter for a period of time and skimming off the white saturated fats is a way of eliminating, or at least lessening, the amount of fatty acids in butter. This is called clarified butter or in India, 'ghee.' It is one of the secrets of delicious French cooking who notably seem to have a lower incidence of cardiovascular disease despite their seeming high fat diet.

Linoleic and linolenic acid are essential fatty acids important for their ability to counteract cancer. Linoleic fatty acid inhibits the ability of macrophages and natural killer cells (NK) to kill cancer cells. Linolenic fatty acid is found in monounsaturated fatty acids such as olive oil, canola oil, fish oils and flaxseeds for instance.

Because fats and sterols are components of hormones, people with hormone sensitive cancers should limit their fat intake, especially from meat and dairy. Instead they should supplement their diet with unsaturated fats from fish, flax, evening primrose or borage seed oils.

Daily Diet for Cancer Patients

Following is an approximate guideline for achieving a balanced healthy diet:

- 40 to 50 percent complex carbohydrates in the form of whole grains, especially brown rice and barley.
- 20 percent protein primarily from beans and other legumes and fish.
- 30 percent vegetables, especially green vegetables including cruciferous vegetables, garlic and onions but other vegetables as well (not so much potatoes, however, since we are using the whole grains as a more wholesome, fiber-rich complex carbohydrate. This would include two 8-ounce glasses of non-acid vegetable juice (carrot, celery, beets, greens – one can also add a clove of garlic and a piece of fresh or dried turmeric and ginger) and at least five shiitake mushrooms as part of the diet.
- 5 to 10 percent would include seasonal fruit, omega-3 oils from fish, flaxseed, fish oil, sesame oil, ghee or olive oil.
- Eight to ten 8-ounce glasses of filtered water, green tea or other anticancer teas such as burdock root tea, dandelion root tea and/or red clover tea.

Macrobiotic Diet

The above diet plan is a modified version of the Japanese macrobiotic diet as promoted by George Ohsawa in the mid 20th century and more recently, Michio Kushi and Herman Aihara. It is a primarily vegetarian, whole grain based diet based on the Asian principles of balance embodied by the theory of Yin and Yang.

The macrobiotic diet has been associated with documented cases of complete remission of various types of cancers. If properly executed, it is possible to derive balanced nutrition following a macrobiotic diet based on the use of whole grains, beans and vegetables. However, as with all dietary systems, there is an implied risk in over-rigidity to a "one diet for all" approach. This can be seen in the results of many macrobiotic adherents who, becoming too rigid in their dietary patterns, have exhibited devastating long-term-effect cachexic (protein deficiencies) tendencies. Admittedly this may be from a fundamental misunderstanding of the most fundamental concept that essentially speaks of achieving balance without any necessity to slavishly use only the prescribed foods but essentially with whatever is at hand.

In fact, the traditional principles of yin-yang balance extends beyond the realm of food to include balance between all the elements of life, which would include selected foods with seasonal and climatic differences, physical activity, and heredity. Therefore any food or experience can and should be included in a macrobiotic diet whose yin-yang principle is primarily directed to forming a theoretical basis for classifying foods, herbs, physical activities, season and all other factors on a single continuum.

This being said, some of the characteristic foods frequently encountered as part of the macrobiotic diet are the use of whole, organic, foods grains, brown rice, tofu, tempeh, seaweeds and the enzyme-rich broth known as miso soup. Concurrently one should avoid the use of refined and highly processed foods as we previously mentioned. Certainly this is not in opposition to the basic principles of sound nutrition.

Paradoxically the promotion of brown rice as the 'founding principle of macrobiotics' meets with disagreement among most traditional Chinese doctors. They believe that white rice is easier to digest and that this may be very important for someone who is sick. Further, by adding even a little animal protein to rice such as fish, chicken or eggs, whatever is lacking from white rice is supplemented by the chicken and small amounts of peas and carrots that is traditionally included.

Another principle of the macrobiotic diet, which is in agreement with all Asian traditions, including the Chinese, is that foods are better assimilated when they are properly cooked and prepared. This is, however, in distinction to those who promote a more aggressive detoxification diet based on the use of raw vegetable, fruit and juices. Besides the Chinese and macrobiotic theory that raw or uncooked foods are too cooling or yin, the basic reason for cooking food is to begin the process of breaking down food into its respective nutrients outside of the body for better assimilation. Some argue that important nutrients such as vital digestive enzymes are lost in the process of cooking foods. However, traditional cultures believe that cooking foods enhances more complete absorption and utilization of food nutrients. Probably more vitamins and nutrients are preserved with light cooking along with the addition of small amounts of chopped raw cucumber or onion.

However, for serious diseases where malabsorption is a serious issue, traditional Asian medical systems, including Japanese, Chinese and East Indian as well as other traditional food cultures throughout the world, advocate long cooking of food. A dish used as a traditional breakfast food in China and for convalescence is made by combining one part by volume of glutinous white rice with seven to ten parts water. This is then slow cooked over 6 to 8 hours to make an easily digested porridge called "jook" or "congee" in China. It is a valuable traditional porridge to which can be added small amounts of legumes, meat, vegetables, mushrooms and various medicinal herbs. It is the most valuable way to give herbal tonics to cancer patients. This is discussed further in the section on Grains.

Foods to Include in the Daily Diet

Foods high in beta-carotene

These include yellow-orange vegetables such as carrots, yams, squash, pumpkin, paprika, cayenne pepper and turnips. Carotenoids other than beta-carotene include canthaxanthin, phytoene, lutein, xanathophylls and lycopenes, many of which, according to herbalist Donny Yance AHG, may offer greater anticarcinogenic effects than beta-carotene. He further states that carotenoids have antioxidant properties, protecting phagocytes, lipids and the cells against oxidation, strengthening the immune system, increasing the production of certain interleukins, and with their special effect on the skin, protect against cancer causing sun damage.

Cruciferous vegetables

Vegetables in the cabbage family (cruciferae) contain high amounts of anticancer constituents called indoles and isothiocyanates. They are also high in vitamins A, C, E, beta-carotene, anti-carcinogenic minerals and fiber. Because when eaten raw, these vegetables contain a high amount of thyroid-lowering agents, they should always be cooked. Some vegetables in this category include cabbage, collards, kale, broccoli, Brussels sprouts, cauliflower, mustard greens, turnips and radishes.

Dark leafy green vegetables

These are high in chlorophyll and other anti-carcinogenic compounds and should be eaten daily, both raw and cooked. Again, this is a place to include uncultivated herbs such as dandelion, chicory, chickweed, malva, watercress, nettles and mustard greens. In addition romaine lettuce, arugula and spinach are valuable.

One of the most powerful wild greens, purslane is a prized delicacy in many other countries including Central America and France. Purslane is high in omega-3 fatty acids and antioxidants as well as vitamins E, C, K, beta-carotene, glutathione and psoralens. Psoralens have powerful antioxidant properties, which besides fighting cancer are particularly beneficial for normalizing skin pigmentation.

The greens with a bitter flavor such as dandelion and chicory more powerfully stimulate detoxification, especially from the liver. They are also potassium rich foods. They can be served steamed or lightly sautéed with a little olive or sesame oil.

Garlic and onion family vegetables

In preparing these greens we can add chopped garlic, which is high in anti-carcinogenic sulfur compounds including allicin. Other foods that contain similar compounds to a lesser extent include onions, leeks, chives and shallots.

Mushrooms

Traditional people around the world have always valued the health benefits of edible mushrooms. Mushrooms are high in minerals, especially potassium, which is important to regulate intracellular fluid and the corresponding absorption of nutrients into the cell. All mushrooms have potent health giving, anti-carcinogenic properties but the one that is the most practical to use regularly is the shiitake mushroom (*Lentinus edodes*). These can be economically purchased dry by the pound in Chinese grocery stores and pharmacies as "Black Mushrooms." They can then be soaked and reconstituted in water before using. Shiitake mushrooms are high in B1, B2, B12, niacin and pantothenic acid. B vitamins are necessary for cell energy and hormone production.

They also contain high amounts of protein, enzymes and 8 essential amino acids and have been found to be useful for cancer, heart disease, AIDS, flu, tumors, viruses, high blood pressure, obesity and aging. Lentinant, a polysaccharide found in the root and cell wall of shiitake, has a triple helix structure, a shape considered an important component for the healing properties of shiitake. Lentinant stimulates the production of T-lymphocytes and macrophages that ingest foreign invaders. It also helps the production of interleukin[4] 1 and 2, known to inhibit the growth of cancer and viruses.

In Japan, lentinan, the polysaccharide found in shiitake is an approved drug used together with chemotherapy to treat cancer patients. Research has substantiated that it increases the lifespan of cancer patients and may also prevent the recurrence of cancer after surgery.

Best of all the oral ingestion by animals and humans has found shiitake to possess strong antitumor activity, stimulating the body's immune system

---

[4] Interleukin-1 is a substance from monocytes and macrophages which are important in initiation of the immune response for various acute inflammations and infections. Interleukin-2 is a lymphokine that stimulates the growth of T-lymphocytes. When this combines with the immune system's T-lymphocytes, they produce together lymphokine-activated killer (LAK) cells that lyse or dissolve cancer cells.

to fight abnormal cells. It also helps the body produce more interferon[5] to defend itself from viruses and other harmful matter. Shiitake is also very beneficial for the cardiovascular system, in the treatment of HIV and the treatment of viral/bacterial infections.

Fruits

Apples, grapes (with the seeds), apricots, peaches and berries all have powerful anti-cancer properties. The seeds of apples, peaches, loquat and apricots have cyanogenic glycosides, which is a potent source of the anti-cancer vitamin B17, and better known as laetrile. In large dosage they should be considered toxic, however apricot or peach seeds taken at the doses of 5 to 10 seeds two or three times a day, offers potent anticancer properties. Generally loquat leaves are steeped in boiling water to make an anti-cancer tea in both Japan and Cyprus. The seeds can also be eaten but in a smaller amount as they are high in cyanogenic compounds. Berries such as raspberry, blueberries and strawberries have various antioxidant and cancer fighting compounds and are a welcome additional to the daily diet. Off-season they can be purchased frozen which has the advantage of making their constituents more bioavailable as a result of their being frozen. Dark grapes contain the anticancer compound resveratrol, which makes them useful as part of the anticancer diet. The seeds are a potent source of one of the most powerful antioxidants, pycnogenol.

The peel of citrus fruits contains D-limonene, which has powerful anticancer properties. Citrus peel has been prescribed as a monotherapy for individuals with pancreatic and large intestine cancer during a research trial in England and has shown statistically significant benefit. Always use organic unsprayed citrus fruits, especially if you are going to use the peel. The anticancer properties of orange, tangerine or lemon rind can easily be added as a zesty condiment to soups, salads and sauces. They are also very beneficial for digestion and assimilation. A variety of citrus peels are used in teas and are an excellent alternative alone or with ginger to counteract the adverse gastro-intestinal reactions to chemotherapy.

Grains

The most balanced grain is brown rice[6] and should constitute a large part of the diet. Other grains are also very beneficial and include millet, quinoa,

---

[5] Interferons are a protein that is formed when cells are damaged by viral or other foreign invaders. Interferons are part of the immune system and have antitumor activity.

[6] The pH of blood is 7.4, which is slightly alkaline. The body must maintain this balance and any slight variation higher or lower can result in severe sickness and death. Brown rice has a similar pH to blood at around 7.4 to 7.5, which is why it is considered the most balanced food.

whole wheat, corn, oats and barley, all containing various anti-carcinogenic compounds and properties.

Barley contains coixenlide, amino acid, saccharides and alkaloids. In Traditional Chinese Medicine, barley is used to drain dampness, meaning it has mild diuretic properties. Dampness associated with joint swelling is one of the causes involved in arthritic and rheumatic conditions as well as cancer. Coix, a type of barley, is used for a variety of cancers but especially cancer of the breast, larynx, uterus and stomach.

Brown rice also has anti-cancer and diuretic properties. If digestion is weak, TCM advocates the use of long cooked white rice for easier digestion and assimilation.

Congee - Chinese Rice Porridge

One of the most assimilable foods is congee, or rice porridge. Traditionally, because it is so easily digested and assimilated, Chinese people use it as a breakfast food. Because of this, congee is made with white rice, which is easier to digest and particularly beneficial for convalescence and for the treatment of chronic diseases such as cancer. The basic recipe is to slowly cook one part by volume of white rice in 7 to 10 parts of water, for six to eight hours (a slow cooker can be used).

For protein supplementation, one can add a good quality soy or whey powder.

There are infinite variations on this basic congee recipe, which should be selected according to individual requirements and needs. One can substitute or mix different grains such as barley for arthritis and cancer. It is also an ideal medium to combine various vegetables or tonic herbs according to one's condition as follows:

- Immune tonic – astragalus root – 9g
- Low energy – codonopsis or Chinese ginseng combined with Poria cocos mushrooms (or shiitake) – approximately 9g of each
- Liver and blood deficiency – lycii berries (high in beta carotene) and Polygonum multiflorum – 9g of each
- Dryness, Yin or wasting conditions – ophiopogon root and Chinese asparagus root – approximately 9g of each
- For general weakness, immune deficiency, emaciation, spontaneous perspiration and loss of appetite – Astragalus root 60g, Chinese ginseng 12g, 90g of white rice, 4 ounces of shredded lean beef, with whole brown sugar (Sucanat) added to taste after cooking.

Congee offers a wonderful opportunity to add grated orange or tangerine peel both for flavor and their anti-carcinogenic properties as desired. Orange or tangerine peel in tea or with congee is good to help overcome the nausea of chemotherapy.

It is not possible to offer all the variations for preparing congee. As one can see, it is the perfect medium for a variety of health giving, easily digested and assimilated food and herb combinations.

Beans and various legumes

Isoflavones are flavonoid compounds that are commonly found in various legumes including soybeans. One of the most important currently is Genistein because of its close molecular resemblance to human estrogen. For this reason it is very important to include beans, especially soybeans, as part of an anti-cancer diet. Fermented soybean products such as miso, tempeh and shoyu tamari go through complex chemical processes that are of particular benefit in the prevention and treatment of cancer.

Protein foods

Cancer is fundamentally involved with mal-utilization of protein. Oncologists generally agree that the actual cause of death in cancer patients is cachexia, a condition of severe weight loss and wasting associated with protein malabsorption. In fact, cancer cells are able to grow by making the amino acids of protein available for their growth at the expense of the body as a whole. Meat, especially red meat, being the most readily assimilable protein, becomes a banquet for cancer cells. Emphasizing the use of plant sources of vegetable protein such as legumes and beans that contain cancer-fighting compounds should be a prominent part of an anti-cancer diet.

Legumes and beans supply high quality protein necessary to rebuild the tissues and maintain a healthy immune system. They are also an important source of insoluble fiber that slows the release of glucose into the bloodstream, keeping blood sugar levels in balance. Sugar itself, on the other hand, speeds up metabolism and is known to promote faster tumor growth. Fiber is also fermented in the colon mostly by beneficial bacteria that produce short-chain fatty acids (SCFA's) that help prevent colon cancer. Legumes also serve as protease inhibitors, which are a protein-splitting enzyme, found to be important to block cancer growth. Finally, legumes are an important source of valuable phytochemicals such as saponins, which tonify the immune system and inhibit the DNA synthesis of cancer cells.

Another important source of protein is from fatty fish such as salmon which, with the skin removed, is a less dense protein than red meat and can also be occasionally used.

Juices

Cancer patients should have one or two 8-ounce glasses of fresh organic vegetable juice each day. A good combination is carrots, beets, celery, garlic and if available fresh burdock root. For a flavor variation one can add an apple as desired.

Green drink

See Chapter Nine on supplements. I also recommend the use of chlorella and/or Green Magma as a twice-daily green drink. Chlorella is a highly nutritive one-celled blue-green algae that is a powerful immune system stimulant that has also demonstrated anti-tumor effects. Research has shown that Chlorella is able to repair the DNA system and increase serum albumin levels.

Beverages

Green tea contains catechin polyphenols that have been shown to have potent anticarcinogenic properties. Other beverages that can be used are red clover tea, the anti-cancer tea described below and roasted root and grain beverages, many of which contain a roasted extract of dandelion root, which is a potent liver detoxifier with anticancer properties.

Detoxification

As with the use of herbs, the dietary treatment of cancer includes strategies for both detoxification and tonification. Usually one begins with detoxification, which involves enhancing the body's ability to neutralize and discharge toxins from all the internal organs, especially the liver and blood. Since in most cases detoxification diets are usually vegetable-based the overall effect, at least for non-vegetarians, is to effect a biochemical change from more acidic to alkaline. Most natural systems for the treatment of cancer emphasize the use of a more vegetable-based diet that avoids refined foods and animal products as much as possible. For many, this has either slowed the progression of a cancer or even caused complete cancer remission.

The danger of such diets is to aggravate progressive nutritional imbalances and protein deficiencies caused by the cancer. Protein derived from beans, soy, whey and fish are easily assimilated non-red meat sources of protein that have known anticancer fighting properties. Cancer patients are encouraged to utilize these as much as possible. To this list, one might add wheat gluten (known as "seitan" in Japan) as alternatives to red meat protein.

Such a diet change may seem radical for most and there is a danger of further creating an emotionally alienated state that may be counterproductive to recovery. When this is likely, one should be careful and allow weekly or less often off-diet indulgences. Another strategy is to discover acceptable compromises such as substituting honey for sugar, tofu or seitan for cheese, etc. or by allowing an occasional weekly indulgence in a favorite food.

The macrobiotic brown rice and beans diet or the mung beans and rice Kicharee diet of Ayurvedic medicine represents a biochemically 'balanced' diet and offers the best opportunity for resolving most diseases dietarily. However, for more stubborn cases such as cancer, alternating this with periods of three or four days on vegetable or fruit juices causes the cells and tissues of the body to alternately expand with the juice fasts and contract with the beans and rice diet resulting in a deeper level of detoxification.

Extracting and Contracting Diets for Detoxification

The Four Day Fresh Vegetable Juice Fast

Organically grown carrots are one of the highest sources of easily assimilable Vitamin A. They also have ample amounts of Vitamins B, C, D, E, G and K. In addition they are a rich source of various minerals, including calcium. Raw carrot juice is one of the most commonly used supplements for the treatment of cancer.

Beets are one of the best builders of healthy red blood cells. Too much at first can cause increased rapid detoxification with attendant dizziness and nausea so that one should use less beet juice in proportion to carrots and other vegetables.

Asparagus is a vegetable that has a long history of use against cancer, which has been confirmed by recent research from Rutgers University that reported that the soapy substances called saponins showed in vitro antitumor activity.[7] The characteristic odor of urine after eating asparagus is due to exotic sulfur compounds excreted in the urine. Asparagus juice can be obtained seasonally or frozen. It is a vegetable that has a cleansing effect through the lymphatic system and the kidneys. It contains the cancer fighting alkaloid asparagine as well as potassium and other anti-cancer vitamins and minerals that act as "Cell Growth Normalizers" on cancer cell division. Asparagus therapy has been used to treat various forms of cancer with several reversals of the disease reported in a number of cases. Asparagus should be an important part of the anticancer diet. One way is to always have cooked asparagus that has been pureed in a blender and then stored in the refrigerator for ongoing use. About 4 tablespoons of this should be taken three times daily alone or mixed in hot or cold water for cancer treatment.

Asparagus is beneficial for regulating the kidneys, glandular problems, diabetes, rheumatic problems and anemia. It dissolves oxalic crystals and

---

[7] Shao et al. 1996

clears the deposit of uric acid caused by the excess ingestion of animal protein. Asparagus is very beneficial to have in the vegetable juice cocktail.

Celery is high in organic sodium, which is useful for maintaining calcium in solution. It is beneficial in removing any toxic byproducts of concentrated sugars and starches in the body. Celery juice helps in the treatment of arthritic and rheumatic conditions as well as dissolving tumors by maintaining the fluidity of the blood and lymphatic system.

Other beneficial vegetables and greens to include in the vegetable juice cocktail include cabbage, brussels sprouts, broccoli, endive, dandelion and burdock root.

A vegetable or carrot juice fast consists of taking one 8-ounce glass of organic fresh pressed juice with one clove of garlic every two hours. This is the sole diet for three days. In addition, the patient is advised to take triphala powder three times daily with one 00 sized capsule consisting of 3/4 parts cascara sagrada bark and a 1/4 part ginger powder. These assist the detoxification process by helping to enhance liver and bowel elimination. Cayenne pepper acts as a natural stimulant that enhances overall metabolism. Two 00 sized capsules of cayenne pepper are taken with a tablespoon of olive oil to further flush bile from the liver and assist the detoxification process. On the fourth day, the fast is carefully broken with the addition of warm vegetable broth, salads with a lemon and olive oil dressing, thin rice or barley porridge.

The Grape Fast

As previously stated fruits, including dark grapes, have potent anticancer properties. Willa Brandt first advocated the Grape Cure as a treatment for cancer around 1927. It consisted first of a water fast for two or three days. This was usually accompanied with a daily enema to promote the cleansing process. After the fast, beginning around 8 AM, up to a half a pound of dark grapes are taken every two hours until 8PM. This may be continued for up to one or two weeks.

Widely promoted by Benedict Lust, who is considered the father of naturopathy and Bernard Macfadden, an early 20th century physical culturist who published several books, the grape cure became widely known as an effective treatment not only for cancer but all chronic degenerative diseases. While there are many positive anecdotal reports, there has never been any serious scientific study to corroborate its effectiveness against cancer.

Recently, a number of anticancer constituents have been discovered in grapes that would substantiate their benefit for the treatment of cancer. One is the presence of powerful antioxidants known as pycnogenols abundantly found in the seeds of grapes and pine tree bark. The other anticancer constituent found in grapes is resveratrol, which helps to prevent heart attacks but also has been found to inhibit cellular processes associated with the growth and proliferation of tumors.

Depending on seasonal availability, four days on the grape diet may occasionally be substituted or alternated with the recommended four-day vegetable juice program described previously.

Kicharee

After completing the vegetable juice fast, one can have either just mung bean and rice Kicharee or a combination with Miriam Lee's Bean and Herb Stew.

In preparing any of the following dishes, never use aluminum pots for preparing either food or herbs. A glass container or good quality stainless steel is the best choice. Use of the microwave is also not recommended for cancer patients. Any of these foods can be stored in the refrigerator for up to three days or frozen for future use. They must always be thawed and taken warm.

Kicharee consists of equal parts mung beans and brown or white basmati rice with the addition of turmeric, coriander, cumin and a dash of salt. First cook a cup each of the mung beans and rice, then sauté approximately one teaspoon each of the freshly powdered spices in a tablespoon of ghee (clarified butter) until they are lightly browned. Then simply mix in the rice and mung beans with the sautéed spices and the kicharee is ready to eat. When making a large amount it can be frozen and stored in daily portions.

Kicharee is considered the most healing food of Indian Ayurvedic medicine and suitable for treating all diseases. It provides complete nutrition, especially when a few tablespoons of yogurt are added. Mung beans are a source of protein that combines detoxifying, acid-neutralizing properties. Rice is considered the most balanced food and helps remove excess water and balance blood chemistry. Variations include substituting or adding barley for rice and the addition of a cooked onion or other vegetables to make a stew.

The recipe on the following page was developed in China by a mother to help heal her daughter of breast cancer. It was passed on to me by one of my esteemed Chinese teachers as a treatment for cancer. While it is best taken with all the herbs, if any of the ingredients are unavailable it can be made with whatever is at hand.

Dr. Miriam Lee's Bean Soup Treatment for Cancer

Contents and Measurements:

Brown rice	10 tbs.	Black beans	1 tbs.
Pinto Beans	1 tbs.	Corn or cornmeal	1 tbs.
Azuki Beans	1 tbs.	Barley	1 tbs.
Pine Nuts	1 tbs.	Millet	1 tbs.
Mung Beans	1 tbs.	Buckwheat	1 tbs.
Split peas	1 tbs.	Oats	1 tbs.
Soya beans	1 tbs.	Peanuts (nip removed)	1 tbs.
Qian-shi (Euryale seed also called Foxnut)	12g	Mai Men Dong (Ophiopogon root)	12g
Bai Guo (Ginkgo seed) with the skin removed (this is the most difficult to obtain and can be omitted)	12g	Bai He (Tiger lily bulb)	12g
Lian Zi (Lotus seed)	12g	Shan yao (Dioscorea batatas)	12g
Fu Ling (poria cocos)	12g		

Preparation: Simmer the entire contents in 18 cups of water. As soon as it comes to a boil, reduce heat and simmer for another 2 hours. (Do not use too high of a flame as this will destroy the nutrients.) Consume over a period of 3 days. Keep unused portion in the freezer. Continue this food therapy for many months. All these herbs are available from a Chinese pharmacy (see Sources in the appendix).

For both the preparation of kicharee and the Bean soup combination, a multitude of variations are possible with the addition of various organic vegetables. For instance, one can incorporate onions and garlic sautéed in a little olive or sesame oil as well as adding other vegetables such as chopped carrots, soaked wakame seaweed, burdock root, cabbage, broccoli, cauliflower, endive, dandelion greens, shiitake or Italian Porcini mushrooms. One will have to experiment with these for flavor. In general only two vegetables should be added for each preparation and flavor is greatly enhanced when these are previously sautéed in a little olive or sesame oil with the basic kicharee or bean soup being stirred in afterwards. Used in this way, these are complete foods, ideal for the treatment of cancer and other serious diseases. In addition, one can alternate these with simple brown rice, cooked vegetables and any of the other recipes presented below. If a little dessert is desired a baked apple, pear or organic apple sauce can be used.

Wheat or Barley Grass

In all anticancer diets, one should incorporate chlorophyll-rich foods derived from the juice of wheat grass, barley grass or a special green algae known in the trade as Chlorella. Chlorophyll is one of the most powerful and basic of all healing substances. It is abundant in all green leafy vegetables and edible herbs but especially grasses such as wheat and barley grass. Often called liquid sunlight, chlorophyll is the direct byproduct of photosynthesis in plants. Chlorophyll from edible greens and grasses is a powerful antioxidant, promoting the purification, oxygenation and generation of blood and forming the basis for tissue repair. Chlorophyll, which is highly concentrated in wheat grass, Green barley grass and the one-cell blue-green algae known as chlorella, has been found to have greater anticancer properties than any other anticancer supplement. Of course, these 'green foods' are very rich in a wide variety of vitamins, minerals and other health-giving constituents as well.

There is an abundance of life giving enzymes from fresh squeezed wheat or barley grass that aid in digestion and assimilation but also assist in the breakdown of tumors.

In fact, all green vegetables and chlorophyll-rich supplements are highly recommended for cancer patients. Whenever possible, potherbs in the form of common edible weeds such as malva, purslane, watercress, amaranth and dandelion greens can be steamed and served up with a little olive oil and lemon juice as a garnish.

Jujube Dates, Shiitake Mushroom and Mung Bean Sprout Soup:

Boil 10 jujube dates with 50g of fresh shiitake mushrooms (or 25g dried shiitakes) and 10g of mung bean sprouts until cooked. Season with high quality rock salt to taste. Consume the entire amount throughout the course of a day. This formula is good for cancers of various kinds.

Pearl Barley, Soybean, Shiitake, Broccoli and Carrot Soup:

Presoak pearl barley and soybeans overnight. Add several shiitake mushrooms, chopped broccoli and carrots, rock salt and sufficient water. Cook until done.

Brown Rice and Green Vegetable Soup:

Daikon radish	250g	Carrots	500g
Burdock seed (crushed)	250g	Shiitake mushrooms	3 pieces
Brown Rice	10 tbsp.	Barley	5 tbsp.
Soya beans (presoaked)	5 tbsp.	Azuki beans (presoaked)	5 tbsp.
Mung beans (presoaked)	5 tbsp.	Dried kombu seaweed	one 4-inch piece

Finely chop the carrots, radishes and mushrooms with a selection of anticancer vegetables such as cabbage, broccoli, chard, spinach, violet leaves, amaranth, purslane, nettles and lamb's quarters as available.

The beans should be presoaked for 8 to 12 hours with the seaweed. Brown rice should be dry fried in a skillet until slightly brown. Various herbs can be added such as Lotus seed, Ophiopogon, organic mushrooms and astragalus root.

Cook in enough water to make a thick soup consistency.

Green Vegetable Soup:

Green turnip and leaves	250g	Carrot	250g
Burdock seed (crushed)	250g	Shiitake mushroom	3 pieces

Finely chop all the vegetables. Add three times as much water as the quantity of vegetables in a pot. Bring to a boil and continue to simmer down for another hour. Drink freely throughout the day as food-medicine.

Roasted Brown Rice and Green Tea:

Stir-fry one cup of short grain brown rice in a pan until lightly browned. Boil eight cups of water. Add the brown rice and a tablespoon of green tea. Continue simmering over a low flame in a covered pot for 5 or ten minutes and then let it stand standing another five minutes. Strain and drink freely throughout the day. The strained roasted rice and green tea can be prepared once more by adding water for a second cooling. Once again, do not use an aluminum pot for preparation. Also, to optimize detoxification, one should not take any protein during, immediately before or after drinking this tea.

Miso Soup:

Miso is made of salt-fermented soybeans either alone or with other substances such as barley. It makes a wonderful stock for many types of soups and has powerful rejuvenative healing properties. Because of the fermented soy, the special soy isoflavones described previously are especially made available in the most delicious form. Miso can be combined with just about any other foods including soy, tofu, vegetables, cabbage, seaweeds such as wakame or kombu, squash, carrots, onions and mushrooms. Mugi miso made with barley and soybeans is the best to use regularly for cancer followed by hatcho miso made with soybeans. Add approximately one teaspoon of miso paste to a cup of water or precooked soup. Have one cup of miso soup daily.

Miso sauce: Combining miso paste, tahini, sesame butter and water can make a delicious sauce. The sauce and can be freely applied to simple foods such as whole grains and vegetables.

For cancer patients, I recommend alternating every two weeks, beginning with the four-day vegetable or grape juice fast with two weeks on the kicharee - Bean soup diet. This program is of benefit for any duration but ideally it should be followed for at least three months.

Raw Foods Vegetarian Diet:

The raw foods vegetarian diet has been found to be effective for some individuals and for the treatment of certain types of cancers. Being an eliminative diet, it is more appropriate for more excess type individuals who tend to have a stockier build and more robust energy. The emphasis unlike that of the macrobiotic diet is on the exclusive use of organic raw vegetables and fruits. There are many variations on this diet including Joanna Brandt's Grape fast as well as other systems involved with fruit and vegetable juice fasting. This approach emphasizes enzymatically rich foods such as sprouted seeds and grains as well as the regular consumption of freshly expressed wheat grass juice. As stated previously, one of the dangers of this diet is the long-term effect of inadequate protein intake. For this and other reasons, this diet can be extremely difficult for many to follow and is definitely not advisable for everyone and certainly not for more that one to three months at a time. For some, however, it can be a useful short-term therapeutic detoxification diet. Of more general value is the regular use of fresh, organic carrot and other vegetable juices, wheat or barley grass juice and the use of grapes, including the whole fruit, the juice and the seeds. With seemingly conflicting dietary regimes being promoted as effective for some in the treatment of cancer, there are a number of common characteristics for all approaches.

First, it is obvious that a low sugar, low saturated fat, vegetable-based diet is generally in common to all anticancer diets. Secondly, wholesome, organic foods are best for all people but especially cancer patients whose immune systems are already compromised by cancer. The success of diets based on the use of raw foods, which by certain advocates includes the use of raw meat,[8] together with the use of fermented foods such as miso soup in Japanese macrobiotics is at least partially due to the increased presence of living anticarcinogenic enzymes.

These are the 'universals' of an anticancer diet. By energetically classifying foods and herbs as heating or cooling, moistening or drying, tonifying or eliminating and according to what organs and physiological systems they primarily affect based on their colors and flavors, traditional healing systems such as Traditional Chinese Medicine, East Indian Ayurvedic Medicine or Tibetan Medicine may further help in 'fine-tuning' a nutritional program based on the innate constitutional needs of each individual. Unfortunately our own Traditional Western Medicine, based on the theories and principles of classifying diseases, herbs and foods following the ancient Greek and Roman theories of Hippocrates and Galen has been relegated to virtual obsolescence as a result of more recent scientific approaches. Science is great at taking things apart and analyzing phenomena bit by bit, but unlike traditional analytical systems it is not so effective in forming an integrative approach based on body, mind and spirit and the integration with lifestyle and environmental influences.

The Energetics of Food in the Treatment of Cancer

Traditional herbal medicine tries to use foods that follow the same therapeutic classification with herbs as much as possible. For instance, if an individual is following an approach of detoxification using herbs such as red clover, dandelion or burdock, then foods that enhance the similar processes of detoxification are also used including green leafy vegetables. If on the other hand tonification or rebuilding is required, that would indicate the use of herbs such as astragalus, dang quai or ginseng, then one would include more building proteinaceous foods such as legumes, soy (especially tempeh), fish and whey.

Traditional herbal medicine classifies both medicinal herbs and foods as stimulating (heating) or sedating (cooling). This describes the stimulatory effect certain foods have on our overall metabolism as well as their drying, moistening, building or eliminating properties. Many times the specific biochemical nutrients responsible for these properties are too complex to attribute to one or another constituent. The first consideration is to evaluate to

---

[8] Aajonu Vonderplanitz, *We Want To Live*, Carnelian Bay Castle Press, Santa Monica, California.

what extent one needs to emphasize building as opposed to elimination and detoxification. In the initial stages, cancer patients may not seem obviously deficient so that detoxification and elimination are emphasized. In later stages with accompanying deficiency and weakness one would emphasize more tonification and rebuilding. The object is to always try to find the most appropriate metabolic balance based on whether an individual needs more warming, cooling, building or eliminating properties.

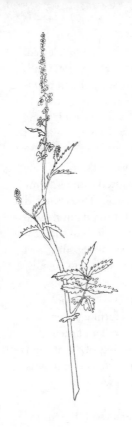

CHAPTER NINE

SUPPLEMENTS USED
IN THE TREATMENT
OF CANCER

There is no question that nutritional supplements such as Vitamins, minerals, antioxidants, essential fatty acids (EFA's) and others have an important role in the treatment of cancer. The problem that faces us is choosing the supplements that are most relevant to the needs of the individual patient.

As with herbs, nutritional supplements have overlapping properties. Thus, the goal is to develop a program using as few packaged supplements as possible while maximizing their nutritional needs through food and herbs. Even given this, it may come down to the fact that a cancer patient will be taking an average of anywhere from 10 to 20 different nutritional products on a daily basis.

In Traditional Chinese Medicine, *zhong liu ke* approximately corresponds to the specialty of oncology. Typically, TCM doctors use large herbal formulas for treating cancer which often consist of more than twenty herbs in a single formula. Therefore it should not be considered unusual that a cancer patient may be taking, in addition to their herbal treatments, from 10 to 20 different supplements on a daily basis.

Hardly a week goes by that we don't hear of some new natural supplement that has anticancer properties. This should not mean that someone with cancer, justly in fear for his or her life, should take every supplement that is advertised. Just as there is heavy-handedness as to how some conventional medical doctors administer their treatments, the same is also possible using so-called natural or alternative medicine. The question is when is enough too much?

Allow me to illustrate: one patient suffering from advanced stages of lung cancer and so weakened that he could not walk unassisted came into my office with a number of complaints unrelated to his cancer. This included chronic indigestion, lack of appetite and constipation. It turned out that he was literally taking 101 supplements each day! I explained to him that taking so many supplements, especially in the form of pills and capsules, was probably a major cause of his indigestion, lack of appetite and consequently, his growing weakness.

As I had to do so many times with new cancer patients, I first took him completely off all supplements except for a single herbal formula taken as a tea. After a couple of weeks, I gradually reintegrated a number of them that seemed most relevant to his condition and suggested a variety of dietary and herbal sources to maximally amplify his nutritional support. The result was that his appetite returned and he was even able to regain a few much-needed pounds of weight lost during his period of digestive stress.

Often if people don't pay dearly for vitamins, minerals and the various other antioxidants, they don't feel that they are getting enough nutrients. What they don't realize is that the amount of various carotenes in freshly juiced carrots, greens, tomatoes, the various sprouts and grasses such as wheat grass or barley grass sprouts are in fact superior to what one would derive from nutritional isolates containing these nutrients. The amount of anthocyanins, the most powerful of all naturally occurring antioxidants, also found in a quarter cup of frozen and thawed blueberries, is superior in both quality and quantity to what one is likely to find in a capsule or pill. Similarly, one can creatively integrate whole foods into the diet such as lightly toasted and crushed silymarin seeds, broccoli seeds, garlic and onions to name only a few to obtain needed supplemental nutrients rather than taking the packaged supplements. For those who have a garden patch, learn the therapeutic and nutritional value of weeds such as dandelion, malva, purslane and amaranth that could be steamed and eaten rather than discarded on the compost patch to reseed themselves anew next year.

Loss of appetite, abdominal swelling and discomfort and gas are all counterproductive to healing and usually signify poor assimilation. Considering that cachexia, or wasting, is the primary cause of death for most people who have cancer, anorexia and indigestion is a condition to be guarded against at all costs. Certainly we don't want to be guilty of inducing this condition through excessive intake of supplements.

Nevertheless, because of possible deficiencies in diet and food quality, a certain number of nutritional supplements may be necessary. At first and for a shorter period, we may develop a "nutritional loading" program using more supplements. After several months a longer maintenance program using less nutritional supplements seems rational. I believe that a cancer patient ideally should commit themselves to a lifetime of healthy eating supplemented by a number of key herbs and nutritional supplements that can be accommodated into a normal lifestyle.

Vitamins, Minerals, Other Antioxidants and Radiation and Chemotherapy

Should cancer patients take supplements including vitamins, minerals, antioxidants and herbs while undergoing conventional medical therapies such as chemotherapy and radiation? With so many cancer patients justly apprehensive of the ravages to their well-being and immune system from cytotoxic (cell-killing) drugs and radiation, many of which that are known in themselves to be a major cause of cancer, it would seem reasonable that they seek any health-giving natural food or substance that would offer some margin of protection while undergoing these therapies. Too often, this clashes with the admonitions of oncologists who, unaware of the vast amount of research and data in support of the use of antioxidant nutritional agents and herbs while undergoing conventional treatment, advise their patients against their use. I have spoken to some patients who were flatly denied treatment by their oncologists if they would not desist from the use of all nutritional supplements and herbs.

The fact is, our body normally makes the most powerful antioxidant, glutathione. So does it make sense that precisely at a time when it is under attack with strong oxidative drugs it should be deprived of the very nutrients that it normally depends on for healing and protection? While my answer is in favor of the use of special foods, antioxidant nutritional agents and herbs, to play the devil's advocate, the answers may not be as simple as one might imagine.

Our first consideration is the use of nutritional supplements in doses that are larger than that found in a normal diet. Generally this refers to mega doses as opposed to a normal to higher dose. For instance, vitamin C, which might be in the range of 1000 to 2000 mg as opposed to a large dose of 3 to 5g, or 20,000 IU's of vitamin A as opposed to 100,000 and 800 to 1000 IU's of vitamin E as opposed to significantly higher doses. While many alternative cancer clinics specifically prescribe higher vitamin doses, these are best administered under supervision rather than through self-prescription. One of the arguments put forward is that excessive doses cause a stress on the system that may actually cause them to adversely work as pro-oxidants.

Secondly, there are a few controversial published studies that suggest that some antioxidants may indeed interfere with chemotherapy and radiation. One study presented at the American Society for Cell Biology in Washington, D.C. in 1999 found that in genetically engineered mice with brain tumors the number of apoptotic cancer cells (cells that self destruct) that were given a diet free of the antioxidant vitamins A and E had only a 3% death of cancer cells as opposed to 19% of the cancer cells deprived of antioxidants. According to Dr. Rudolph Salganik of the University of Northern Carolina, Chapel Hill, vitamins A and E specifically prevent apoptosis (cancer cell death). Paradoxically these findings coincide with another study that found higher rates of lung cancer in smokers who consumed a high vitamin A and E antioxidant-rich diet as opposed to those who had less of these antioxidants. This is a highly controversial idea that suggests that these specific antioxidants seemed to prolong the life of developing cancer cells that might otherwise normally self-destruct. To further test his findings, Salganik and his team are planning further human studies.

In another recent article it is stated how large doses of Vitamin C given during cancer treatments are counterproductive because the cancer cells greedily use it as a way to protect themselves from the harmful effects of radiation and chemotherapy.[1] Logically the implied assumption from this is that those who receive chemotherapy without simultaneously taking Vitamin C have a better prognosis. This seems to further suggest that the antioxidant properties of vitamin C interfere with radiation and chemotherapy. I have always been skeptical of large doses of any nutritional isolate, including Vitamin C, since I think that the excess ultimately places an undesirable burden on the body. In that sense, I might find some agreement with this idea but is there any question that a reasonable amount of Vitamin C, say around 2000 to 5000 mg would indeed be advantageous to cancer patients undergoing conventional medical therapies?

From my perspective, I must admit that it is hard to fully go along with the conclusions of these studies since it seems to suggest that while on the one hand vitamins and antioxidants through one mechanism generally inhibit tumor proliferation and growth, the facts as they stand suggest that on the other hand, they would promote the development of cancer by prolonging the life of cancer cells.

Realizing that antioxidants are widely present in most natural organic foods, especially fruits, vegetables and whole grains, because these occur in naturally complex living biochemical compounds, the amount of any single constituent is less and may be buffered by the myriads of others that are simultaneously present. This seems to support the idea of deriving as many of our nutrients from organic whole foods, or at least in compounds with a number of other isolated nutrients, at the same time.

A third consideration is that a number of chemotherapeutic agents are specifically intended to destroy cancer cells by producing free radicals. As is known, while cancer cells are the primary victims, normal healthy cells are also adversely affected causing hair loss, low blood cell counts and mouth sores. The fear, which is largely theoretical at this point, is that taking antioxidant supplements will limit the ability of the free radical chemotherapeutic agents to damage proteins and other structures of cancer cells that will ultimately lead to their death or the inability to divide and make new cells. Following is a partial list of some of the more common chemotherapeutic agents whose mechanism is based on their ability to produce free radicals.

Chemotherapeutic Agents Producing Free Radicals

- **Alkylating agents**
  cisplatin (Platinol®)
  carboplarin (Paraplatin®)
  chlorambucil (Leukeran®)
  carmustine (BiCNU®)
  cyclophosphamide (Cytoxan®)
  busulfan (Myleran®)
  ifosfamide (Ifex®)

- **Anthracyclines**
  doxorubicin (Adriamycin®, Doxil®)
  daunorubicin (Cerubidine®)
  epirubicin (Ellence®)
  Mitomycin (Mutamycin®)
  BIeomycin (Bleoxane®)

- **Podophyllum agents**
  etoposide (VP-I6, Vespid®)
  teniposide (Vumon®)

As stated, the inference that vitamins, minerals and antioxidants limit the efficacy of chemotherapy or radiation treatment at this point is controversial with proponents on both sides. However, medical evidence against their use by oncologists is primarily based on the theoretical concern that if one administers a substance that is intended to kill cancer cells by promoting free radical damage, the simultaneous use of substances in the form of nutritional antioxidants, would compromise or interfere with the intended use of the chemotherapeutic agent.

So far, there are numerous studies that not only confirm the efficacy and safety of vitamins and antioxidants during chemo and radiation therapy, but actually enhance the effect of the chemo-radiation treatment. I have cited many of these in the discussion of the individual nutrients; however, to provide one of many examples, the chemotherapeutic drug, cisplatin is at least partially intended to promote free radical damage to cancer cells. Therefor, one might be persuaded to not administer any nutrient that would have an antioxidant effect, lest it interfere with the oxidant producing effect of the cisplatin. However, studies cited further in the text have found that the combination of vitamin E, beta carotene (a vitamin A precursor), zinc and selenium not only raises the bodies inherent glutathione levels but improves the therapeutic result of the cisplatin.

Ralph Moss Ph.D., in his book *Antioxidants Against Cancer* (Equinox Press, 2000) summarizes over 450 scientific studies that led him to conclude that "The data supports the idea that dietary antioxidants protect against harmful side effects, without interfering with the cancer-killing ability of conventional treatments."

This conclusion seems to be additionally supported by four published peer-reviewed articles that have summarized the scientific literature on the interaction of antioxidants with radiation and chemotherapy. These articles have concluded that antioxidants do not interfere, and in fact may improve, the ability of these treatments to destroy cancer cells while protecting the healthy ones, as well as reducing their side effects and prolonging survival.[1]

Ironically, about the same time the article was published warning against the use of vitamin C during chemotherapy, the National Cancer institute (NIH) announced a new study. They are initiating the study to compare the efficacy of an alternative-therapy regimen involving a vegetable and whole grain based diet, digestive enzymes, nutritional supplements (I presume antioxidants such as Vitamin C are included) and coffee enemas against those who followed the standard medical protocol. This is a $1.4 million dollar study based on a prior 11 patient study conducted by immunologists Nicholas J. Gonzalez, M.D. and Linda L. Isaacs, M.D. where it was shown that that patients undergoing the alternative protocol lived three times longer than those who did not.[2]

Nutrition is certainly the key. Even the National Cancer Institute (NCI), after years of denying any correlation between nutrition and cancer, have come to 'officially' recommend that all people consume at least 5 servings of antioxidant-rich fruits and vegetables a day. The problem that even if they emphasized 'organic' fruits and vegetables which are known to contain 50% or more denser nutrients than their inorganic counterpart, as a result

---

[1] Prasad, et.al., 1999; Simone, et al., 1997; Lamson & Brignall 1999; Weijl et al., 1997.

of depleted soils from years of over-harvesting, these organically grown foods may still be lacking in adequate nutrients for health. This is one of the major arguments for adding at least a minimal amount of nutritional supplementation to one's daily regime.

To measure the effectiveness of fresh fruit's and vegetable's ability to neutralize cancer causing oxygen free radicals in our body, Dr. Guohua Cao and colleagues in the 1990's devised a standardized Oxygen Radical Absorbance Capacity (ORAC) test at the USDA laboratory at Tufts University, Boston. It was found that the average intake of ORAC from fruits and vegetables was around 1200 per day. However, by increasing to five vegetable and fruit servings (a single serving is about a quarter of a cup), this could increase to 1,640. Ralph Moss points out how a diet concentrating on the most powerful cancer fighting superfoods could boost even this to 6000 per day, thus lowering our risk for cancer as well as other chronic diseases.[3]

The quality of supplements one uses is certainly of importance. In the resources section at the back of the book, I offer a number of quality manufacturers whose supplements my colleagues and I have come to trust and rely upon as being of high quality. I feel that one should, as much as possible, utilize the highest quality nutritional supplements that have been derived from organic food sources rather than synthetically manufactured. I realize that for some of these, this may not always be possible. Increasingly, companies such as Rainbow Light with their *Complete Nutritional Program* are manufacturing Vitamins and supplements that are derived primarily from organic food sources.

It is certainly advisable to engage the assistance of a qualified practitioner in creating a nutritional and herbal program for cancer patients. Increasingly there are numbers of organizations and individuals throughout the country who can be of assistance. A word of caution however: beware of anyone who promises a universal cure for all cancers based on their protocol. Cancer is a multifaceted disease and, in fact, it may be argued that it is many diseases in one. There is no panacea for all cancers. The manifestations of the disease are as different as the millions of people are who have it. Just as surgery, chemotherapy and radiation may be helpful for some with cancer and disastrous for others, so also are the many shotgun approaches, one for all, cancer programs that promise a universal cure.

As of this writing, the hard facts are that most people will not survive most cancers. The question may not necessarily be 'cure' as it is well-being and quality of life that matters. Too many in their pursuit of a 'cure' will completely forsake issues of life quality when, in the end, this may have been the only choice they had to begin with. Beware of exaggerated and puffed-up promises of a cure from sources such as the Internet, public forums and so forth. Remember, just because someone is honest and is unable to promise a cure does not mean that they cannot be of significant assistance and help.

Some of the organizations whose professional register and graduates are likely to have qualified practitioners are listed at the end of the book. I suggest contacting them for referrals.

Vitamins

In the early part of the century it was found that the macronutrients consisting of carbohydrates, proteins, lipids and water were not enough to sustain animal life. This led to the discovery of some thirteen different carbon-containing Vitamins. These are classified as water-soluble and fat-soluble. There are some well-known associations between Vitamin deficiency and cancer. These include:

- Deficiency of choline and B Vitamins and an increased risk of liver cancer.
- Deficiency of Vitamin B6 (pyridoxine) and an increased risk of cervical cancer.
- Deficiency of Vitamin E and an increased risk of cancer generally and leukemia.
- Deficiency of Vitamin A with an increased risk of cancer generally.

The Water-soluble Vitamins

Vitamins that dissolve in water include the B complex Vitamins and Vitamin C. After being absorbed through the blood stream to the liver, they are distributed throughout the body. The darker yellow urine color that occurs after taking certain Vitamins, especially Vitamin C, transpires because their excess is not stored in the body but secreted through the urine. This means that we need to obtain an adequate daily supply of Vitamins either from food or supplementation.

The B Complex Vitamins

The B complex Vitamins are like the "ginseng of Vitamins" because of their ability to increase energy. To do this, they act like enzymes in their capacity to assist in the conversion of carbohydrates to glucose in the body. Other tonifying, ginseng-like effects are in their ability to counteract stress by strengthening the cell membranes, the nervous system and the immune system by stimulating antibody response. Except for a few of the B Vitamins, such as B-12 and folic acid, most B Vitamins are created in the body as a natural process of fermentation in the intestines. B-1 - thiamine, B-2 - riboflavin and B-3 – niacin, along with Coenzyme Q-10, are essential nutrients for both the prevention and treatment of cancer because they facilitate aerobic metabolism.

With all of these benefits and the fact that the two major sources for B Vitamins are whole grains and a healthy gastrointestinal system, our capacity to derive and absorb them is diminished with a diet of refined foods and as a result of aging. Further, as a class, all the B Vitamins are synergistically interdependent upon each other for absorption so that in most instances it is better to take them together rather than separately.

As part of their normal life cycle healthy flora of the intestines manufacture B Vitamins together with the conditions that favor their absorption. For this reason, supplements such as acidophilus and other beneficial bacteria are vitally essential to all levels of health. Traditionally, people would consume fermented vegetables and dairy products such as sauerkraut in Europe, Kim Chee in Korea and miso paste in Japan to replenish these bacteria. In Northern Europe, fermented dairy in the form of yogurt is also used. It is now possible to take supplements with these favorable bacteria. These in turn become one of the major sources for many of the B Vitamins. Other sources include brewer's yeast, almonds, wheat germ, nuts, beans, other legumes and whole grains as well as sea vegetables.

Thiamine – Vitamin B1

Thiamine assists in the production of energy through the breakdown of food and helps to maintain a healthy nervous system. Subclinical deficiency of B1 can cause low energy and is associated with various personality disorders ranging from a tendency towards irritability, to schizophrenia and even Alzheimer's disease. It is also an important nutrient for diabetics because by strengthening the nerves, it helps to prevent diabetic neuropathy. Sources of Thiamne: egg yolks, fish, pork, poultry, legumes, brown rice, whole grains, wheat germ, nori and wakame sea vegetables.

Riboflavin – Vitamin B2

Like thiamine, riboflavin is also involved in helping to release the energy from food. Furthermore, it is vital for the absorption of pyridoxine or Vitamin B6. This B Vitamin is necessary for cancer patients to combat the effects of chemical pollutants and free radicals by releasing the powerful antioxidant properties of glutathione. A deficiency of B2 may result in a number of conditions including cataracts, diabetes, the recurrence of malaria symptoms, sensitivity to light, skin disorders and cracks around the corners of the mouth and nose. In their book, *Nutritional Therapy in medical Practice*, Drs. Alan Gaby, M.D. and Jonathan Wright, M.D. state, "deficiency of impaired utilization of riboflavin may result from the administration of Adriamycin, phenothiazines, dilantin, imipramine or amitriptyline," thus specifically necessitating the supplementation with this nutrient.

Riboflavin is derived from dairy products, egg yolks, whole grains, meats, seafood, hiziki seaweed, nuts, seeds and legumes.

While the need for Vitamin B2 is based on weight, growth, caloric intake and metabolic level, on the average, 10 to 50 mg daily would offer a large buffer of safety.

Niacin – Vitamin B3

Niacin, or nicotinic acid, has 'cayenne-like' blood and energy stimulating properties. For over four decades, it has been recognized as one of the most effective ways to lower LDL cholesterol and triglycerides while raising beneficial HDL cholesterol in the blood. By so doing it has been shown to reduce the incidence of nonfatal heart attacks while prolonging the survival rate of heart attack survivors.

Niacinamide is a synthetic form of niacin and while it has no cholesterol lowering abilities it has a special effect in reducing the insulin requirement of diabetics for which it was widely used in the 1940's. It also has been shown to be an effective nutrient for osteoarthritis.

Sources for all forms of niacin include meat, poultry, dairy products, seafood, brewer's yeast, brown rice, wheat bran and various nuts and seeds.

Niacin needs are based on caloric intake. We need about 6.6 mg per 1,000 calories with a minimum of 13 mg per day. From 25-50 mg per day seems to be adequate so long as appropriate protein requirements are met.

Inositol

Inositol is a time released, non-flushing form of niacin. Unlike niacin, it has a general calming influence. It also helps to reduce cholesterol levels and prevent hardening of the arteries and is useful for helping to remove fats from the liver. A deficiency can cause arteriosclerosis, constipation, hair loss, cholesteremia, irritability, moodiness and skin eruptions.

Inosital is found in brewer's yeast, fruits, lecithin, legumes, whole grains, meats, dairy, unrefined molasses, raisins and vegetables. Large amounts of caffeine may lower inositol levels. There is no known daily requirement because it can be made in our bodies. However, a therapeutic dose might be around 500 mg.

Inosital Hexaphosphate (IP6) – an important cancer fighter

Inositol hexaphosphate (IP6), also known as phytic acid or phytate, is involved in the regulation of all cells in the body. It enables cellular assimilation and elimination and also is a protective function. In the treatment and prevention of cancer and other serious diseases, IP6 helps to prevent genetic mutations and DNA damage, increases anticancer natural killer cells, and has further demonstrated potent antioxidant properties.

When taken with inosital hexakisphosphate (phytic acid), commonly known in the trade as IP6, it has a synergistic ability in the prevention and inhibition of various forms of tumors and cancer, including cancer of the colon, breast, prostate, liver and other types.

While inosital is found as part of the fibers from whole grains, IP6 is specifically derived from the bran of brown rice. The combination of both inosital and IP6 is an important detoxicant and anticancer agent. (This is a potent argument for the use of whole grains, depending on digestion, as opposed to refined grains. It also shows the wisdom behind the macrobiotic brown rice diet and the Ayurvedic kicharee diet.)

I regularly prescribe IP6 as a supplement for all cancer patients. As a normal dietary supplement one would take IP6 + inositol to a total of 1-2g, or 1000 to 2000 milligrams, in a divided dose twice daily. Ideally because of the interaction with proteins that might neutralize some of its effectiveness, it should be taken between meals. For those who are at higher risk for cancer double that amount may be useful. For those with existing cancers the dosage should be up to 5 to 8g daily.

Pyridoxine – Vitamin B6

Pyridoxine is important for fat and protein metabolism. It is vital to the immune system of cancer victims, since a lack of pyridoxine reduces the number of lymphocytes necessary for fighting disease. It is almost always deficient in those who are ill and it has been correlated with a compromised immune function. Other uses include its value for maintaining healthy brain function, the growth of red blood cells and skin health. Similarly, women who are on oral contraceptives require higher doses of B6. As the 'diuretic Vitamin' and because of its ability to remove 'dampness' or fluid retention according to TCM theory, it is useful for a wide range of conditions including asthma, PMS, nausea from pregnancy and candida overgrowth. It is one of the first treatments that should be tried for the relief of carpal tunnel syndrome. Even as little as a daily 200 mg supplementation of B6 has significantly reduced the pain. If this isn't effective, then one should try the activated form of B6 called pyridoxyl-5-phosphate (P5P). Taken with magnesium it has been found to be helpful for autistic children with significant improvements in auditory response.

Like other B Vitamins, food sources for pyridoxine include whole grains, nuts, legumes, bananas, meat, fish and poultry. The average daily requirement of B6 is a minimum of 2 mg for adults per 100g of protein consumed. For children it is 0.6 to 1.2 mg per 100g of protein.

Folic Acid

Folic acid is one of the B Vitamins that must be externally derived from food. In various nutrition surveys, it ranks as the number one Vitamin deficiency in North America.[4] It is vital for healthy gums, red blood cells, skin, the gastrointestinal tract and RNA synthesis. Folic acid enables the process of healthy cell division while a lack of it can be a cause of anemia and a degradation of the intestinal lining, impairing intestinal absorption of nutrients. Even a mild deficiency of folic acid has been implicated in the development of precancerous cervical dysplasia. According to herbalist Donald Yance, AHG, "a deficiency of dietary Folate intake may predispose individuals to cancer as a consequence of disruption of DNA synthesis, repair, and methylation; diets deficient in methyl groups may result in the activation of oncogenes and inactivation of tumor suppressor genes." A recent study showed an inverse association with folate and methionine intake, and breast cancer risk in women with relatively high intake of alcohol.[5]

A lack of folic acid represents one of the most prevalent deficiencies that most people have. It is derived from only the freshest vegetables and much of folic acid is lost the first day it is picked. Of course, both cooking and even exposure to light will greatly diminish the presence of folic acid. This is only one of the reasons that people throughout the world favor the use of the freshest vegetables.

According to Donald Yance, the consumption of alcohol as well as many over the counter drugs puts a high demand on the liver, particularly with regards to methylation function. Folic acid, B 12, B 6, methionen, choline and SAMe are all important nutrients for proper methylation function. Methotrexate, one of the most common chemotherapy drug,s is also known to disrupt methylation.

It has been known for decades that a lack of either folic acid or Vitamin B 12 causes pernicious anemia and even as little as 400-800 mcg is enough to overcome anemia. However, taking too much folic acid alone could mask a Vitamin B 12 deficiency; therefore, it is a good idea to take both simultaneously. Finally, it is well known that pregnant women or women trying to become pregnant should take a daily supplement that contains at least 800 mcg of folic acid as it has been proven to prevent spina bifida, one of the most serious but common types of birth defects.

Cobalamin – Vitamin B12

Vitamin B12 binds with intrinsic factor (IF) in the stomach to from the IF-cobalimin complex, which is absorbed in the small intestine. It is essential for the metabolism of protein, fat and carbohydrates. A lack of IF in the stomach lining of older people and strict vegetarians may put them at risk for

B12 deficiency. Symptoms of B12 deficiency are perni[illegible]us deterioration, confusion, depression and other cognit[illegible] B12 deficiency is well known among vegetarians, people [illegible] diet and the elderly and can cause irreversible nerve dama[illegible] B12 is extremely important.

B12 has a generally tonic effect on one's vitality and circulation. It has been found that individuals suffering from bursitis were relieved with a shot of B12 whether there was B12 deficiency or not. For patients undergoing chemotherapy and radiation, an injection of B12 into certain acupuncture points, including Stomach 36 (located approximately 3 inches below the patella about one inch from the anterior crest of the tibia), Spleen 6 (3 inches above the tip of the medial malleolus, posterior to the tibial border) and Conception Vessel 6 (1 1/2 inches below the umbilicus on the midline of the abdomen) or Conception Vessel 4 (3 inches below the umbilicus on the midline of the abdomen), has a powerful and immediate recuperative effect and should be part of the standard of care for all cancer patients.[2]

Vitamin B12 is primarily derived from animal protein sources including all meat, fish, eggs, microorganisms, yogurt and milk. There are amounts of B12 in certain fermented foods such as tempeh and yeast. It is also interesting that an overly sterile food environment does not allow for bacteria and even small insects to be present that might otherwise engender B12 as an introduced byproduct. For an adult the average daily dosage is small, from 3 to 4 mcg. For pregnant and lactating women as well as infants 10-20 mcg represents a good insurance level.

Biotin

An essential part of enzyme systems, biotin is closely associated with B12. Biotin is one of the coenzymes that participate in the metabolism of fat. At the same time it is necessary for the production of fat and the synthesis of fatty acids. Thus biotin is used to normalize fat metabolism. It is also useful for helping to reduce blood sugar of diabetic patients. It is available from foods in only trace amounts and therefore is often deficient. It is found in egg yolks, liver, brewer's yeast, unpolished rice, nuts and milk. However, the friendly

[2] Medical doctors and health practitioners might consider giving B12 injections following chemotherapy and radiation. From 5 to 10 C.C. are divided between a selection of acupuncture points stomach 36 spleen 6 and/or conception vessel 4 or 6, which can be found in any standard acupuncture text or chart. For instance, one might choose Conception vessel 4 or 6 combined with a bilateral treatment of either Stomach 36 or Spleen 6. In China various tonic and blood moving herbs are used such as injectable forms of ginseng, codonopsis, dang gui, salvia milthiorrhiza, astragalus, etc. This can have an immediate beneficial effect on a patient's recovery from chemo or radiation therapy and is also used generally for tonification and pain relief.

bacteria acidophilus produce biotin. The dosage range is between 150-300 mcg depending on how efficient the intestinal flora is in producing it.

Pantothenic Acid – B5

Pantothenic acid is needed for optimal food digestion to maintain energy and promote wound healing. It is also necessary for the manufacture of adrenal hormones and neurotransmitters and those who are under stress. It is required by all cells in the body and is especially concentrated in the internal organs. It plays a vital role in the formation of antibodies, aids in Vitamin utilization, and helps to convert fats, carbohydrates and protein into energy. Pantothenic acid is found in whole grains, eggs and milk and manufactured by bacteria in the intestines. The average dosage for children is around 5 mg and around 10 mg for adults. However, many feel that the minimum needs may be more around 50-100 mgs. A therapeutic dose is approximately 250-500 mg.

Other B Complex Vitamins

Other B complex Vitamins include para-aminobenzoic acid (PABA), B13 (orotic acid) and B15 (pangamic acid). Briefly, PABA is part of the folic acid molecule and is used to support folic acid. It is also used to assist as a sunscreen and to normalize hair color and growth. It is found in liver, brewer's yeast, wheat germ, whole grains and molasses. It is synthesized in the intestines and can be stored in the tissues of the body.

Orotic acid is not fully recognized as a Vitamin. They are considered by some as transporter salts of minerals into the blood from the GI tract. It is found in dairy products, root vegetables, carrots, beets and Jerusalem artichokes. The body is also able to make orotic acid from its amino acid pool.

Pangamic acid is a controversial Vitamin because based on usage in European countries, especially the Soviet Union, there are many claims for a multitude of diseases and symptoms including diseases associated with aging, drug addiction, alcoholic addiction, mental problems, senility, autism, schizophrenia, heart disease, hypertension, diabetes, skin diseases, liver disease and chemical poisons. Because of all of these wide claims, the FDA heavily regulates it in the US. Soviet scientists have found that pangamic acid can reduce the buildup of lactic acid in athletes. In the US it is marketed as dimethyl glycine (DMG) and best used in supplemental doses of 50 – 100 mg taken twice daily with Vitamins E and A especially after a heavy physical workout to reduce the buildup of lactic acid.

Vitamin B 17 (laetrile-amygdalin)

B17, or laetrile, is specifically considered to be the anticancer Vitamin. It is widely derived from apricots and peach seeds, apple seeds, loquat leaves an the pits of cherries and plums. Mentioned elsewhere in this book, the basis for the use of laetrile for the treatment and prevention of cancer is that cancer cells specifically lack the enzyme rhodanase necessary to inactivate the cyanide molecule of the laetrile compound. Another enzyme, beta-glycosidase, actually assists in releasing the cyanide that specifically targets cancer cells. Based on the work of Dr. Sugiura at Memorial Sloan-Kettering hospital in 1974, laetrile was able to stop the growth of small tumors and reduce the proliferation of breast cancer in laboratory animals. While 80% of the laboratory animals that did not take laetrile developed lung metastasis, only 20% who were given laetrile did.

Vitamin C

Vitamin C is one of the most important of all the antioxidant and immune enhancing nutrients needed by the human body. By protecting the cells from the damaging effects of free radicals, it plays a vital role in virtually all degenerative diseases including, of course, cancer. It is also needed to maintain healthy gums, skin and the connective tissue throughout the body. As if this were not enough, it prevents the deterioration in the body of Vitamins B1, B2, B5, folic acid and Vitamins A and E.

While most mammals are able to convert glucose to Vitamin C in their livers, humans lack an essential fourth enzyme to accomplish this and must depend on external sources from fresh fruits and vegetables for their daily requirement.

There have been nearly a hundred well-documented studies that have demonstrated the protective effect of Vitamin C in the prevention of cancer. All of these have been based on the relationship of Vitamin C to the immune system and its primary antioxidant and defense against cancer.[8] Besides serving as a powerful antioxidant itself, Vitamin C also activates two other powerful antioxidants, Vitamin E and glutathione.[9] Because of these effects, there is a direct relationship of diminished cancer risk with the amount of Vitamin C consumed.[10,11] A minimum daily dosage of 500 mg is required, however for cancer it has been customary to increase the dose to 'bowel tolerance,' which is the amount at which the bowls become loose after which the Vitamin C dose is accordingly reduced.

Probably the best way to take Vitamin C is in smaller amounts throughout the day. Because it is water soluble, like other water-soluble Vitamins excess will cause frequent urination. From a balanced perspective, this may not be good for the overall well being of the body and the sustaining dose of 500 to 2000 mg is probably adequate for all people and conditions.

Vitamin C is found in all fresh vegetables and fruits. In its organic form, it is sensitive to both heat and aging. The only exception is the Amla fruit (myrobalan emblica) that grows in India. It is the second known highest source of Vitamin C (acerola berries are first) but uniquely because of its tannins that bind and hold the Vitamin C stable, it is practically impervious to cooking and aging. It is one of the most important botanicals in the East Indian Ayurvedic tradition and a key ingredient in traditional formulas such as triphala and Chyavanprash.

Fat-soluble Vitamins

Vitamins that dissolve in oil or fat include Vitamins A, D, E and K. They are more heat-stable than the water-soluble Vitamins B and C and are stored in the fatty tissues of the body.

Vitamin A and Beta-carotene

Some believe that Vitamin A can be toxic in dosages over 15,000 IU's, however, practical experience has demonstrated a tolerance to as much as 50,000 IU's. This is especially true for some individuals who have damaged livers. The potential toxicity of Vitamin A, however, is somewhat mitigated by using it's antioxidant precursors, beta-carotene, and the other carotenoids as well as taking Vitamin A together with Vitamin E.

A lack of Vitamin A will decrease cancer antibody formation while taking it as a supplement will increase anticancer properties of T-cells, Natural killer cells and macrophages. Vitamin A and its precursor, Beta-carotene is naturally found in orange and yellow vegetables including carrots and yellow squash. Beta-carotene is also generously found in a wide variety of green leafy vegetables. Vitamin A itself is found in liver, eggs, butter and fortified dairy products.

In nature, beta-carotene supplies the many colorful pigments of plants, birds and fish; however, its conversion into Vitamin A allows our body to see them. This is because beta-carotene as the precursor of Vitamin A is essential for eyesight as well as healthy skin and intestinal tract. In the early 1900's it was known as the "infection-fighting Vitamin" since it was found to be valuable in helping to protect the body from toxicity and pollution.

Far from being a subservient precursor, beta-carotene has its own distinctive effects in boosting the immune system, preventing clogged arteries, maintaining thyroid function and cancer prevention. For this reason, for optimal health, both nutrients should be supplemented.

Because Vitamin A is stored in the fatty tissues of the body, an overly high dose of around 15,000 IU's daily may pose a risk to health. This is especially true for those with liver damage such as alcoholics. Further, those who take high amounts of Vitamin A, even in the form of carrot juice, may develop an orange-yellow complexion, which is harmless and vanishes after ceasing to take high doses of these nutrients. Authorities differ as to the safe upper range of Vitamin A supplementation. To prevent the adverse free radical effects of environmental pollutants and tobacco, one should take at least 25,000 IU's of Vitamin A daily but for most others around 10,000 IU's is sufficient. Those with low thyroid function lack the ability to convert beta-carotene into Vitamin A and should supplement this Vitamin in either food form or a Vitamin supplement. This should be accompanied with the intake of Vitamin E to protect Vitamin A from oxidation.

There has been increasing concertn over the possible risk of liver damage resulting from a high intake of Vitamin A. Because of this pregnant women should not ingest more than 8,000 IU's daily. Others should not take long-term high doses of Vitamin A without medical supervision. Therapeutically, micel Vitamin A is the best form to use.

Beta-carotene does not carry the precautions of Vitamin A and optimal daily supplementation ranges from 25,000 to 100,000 IU's daily. Ideally beta-carotene should be derived from natural sources such as carrot and other vegetable juices.

In one study by J.P. Allard, quoted in the April, 1994 *American Journal of Clinical Nutrition*, beta-carotene taken as a supplement has been found to reduce the number of free radicals in tobacco smokers. Two months previous in the same journal Dr. Kumegaki found that "beta-carotene supplements prevent radiation-induced free radical damage to chromosomes in human lymphocytes."

Many oncologists warn their patients to not take antioxidants and beta-carotene since it may compromise the efficacy of chemotherapy. This controversy, according to Dr. James Marshall may be based on the tendency for a synthetic or all-trans form commonly used in most supplements to be used. In fact nothing could be further from the truth. The naturally occurring form contains about 50% trans-isomer and several other forms of which the most prevalent is 9-cis-beta-carotene (2.3).[12] An important 1996 study found that taking beta-carotene offset the potential heart damage of the drug Adriamycin. Further, it seemed to enhance the cancer cell destroying properties of the drug.[13] This same study found the combination of beta-carotene with melphalan and etoposide highly effective, again enhancing the cancer cell killing effects of the drugs while benefiting the immune system. Another study conducted at Harvard University found that the combination of Vitamin E and beta-carotene taken together reduced the toxicity of the drug, cisplatin.[14]

Lycopene

Other carotenoids have also been found to possess anticancer properties. Lycopene, found abundantly in cooked tomatoes, is an even more potent antioxidant than either alpha-carotene or beta-carotene according to studies presented by Dr. Yoav Sharoni and Joseph Levy of Ben Gurion University in Israel. This is especially true of fast growing cancers where lycopene interferes with the complex method of cellular communication between cancer cells and, as a result, they found that both cell growth and cell movement are slowed in breast, lung and endometrial cancer cells. They also found that lycopene increased the process of human cell differentiation into specialized organ cells such as (liver, heart, pancreas, lung, etc.) Other studies have shown that the combination of the antioxidants Vitamin E, selenium and lycopene all significantly slowed and reduced the risk of prostate cancer.

Interestingly, lycopene is better absorbed from cooked tomatoes than from raw tomatoes, tomato juice or salsa because cooking breaks down their cell walls. Further, lycopene being a fat-soluble substance is ideally consumed with some fat or oil in order to be absorbed through the intestines. Thus, the use of cooked tomatoes with fish or in a recipe with olive oil is superior to taking them alone.

Other Important Carotenoids

There are literally hundreds of carotenoids, most of which are involved with the green, red or yellow-orange color of plants. Undoubtedly more will be discovered to have potent antioxidant properties. Other important carotenoids that have been found to be effective against cancer include alpha-carotene, lutein and zeaxanthin. Various studies on experimental mice have found Lutein, a carotenoid that is five times more available from vegetables than beta-carotene, to be effective in suppressing and slowing the growth of breast and colon cancer in mice.[15,16]

Vitamin D

Vitamin D, also known as the "sunshine vitamin" is manufactured in the skin when it is exposed to the ultraviolet rays of the sun. It is then absorbed through the intestinal walls. It is finally transferred to the liver or kidneys and changed into an active form of Vitamin D. Vitamin D helps to regulate calcium and phosphorus utilization and thus plays a pivotal role in bone formation and the prevention of osteoporosis.

Because Vitamin D binds with calcium when it is absorbed through the colon, they don't change as quickly and cells that are less likely to change are also less likely to become carcinogenic. As for preventing breast and prostate cancers, Vitamin D seems to inhibit the proliferation of hormones such as estrogen so that these hormonally driven cancers are suppressed.

Fair skinned people require as little as 20 minutes per day in the sun while dark skinned individuals may require up to an hour to receive their full daily Vitamin D supplementation. It is naturally found in fortified cow's milk, soymilk, egg yolks, butter, deep-sea fish, fish oils, sea vegetables and ergosterol in plants. Vegetal sources of Vitamin D, however, are negligible so that vegetarians need to be aware of receiving adequate daily sunlight exposure. The intake of fish liver oils, especially during the winter months or in areas where there is less sunlight may be an important source of Vitamin D. For the elderly, less exposure to sunlight increases their risk of osteoporosis and other degenerative conditions associated with calcium uptake such as eyesight and hearing, since the small bones of the ear are especially prone to deficiency of Vitamin D.

An excess of Vitamin D can be toxic and this is implicated in the incidence of skin cancer as a result of overexposure to sunlight. Vitamin D toxicity is associated with the intake of high doses of more than 1,000 to 1,500 IU's daily for a month or longer, more than 600 IU's in children and 400 IU's in infants. Excessive Vitamin D intake interestingly exhibits symptoms similar to overexposure to sunlight including thirst, nausea, diarrhea, weakness and headaches. Vitamin D is best utilized with Vitamin A. The average daily dose is approximately 400 IU's or 10mcg per day. For infants, pregnant women and lactating women, higher Vitamin D intake may be necessary.

Vitamin E

Vitamin E actually represents a range of tocopherols and the best quality Vitamin E should reflect this. It is often added to cooking oils to prevent oxidation. Similarly, herbalists add it to oils and salves to prevent spoilage and rancidity. All of this attests to the fact that it is indeed one of the most powerfully effective antioxidants useful to protect the body from free radical damage as a result of radiation toxicity and from certain chemotherapy drugs. Optimal amounts of Vitamin E have been shown to tonify the immune system as well as reduce the risk of cardio-vascular heart disease and cancer. It also improves the action of insulin in diabetics. Those who are involved in aerobic exercise are protected from free radical damage in conjunction with Vitamin E supplementation.

In one Finnish study, 36,000 adults were observed over a period of eight years. Of these, 766 developed cancer and it was found that in people with low blood levels of Vitamin E their risk of cancer was increased by one and a half times.

Vitamin E has also been found to strengthen the nervous system and prevent or slow the occurrence of Alzheimer's disease.[17]

Both Vitamin E and A, being fat soluble unless taken with oils, are best absorbed when taken in the "micellized" or water-soluble form. The widespread use of refined vegetable oils not only does not offer your body adequate amounts of Vitamin E but also actually depletes its reserves. Because of this it has been found that the average American receives about 12 IU's daily [18, 3] while the optimal daily amount is from 100 to 800 IU's daily. Vitamin E is naturally found in unrefined vegetable oils, whole grains, egg yolk and nuts.

Tocotrienols

Tocotrienolsis is a form of Vitamin E that is found in palm oil, rice bran oil, olive oil and other foods. They have been found to inhibit the development and growth of non-estrogen receptive breast cancer cells.[19] They have also been found to inhibit melanoma and leukemia cells. How much to take seems to be a matter of debate and conjecture. Cost and bioavailability is also a factor. They should probably be included with Vitamin E tocopherols or only used if one is fighting an active cancer.

Vitamin K

Over the last thirty years, evidence has been accumulating concerning the anticancer effects of Vitamin K.[4] It has been found to inhibit several different types of cancers including cancer of the breast, ovaries, colon, stomach, kidneys, and squamous cell carcinomas of the lungs.[5] Known as the "clotting Vitamin," Vitamin K is also necessary for the regulation of calcium and bone development. About half of the daily requirements are manufactured in the intestines by beneficial bacteria. The other half is derived from dark leafy green vegetables, from milk, soybeans and eggs.

Any substance that destroys the healthy intestinal bacteria such as long-term use of antibiotics creates a need for Vitamin K supplementation. On the other hand, those who are taking blood-thinning medications should consult a qualified health practitioner for advice about Vitamin K supplementation. Vitamin K-1 is the natural form of Vitamin K and does not cause blood clotting. Rather, it seems to have a regulating effect, assisting or preventing clotting as needed. Approximately 300 mcg per day is probably an optimal dose for the average adult. Newborns and infants require a higher amount to prevent bleeding. Alfalfa leaf is a good source of vitamin K.

---

[3] "Vitamin E Status of U.S. Children." Adrienne Bendich, Ph.D., *Journal of the American College of Nutrition*, 1992; 11: (4) 441-44

[4] Chlebowski, R.T., et al., *Cancer Treatment Reviews*, vol. 12, p. 49, 1985

[5] Yance, Donald, *Herbal Medicine Healing & Cancer*, p. 186

Minerals and Cancer

There are two types of minerals needed by the body. Those that are needed in large amounts are called *macro-minerals* while those that are required in trace amounts are called *trace minerals*.

Minerals exist as both ions (carrying an electrical charge) and salts. Metals form positive ions and include sodium, potassium, magnesium and calcium. Nonmetals form negative ions and include chloride, sulfur, phosphorus and bicarbonate. Salt (sodium chloride) is a combination of both a positive metal and a negative nonmetal.

Salts, mainly in the form of calcium and phosphates, are found in bones and teeth.

Cancer patients can be mineral deficient do to a deficient diet, radiation therapy, absorption interference from negative drug interactions or tumor growth requirements and loss of minerals as a result of diarrhea or vomiting.

The Macro Minerals

The seven-macro minerals are calcium, phosphorus, magnesium, sulfur, sodium, potassium and chloride.

Calcium and Phosphorus

These two minerals are discussed together because they are very closely related. Both are found in abundance in the bones at the ratio of approximately 2.5% to 1% phosphorus.

Calcium represents the single most abundant mineral in the body at around 39%. 98% of this is stored in the bones while 1% is in the teeth. The remaining 1% is stored in other tissues and circulated where its presence triggers vital metabolic reactions.

Calcium activates certain enzyme systems, such as choline acetylase, which helps to generate acetylcholine, which is necessary for the production of energy. Circulating calcium is needed for muscle contraction and to help regulate the heartbeat. Similarly, calcium is essential for nerve transmission assisting in the activation of various neurotransmitters, such as seratonin and nor epinephrine. Other vital uses for calcium include its role in facilitating cell division as well as helping to convert fibrinogen to fibrin to help blood coagulation.

There are several factors that enhance calcium and phosphate absorption:

- Sufficient hydrochloric acid in the stomach.

- The presence of fat in the digestive system that slows digestion, giving more time for calcium absorption.
- Protein tends to favor the intake of calcium.
- Vitamin D, mostly from the sun, helps the intestines absorb calcium.
- Growth needs: As the body grows, more calcium is needed and therefore it is better absorbed; however, with aging, absorption decreases which, along with a waning of other self-maintaining metabolic problems, results in the danger of osteoporosis in the elderly.

Phosphorus is abundant in meats of all kinds, fish, dairy and eggs. Even fruits and vegetables and whole grains contain a certain amount of phosphorus. Therefore, obtaining a sufficient amount of phosphorus is hardly ever a problem. Conversely, too much phosphorus from prepared foods and sodas tend to leach calcium from the bones and tissues of the body.

Protein tends to favor the absorption of calcium. However, high protein intake also requires that higher amounts of calcium be taken in as well.

Contrary to popular opinion, dairy may not be the best source of calcium. In fact there is twice as much calcium weight for weight in turnip greens, kale or collards than in a comparable amount of milk. Other sources for dietary calcium besides dairy products include fortified soymilk, tofu, corn tortillas, collard, turnip greens, kale, broccoli, sesame seeds, small bones of animals and sea vegetables.

Supplementally, calcium orotate is the best to use for bone recalcification. As such it is particularly useful for metastatic bone cancer. If there is pain, one should combine calcium with blood moving herbs, such as salvia milthiorrhiza, or better yet, a combiation of guggul and boswellia. I use Planetary Formula's Willow Aid that contains these two botanicals with others in an effective formula that relieves pain by promoting blood circulation. The absorption of calcium is dependent on a number of factors, including Vitamin D and phosphorus. The average daily supplemental intake of 1,000 mg of calcium in a ratio of 1,000 to 2,000 mg of phosphorus is recommended.

Magnesium: The anti-stress vitamin

Magnesium is abundant in various vegetables and is even responsible for the green color of chlorophyll. Whole calcium is responsible for muscle contraction while magnesium is responsible for the relaxation phase. Magnesium deficiency is fairly high, especially in those who eat a diet of mostly refined foods, who cook or boil all foods, drink soft water, in alcoholics and in food grown in magnesium depleted soil. Its absorption is also decreased with serious diseases or injuries. Symptoms of magnesium deficiency include fatigue, nervousness, spasms, irritability, tension, anorexia, and mental confusion and rapid and/or irregular heartbeat. Other symptoms include numbness, tingling, spasms, muscular contraction, hallucinations and constipation.

One of the side effects of many chemotherapeutic drugs is depletion of magnesium reserves. For this reason, supplemental magnesium taken alone or in combination with calcium and potassium is recommended at least for some time before and after undergoing chemo or radiation therapy.

Sources of magnesium include nuts, brewer's yeast, soybeans, dried apricots, sea vegetables, collard greens, kale, cabbage, broccoli, whole grains and molasses. The current recommended daily dose is from 300-500 mg for adults, 350 mg for men and 300 mg for women, increasing during pregnancy and lactation to around 450 mg. This is considered low by many authorities that feel that the amount of daily magnesium requirement should be at least doubled.

Potassium

Potassium deficiency is associated with low tissue oxidation. Because oxygen is vital for the treatment and prevention of cancer, increased amounts of potassium are associated with decreased cancer risk. The ratio of sodium to potassium is important for the transference of energy to and from cells. Cancer is associated with a higher rate of intracellular sodium and a corresponding lower rate of potassium. This is one of the mechanisms for what the Chinese describe as 'yin deficiency' with a lack of sufficient intercellular fluid because of a corresponding lack of sodium absorption. Having sufficient potassium allows for a proper balance of intracellular potassium and intercellular potassium.

Edema is a common indication of potassium deficiency with swelling of the ankles being a positive sign of low tissue oxidation edema. The cerebellum of the brain is also affected with associated memory loss and poor mental function. Weak bowel peristalsis with associated constipation may also be an indication. Other signs include dry skin, skin eruptions, depression, diminished reflexes, nervousness, insatiable thirst, heart arrhythmias, high cholesterol, insomnia, low blood pressure, muscular fatigue and weakness.

Potassium sources are primarily found in greens, vegetables and whole grains. Because potassium is found on the exterior portion of the grain, when these grains are milled it is lost along with the bran. As with many vitamins and minerals, there is no specific RDA for potassium but at least 2 to 2.5g per day are needed or from 0.8-1.5g per 1,000 calories consumed.

Sulfur

Sulfur is usually found as part of larger compounds and it is readily available in protein foods including meats, fish, poultry, eggs, milk and legumes.

Other foods include onions, garlic and cabbage-family plants. In the body the highest concentrations are in the hair, skin and nails. It was commonly used in the 19th century as Grandma's "Spring Tonic," which consisted mainly of blackstrap molasses. This acted as a mild non-dependent laxative and had the most noticeable effects in making the skin clear. It is a detoxifying agent that combines with more toxic substances, rendering them harmless before excreting them.

Cystine, a disulfide amino acid, comprised of two cysteine molecules, is synthesized in the liver and involved in a number of metabolic pathways. In hair, it combines with methionine to become a form of sulfur accounting for the characteristic smell when hair or feathers are burned. Cystine is part of other important bodily chemicals including insulin for carbohydrate metabolism, and heparin, which acts as an anticoagulant.

Taurine, another lesser-known amino acid produced from sulfur-containing cysteine is responsible for active electric transmission to the brain and heart and to help stabilize cell membranes. Taurine has a variety of other duties and functions as an antioxidant and detoxifying agent and will be discussed at length later. Sulfur is also important for cellular respiration, helping the utilization of oxygen in the cells.

The Trace Minerals

There are numerous trace minerals including iron, zinc, copper, selenium, chromium, iodine, manganese, cobalt, arsenic, boron, molybdenum, nickel, silicon, vanadium, cadmium, lead, lithium, bromine, fluorine and tin. Of these lead and cadmium are poisonous in excess amounts.

Most of these must be taken only in small amounts, as larger amounts are toxic. Trace minerals are found in whole grains and deep-rooted vegetables and herbs. Their presence in food depends on the condition of the soil.

Manganese

The word manganese is derived from the ancient Greek word for magic because of its seemingly magical healing properties. It is essential for growth, reproduction, wound healing, brain function, and sugar metabolism, insulin and cholesterol regulation. As such, it has a place in the treatment of a number of diseases including diabetes, heart disease, rheumatoid arthritis, osteoporosis, cataracts and epilepsy. It has a special function in the treatment of cancer because it is required to form SOD (superoxide dismutase), an enzyme that protects the cells of the body from free radical damage. It can also counterbalance the negative effects of excess iron. Manganese is best absorbed when it is taken with zinc at the dose of approximately 35 mg with 100 mg of zinc.

Iron

Iron is the most well known of all the trace minerals. There is approximately 4g, or a tenth of a teaspoon, of iron in an average 150 lb. individual. As the active component of hemoglobin, it is essential for carrying oxygen throughout the body and carrying carbon dioxide back to be exhaled through the lungs. Therefore, iron is essential for the vitality and energy based on healthy red blood cells. It is also important for certain enzyme functions as well.

Iron is especially needed during growth, pregnancy, lactation, for blood loss and for menstruating women. It is found in a wide variety of foods and is abundantly available from red grapes, red meat, blackstrap molasses and sea vegetables to name a few sources. Iron requires sufficient hydrochloric acid, citrus fruits, vegetables, copper, cobalt and manganese for absorption. One simple way to obtain iron is to cook at least some foods in iron cookware. It is decreased with low hydrochloric acid, antacids, calcium, the phytates of grains, oxalates in leafy vegetables, soy protein, coffee and black tea. The approximate required daily amount of iron is different for men than it is for women and growing teenagers. This is because of the monthly blood loss of women and the accelerated growth rate of teenagers. Vitamin C also improves one's uptake and utilization of iron. There is also a problem from taking too much iron as it causes hemosiderosis, a disease caused by an excess of iron deposited in the liver and tissues of the body.

As stated, women and vegetarians are more prone to symptoms of iron deficiency anemia. I have personally found many who, by traditional Chinese diagnostic indications appear as blood deficient or anemic; however, this is not corroborated with laboratory blood tests. By giving them a diet with sufficient animal protein, bone marrow soup broth and an herbal blood tonic formula frequently containing the herb dong gui (*angelica sinensis*) the symptoms of anemia eventually were resolved. Standard blood tests may quantify the number of red blood cells in the blood but issues such as how the body utilizes blood nutrients may not show up in a routine blood test for anemia.

Iron supplements commonly recommended by medical doctors for anemia may not help in treating the anemia and further contribute to the formation of free radicals. Cancer cells can benefit from excess blood iron because it will bind with oxygen free radicals and assist their circulation.

Natural sources of iron that will not create excess include kelp, seaweed, brewer's yeast, wheat bran, sesame and pumpkin seeds, leafy green vegetables, wheat germ, liver and red meat. Yellow Dock root (*Rumex crispus*) actually contains little iron but works to release iron from the liver. Syrup of blackstrap molasses, kelp and yellow dock makes an excellent iron tonic if needed.

The RDAs for iron vary according to age, gender and growth cycle. The average adult male requires about 10 mg daily while the average adult woman and teenager is around 18 mg. Pregnant and lactating women require from 45-60 mg of iron. The propensity for taking too much iron as part of one's diet is negligible so that one probably should not take a multi-supplement with iron. If it is needed then one should take a separate supplement.

Lactoferrin deficiency and iron malabsorption

Lactoferrin is an iron-binding protein used to assimilate iron and then carry it to whatever areas of the body it is needed. Lactoferrin binds to circulating iron, which in turn is used by bacteria for its proliferation. Often anemia is caused not so much as a result of a lack of iron in the diet, but by poor assimilation and utilization of iron.

Many people have a condition of poor iron assimilation based on a deficiency of lactoferrin. Taking this together with B 12 and folic acid will help in the overall assimilation of iron. For anemic individuals, about 4 capsules should be taken before retiring each night.

Zinc

Zinc has become one of the more important trace minerals because of its well-known positive effects on the immune system as well as wound healing. Thus, this trace mineral is essential for patients who are recovering from surgery, radiation or chemotherapy. Zinc plays a pivotal role in increasing T-cell and Natural Killer cells vital to the immune system. Because people with cancer have problems with sugar metabolism, zinc is needed to help utilize increased insulin demands. Zinc supplements are generally taken between meals to facilitate their better absorption.

It is a controversial issue whether one should take zinc with the metal-based chemotherapeutic drugs, cisplatin and carboplatin. According to Ralph Moss, this seems to be largely hypothetical and in fact a number of studies thus far have generally not supported this thesis and have even demonstrated the opposite.[6] However, Moss goes on to say that it is better to err against caution and avoid zinc supplements while taking either cisplatin or carboplatin.

In general zinc should be taken at a different time from other supplements and not with meals. A number of foods including dairy, soy and whole wheat may interfere with its absorption.

Foods that are high in zinc include: whole grains, nuts, shellfish (especially oysters), split peas, lima beans, anchovies, sardines, egg yolk, turnips and potatoes. The RDA for zinc in adults is approximately 15 mg. Pregnant or lactating women typically require higher amounts of up to 25 or 30 mgs.

---

[6] Moss, Ralph, *Herbs Against Cancer*, pub. Equinox Press, 2000

Iodine

Low iodine intake is endemic throughout the western world. As a result one of the most common conditions associated with this deficiency is low-thyroidism or hypothyroid. Because the thyroid is the master gland regulating and controlling metabolism throughout the body, low thyroid function is often associated with a variety of other 'hypo' conditions such as low adrenal function, hormonal imbalances (including low estrogen) and so forth. Because of this, there is an association between low thyroid and an increased risk of female reproductive cancers including cancers of the breast, cervix, ovaries and endometrium.

Laboratory thyroid tests often fail to indicate low thyroid, causing a subclinical condition that is only determined by various clinical signs. These include low basal metabolism temperature, coldness, dryness of the skin and hair, low energy, hormone imbalances, mood swings, pear-shaped body.

While iodine in salt certainly attends to the clinical signs of low thyroid, the fact that the salt is refined, devoid of associated minerals and only contains a minimal amount of iodine may only serve to mask the clinical manifestations (based on lab tests) of low thyroid. Traditional people around the world have learned to include daily amounts of various edible seaweeds as part of their diet. Many in western countries do not normally include sea vegetables as part of their daily diet. For these it must become an acquired taste. However, adding sea vegetables to soups and various dishes can make a wonderfully savory and delicious adjunct to soups and other dishes. Some forms of seaweed can be soaked and added to salads. I regularly add about a 4-inch piece of kombu (kelp) when presoaking beans. I then cook the kelp and beans together. So far, no one has been able to detect that the kelp adversely affected the familiar flavor of beans. I also add a variety of seaweeds such as Japanese wakame (one of the seaweeds with the greatest cancer inhibiting potential) to soup stocks for other purposes and of course to traditional miso soups.

Only seaweeds from unpolluted ocean sources should be used. One that I most commonly recommend is a capsule of a hand-harvested seaweed supplement called Ocean Herbs. I also use kelp tablets from Japan and recommend two or three doses daily of either of these.

Western herbalists had a wide range of indications and uses for kelp seaweed or potassium iodide. These include any type of glandular swelling, enlarged spleen, liver, lymph glands and, of course, goiter. Potassium iodide is traditionally included in the Hoxsey herbal formula used as a blood purifier for the treatment of cancer.

The psychic mystic of the early part of the 20th century, Edgar Cayce, is one whose gifts were genuine. The many treatments and remedies he arrived at have been studied and confirmed for their safety and efficacy and found to be valid. One common recommendation he gave for individuals complaining of enlarged glands, tonsillitis, fibrocystic breast disease, fibroid tumors, ovarian congestion and pain is a potassium iodide preparation sold as Atomidine. The dosage is 1 to 6 drops daily.

Measuring and averaging basal metabolic temperature over a period of several days is one way to determine high or low thyroid and thus monitor iodine dosage.

To measure basal metabolic temperature, place a thermometer under the armpit first thing upon awakening and without stirring each day. The basic temperature should measure 97.6 on the average. A higher or lower temperature is indicative of thyroid function. If it is higher, it indicates a hyperthyroid condition for which combinations of seaweeds are taken with anti-inflammatory herbs such as barberry root, dandelion root and/or bugleweed. A subnormal temperature indicates a low thyroid condition. For this one may consider a Chinese warming, yang tonic such as Zhen Wu Tang, also known as True Warrior Decoction. However, gradually increasing the number of daily drops of Atomidine to as much as 6 drops daily may be effective as well.

Other natural sources of potassium iodide include eggs (providing they are from free range hens), apricots and one of the most potent of all, blackstrap molasses.

Copper

Copper is important for many functions, but especially to make hemoglobin. Found in most enzymes, copper plays an important role in superoxide dismutase (SOD), an important oxygen-free radical metabolism and in this way it exhibits mild anti-inflammatory properties. Like other metals in the body, copper is important as an electricity conductor and thereby has an important effect on the nerves. Both copper and zinc are important for converting T3 to T4 for normal thyroid function. Being part of the anti-histamine enzyme, histaminase, copper is also involved in neutralizing histamine in the body.

A deficiency of copper results in several deficiencies including anemia, fatigue, and labored respiration because of impaired oxygen delivery to the cells. It also causes a weakening of the immune system due to lowered white blood cell count and possibly impaired thymus hormone production. A high level of Vitamin C and zinc decreases copper absorption so that those taking these supplements should supplement copper at a different time. When taking zinc one should always supplement copper at the ratio of 15-30 mg zinc to 2 mg copper. Copper is found in whole grains, especially buckwheat, liver, other organ meats, legumes, nuts and shellfish. Like zinc, copper is especially high in oysters.

A word of caution, while a deficiency of copper is not good, excess has been associated as a nutrient used by cancer during the metastatic process.

Selenium

If there is one mineral that is important for cancer patients to take, it is selenium. The primary function of selenium is to convert the hydrogen free radical to harmless water. Studies have shown that there are lower levels of this mineral in cancer patients and that in areas where the selenium level is high in the soil, there are fewer cancer deaths.[20] Animal studies have shown that selenium specifically inhibits and slows the growth of tumors and that it has a directly toxic effect on tumors. Its antioxidant and immuno-stimulating effects are similar, though not exactly the same, as Vitamin E, both having anti-aging and longevity effects and generally working to protect the cell membranes.

An experiment to find whether increased selenium intake would prevent skin cancers was conducted at the University of Arizona under the direction of Dr. Larry Clark and his colleagues. Over a thousand people of advanced age who were previously at risk for skin cancers were prescribed 200 mcg of selenium daily over a period of ten years. Interestingly, they found no affect on the incidence of skin cancer, but there was a 37% drop in other life-threatening cancers and a 50% reduction of deaths from cancer generally. Other statistics showed 46% fewer lung cancers, 67% fewer esophageal cancers, 62% fewer colon cancers and 72% reduction of prostate cancers.[21]

Other studies have found that the combination of beta-carotene, Vitamin E and selenium, all among the most potent antioxidants, were responsible for significantly fewer cancers, deaths from cancer and strokes.

Selenium given to rectal cancer patients in conjunction with the chemotherapeutic drug, 5-FU and radiation exhibited a protective effect on overall quality of life.[22] Other studies involving the use of the chemotherapeutic drug cisplatin, found that selenium had not affected the anticancer effect of the drug.[23] As previously mentioned, selenium is a vital cofactor for the production of glutathione peroxidase, the most important enzyme for the body's defense against free radicals.

Normal supplementation should be about 200 mcg per day. In order to get that much selenium in one's diet it is necessary to consume the equivalent of about two acres of parsley daily. It is important for cancer patients to supplement this mineral. However, an excessive dosage of selenium can be toxic, thus the safest and best levels of supplementation for cancer patients are around 700 mcg daily. Sources include brazil nuts (the most concentrated source of selenium), swordfish, salmon, tuna, lobster, shellfish, sunflower seeds, barley, brown rice, Swiss chard, broccoli, garlic, onions, mushrooms and brewer's yeast.

Molybdenum

This trace mineral helps in the detoxification of carcinogenic chemicals from the body. It was found to inhibit cancers in rats with esophageal cancers.[24] In China it was shown that a molybdenum deficiency in the soil was responsible for the highest known incidence of esophageal cancer. Whole grains, many vegetables and legumes are good sources of molybdenum so long as it is present in the soil. It is mostly useful for cancer prevention. The RDA is not known, but in general 150-500 mcg is acceptable for adults, while 50-300 mcg is acceptable for children.

Chromium

Chromium, once considered a toxic mineral, was found in 1957 to be the most essential part of glucose tolerant factor (GTF). Both GTF and chromium are vital to the metabolism of carbohydrates and in the regulation of sugar and insulin levels in the blood. Besides altering protein metabolism to suits its needs, cancer also alters the metabolism of carbohydrates causing high blood glucose levels. By helping to stabilize blood glucose levels, chromium in the diet inhibits the utilization of sugar as fuel for developing cancer cells.

Of all the food sources of GTF chromium, brewer's yeast is the highest. Other good sources include whole grains, shellfish, chicken, wheat germ, bran and many different vegetables, especially potato skins, as well as beets and mushrooms. Because only about 2 percent of what we ingest is absorbed, a safe supplementation range is between 200-300 mcg for adults with children taking somewhat less accordingly.

Vitamin and mineral supplementation for cancer patients

In general, I recommend that all cancer patients take a good quality multi-Vitamin such as Source Natural's Mega-Vite 85 or Ultra Multiple or Rainbow Light's food based Advanced Nutritional System. These supplements will supply a basic supply of Vitamin and mineral supplementation for general purposes. In addition, I would supplementally add selenium and a good seaweed supplement such as kelp tablets. I use Katsu Chewable Kelp Root Tablets distributed by Kenshin Trading Company (Torrance, California) or Kelp tablets by Thompson Nutritional Products.

I would also add supplemental Vitamin E, C and selenium, which is usually not present in therapeutic amounts for cancer patients in a multiple Vitamin and mineral compound.

Free Radicals and Antioxidants

Free radicals

Free radicals are molecules that have become destabilized with an odd number of electrons. This causes them to behave erratically and multiply by seeking out and robbing electrons from healthy nearby molecules as they spread their destructive influence with the ongoing creation of new free radicals. Interestingly, when in balance free radicals also play a positive oxidative role that help to kill invading pathogens and thereby prevent inflammation. Negatively, however, free radicals are implicated as one of the most common causes of aging, degenerative diseases, including heart disease, arthritis, cancer and immune deficiency diseases. According to an article in the *New York Times*, April 28, 1988, "Free oxygen radicals, the main type formed in living organisms, have been implicated in more than 60 disorders, including heart disease, cancer, Alzheimer's disease, cataracts and rheumatoid arthritis."

Free radicals are created as a result of a number of damaging stress factors including exposure to radiation, chemical injury, aging, death of bodily microbes, inflammatory damage, tumor destruction and as common physical and emotional stress. In fact, our bodies cannot live without free radicals since they help in the destruction of various pathogens. The problem comes from the amount of free radical exposure that can overwhelm the body's natural control mechanisms to cause a destructive chain reaction. This adversely affects lipids, carbohydrates and proteins, but especially cellular membranes and DNA, which in turn set the stage for a wide variety of adverse conditions. These may range from aging to various chronic degenerative diseases, including cancer, heart disease and arthritis. In terms of their ability to cause cancer, free radicals are implicated and involved in every stage of the complex disease known as cancer from its initiation phase to all further stages of growth and proliferation. Following is an outline of how free radicals cause cancer:

1. Free radicals damage DNA that initiates and causes cell mutations which, if allowed to go unchecked, develop into cancer.
2. Free radicals activate cancer genes called oncogenes.
3. Free radicals suppress the immune system, incapacitating the body's defenses against cancer.
4. Free radicals activate carcinogens that allow them to initiate the development of cancer.
5. Free radicals can damage cell membranes, inactivating their capacity for cell growth and proliferation.

Antioxidants

Antioxidants consist of a variety of endogenous substances created by the body itself, or taken in the form of various nutrients, such as Vitamins A, C, E, the family of antioxidant carotenoids, flavonoids from fruits and vegetables, enzymes such as Coenzyme Q-10 and alpha-lipoic acid and various enzymes created by the body specifically to fight and control free radicals including the enzymes catalase and glutathione peroxidase. In addition, the mineral selenium is also needed for the body to form glutathione.

Professor Bruce Ames Ph.D., of the University of California at Berkeley estimates that every cell of the body endures about 10,000 free radical hits each day with much of it being to the DNA or the body's genetic material. The older we get the more frequently do cell mutations occur. Indeed it is clearly understood that free radicals are implicated in all stages of the aging process and that their control is one of the primary keys to longevity. For instance, the accumulation of wrinkles, thickening of the skin and the small skin tags that accumulate as many age are actually the result of cell mutations from accumulated free radical damage. We often notice the thickening and wrinkling of the skin associated with smokers and drinkers and the development of varicosities and so many other changes that are all associated with free radical damage. It is hard to believe, but over an average seventy-year period it is estimated that the body produces approximately 70 tons of free radicals. Because excessive amounts of physical exercise also causes free radical damage leading to a variety of age related conditions, it is imperative that athletes and those who indulge in a great deal of physical stress add antioxidant supplements to their diet.

While free radicals are able to damage all substances and tissues of the body, those that are most commonly affected are fats. The reason is because fats are most prone to peroxidation. Lipid peroxidation sets off a chain reaction of free radical proliferation that continues throughout the fatty material of the body until it is stopped by an antioxidant. This is one of the reasons the intake of fats, especially saturated and/or transfats that tend to accumulate in the body, is linked to the development of arteriosclerosis as a result of lipid buildup in the veins and arteries and the development of breast cancer. Free radicals can also damage proteins, which sets up the various benign mutations described above. However, they can also cause malignant mutations that lead to cancer.

"Antioxidant" as a term was first used in the 1920's and it designated any substance that counteracts the effects of radiation. The damaging effects of oxidation might manifest as rust on metal, rancidity of oils and the degradation of stored foods to the adverse effects of stress, injury, disease and environmental toxins on living organisms. In fact, oxidation is implicated as a major initiating component for all degenerative diseases including the process of aging.

Any substance that is adversely affected by exposure to oxygen is liable to oxidation or free radical damage. Damaged cells utilize more oxygen in the body, which in turn naturally convert to the free radical hydrogen peroxide. The build up of hydrogen peroxide is capable of causing extensive cell damage if it is not naturally converted to water, for the mineral selenium is needed.

There are two parts to antioxidants: (1) enzymes and substances created by the body that serve as endogenous antioxidants, and (2) nutrients that directly exert antioxidant function or are necessary for the body's production of endogenous antioxidants. In terms of endogenous free radical control, we must look to the body's own process that involves superoxide dismutase (SOD), catalase and glutathione.

The free radical superoxide dismutase is formed as part of cellular respiration by the mitochondria. In other words, it is a natural byproduct of their normal consumption of oxygen and water. Superoxide dismutase (SOD) converts into hydrogen peroxide and this in turn is converted to water by the enzymes, catalase and glutathione peroxidase (an enzyme dependent upon the presence of selenium). This forms glutathione, an enzyme found in many foods. When combined with the amino acid N-acetyl cysteine, it increases the levels of glutathione peroxidase. This enzyme is used to counteract free radicals in the liver, lungs, heart and blood before they can cause damage.

As just stated, superoxide dismutase (SOD) is used to prevent damage by the superoxide free radical. If this radical is not deactivated by SOD into its peroxide form, it further degenerates to the most deadly hydroxyl radical. In order for SOD to work in the mitochondria, it requires manganese. It also requires copper and zinc to work in the cytoplasm. Catalase, requiring the presence of iron, completes the reaction of SOD by converting peroxide into oxygen and water.

Glutathione peroxidase has many other benefits for the treatment of cancer including its ability to promote DNA repair, the activation of T-lymphocytes and a variety of other properties that are favorable to combating cancer. It has a special effect in deactivating free radicals of cells of the liver, lungs, heart and blood. When oxygen free radicals attack the unsaturated fatty acids of cell membranes, the cell membrane becomes more permeable. This in turn leads to a mineral imbalance of calcium, magnesium, sodium and potassium. Glutathione requires the presence of selenium, Vitamin B2 (Riboflavin) and Vitamins C and E to maximize its cancer preventing properties.

By recommending a diet that includes five portions of fruits and vegetables daily, the National Cancer institute (NCI) has acknowledged the power of antioxidants for the prevention of cancer. Of course, this may not reflect the vitally important aspect of food quality based upon whether it is organic, grown on mineral-rich soil, or nutrient altered and/or deprived by being grown with the use of synthetic fertilizers, herbicides, pesticides or through genetic modification.

Few people are able to achieve more than two or three servings of fresh fruits and vegetables per day, and those that are most often deprived are children. The fact that there are so many environmental causes that generate free radical damage every day, which account for up to 70% of all cancers,[25] suggests that antioxidant-rich foods and supplements may afford the greatest margin of cancer protection that we have.

For those who have cancer, the use of antioxidants in conjunction with conventional cancer therapies such as surgery, radiation and chemotherapy has been found to play a vital role in minimizing damage to the blood, bone marrow, immune system, liver and other vital organs. It has also reduced various distressing side effects such as mouth sores and hair loss. In a surprising number of instances, solid research has confirmed that certain antioxidants are actually able to enhance the effects of conventional therapies.

While the evidence as to the direct curative powers of antioxidants against cancer remains largely inconclusive, increasing numbers of studies, mostly on in-vitro cancer cells and in live animals such as mice and rats but also in increasing numbers of human studies are showing compelling evidence for using antioxidants when treating cancer.

Superoxide dismutase naturally occurs in barley grass, broccoli, brussels sprouts, cabbage and wheat grass. In addition, many herbs have powerful antioxidant properties including garlic, milk thistle, turmeric and the various medicinal mushrooms such as reishi mushrooms as well as a wide variety of fruits and vegetables, wheat and barley grass, dark green leafy vegetables, berries, grape seed extract, ginkgo and green tea. Many vitamins and minerals previously discussed also serve as antioxidants

Usually these are taken with the addition of a few of the specific antioxidants discussed below such as lipoic acid, N-acetyl cysteine (NAC) and glutathione even though this latter antioxidant is poorly absorbed orally.

Both superoxide dismutase and catalase are supplementally available. When taking superoxide dismutase, be sure it is enteric coated so that it passes through the stomach to be directly absorbed in the small intestine.

Glutathione

Glutathione (GSH) is a complex tripeptide enzyme consisting of three amino acids found in almost every cell of the body. Glutathione-S-transferase (GST) is a family of protein enzymes active in Phase II detoxification. N-Acetyl cysteine is a precursor of GST. Glutathione peroxides is the oxidized form of glutathione.

Glutathione is an antioxidant molecule naturally produced by the body and is undoubtedly the most important antioxidant. It functions as an enzyme working with the liver and the lungs to help detoxify the body both intracellularly and extracellularly.

It is a well-known fact that glutathione levels tend to diminish with age. By the age of forty it is estimated that there is as much as a 20 to 30% decline in glutathione levels. By the age of 65, half of all people show a deficiency of glutathione, which is considered by many to have a direct correlation with all age related diseases, including cancer. Further, any stressful disease such as cancer as well as chemo and radiation therapy depletes the body's store of glutathione.

Glutathione works by directly neutralizing the hydrogen peroxide in lipids and through an amazing process of reconverting the hydroxyl radical to water and finally back into glutathione itself. The fact that this process is potentially available to every cell of the body makes glutathione the most powerful of all antioxidants.

As a cancer fighter, glutathione helps neutralize and detoxify the body's exposure to carcinogenic chemicals that can have a cumulative effect over time. It can repair what is often regarded as non-repairable damage to cells, protecting the mitochondria and regulating normal DNA replication. One 1996 study found that glutathione was superior to 5-FU, a popular chemotherapeutic drug, in inducing apoptosis (cell death) in various cancer cells, including small cell carcinoma, colon carcinoma, neuroblastoma, mammary carcinoma and leukemia.[26]

Strangely, there seems to be a higher concentration of glutathione in cancer cells as opposed to normal cells. This serves to protect the cancer cells from attack, especially from the poisons of chemotherapy (which also leaves the normal cells with less glutathione and, therefore, more open to attack).

This has led to the popular misconception that the use of antioxidants may conflict with the efficacy of chemo and radiation therapy. In fact, the opposite is true. An Italian study used 2,500 mgs of chemo and radiation therapy in combination with the chemotherapeutic drugs, cisplatin and cyclophosphamide on 20 women diagnosed with advanced ovarian cancer. The favorable response rate was 55%, leading to the conclusion that glutathione had no negative impact on the intended use of these drugs. Further, their therapeutic results were significantly improved with the use of glutathione.[27] In fact, the opposite is true. When we feed the body what it needs to create glutathione it will boost the total amount of glutathione needed by the body and the imbalance seems to resolve itself.

An important study quoted in Donald Yance's book involved the use of glutathione together with cisplatin, another popular chemotherapeutic drug, for the treatment of ovarian cancer. It revealed that women receiving glutathione experienced significant benefit in the most common symptoms associated with the drug depression, nausea, peripheral neuropathy, hair loss, indigestion and shortness of breath. It was further found that concurrently taking glutathione with cisplatin allowed for a higher safe dose of the drug, thus improving its efficacy.[28]

Ultimately glutathione needs to be made by the cell itself because it cannot be absorbed by the body intact. In order to do this, we must give the body what it needs to synthesize its own glutathione. This includes glycine and glutamic acid, which are commonly available. However, the limiting factor is cysteine. First off, cysteine is an amino acid rarely found in foods and secondly, any direct intake of cysteine is toxic. However, cystine is a compound commonly found in milk whey. It consists of two molecules of cysteine, which are bound together by a disulfide bond. When this enters the cell, the bond breaks so that the cysteine in the cell can combine with other elements to form glutathione.

Immunocal™ is a whey protein that simulates the protein in human milk and provides effective quantities of cellular cysteine for the production of glutathione. Taking a combination of N-acetylcysteine (NAC), lipoic acid, selenium and Vitamins C and E together will also effectively raise glutathione levels.

Lipoic acid

Lipoic acid (alpha-lipoic acid, or ALA) is an antioxidant amino acid beneficial for the whole body, especially the liver. It is a powerful detoxifier able to neutralize toxic metals in the body such as lead, mercury and cadmium. Copper and iron are essential minerals for the body, but in excess they generate free radicals. Lipoic acid neutralizes these through a binding process called chelation.

The buildup of lactic and pyruvic acid in the tissues comes about with increased oxidative stress associated with physical and emotional stress. This can promote tumor growth and metastasis. Lipoic acid, as part of its detoxifying properties, has been found to be useful in reducing the build up of lactic and pyruvic acid.

Lipoic acid also acts as a coenzyme for the production of energy. It generally improves metabolism while it protects the body from harmful oxidative stress that leads to the development of free radical damage.

German research has found that lipoic acid activates the immune system by stimulating T-cells, preventing oncogene activation and regenerating glutathione.[29] It is able to function anywhere in the body because it is both water and fat-soluble, making it known as the 'universal antioxidant.' Because of these considerations it is considered the ideal anti-aging antioxidant of great value for a wide variety of diseases including diabetes, liver and kidney diseases, retinal disease, cataract, peripheral nerve and heart damage, artherosclerosis and, of course, cancer. Taken with glutathione it has potent detoxifying, antioxidant, cell protecting properties and as such should be routinely taken prophylactically with chemo or radiation therapy.

European studies have found lipoic acid to be an even more effective liver protector than milk thistle seeds for individuals exposed to deadly amanita mushroom poisoning. For all types of hepatitis and liver cirrhosis, as well as the many drugs that are known to damage the liver, lipoic acid has been able to greatly assist in the regeneration of liver cells and the normalization of liver enzymes. Both for diabetic neuropathies as well as chemo or radiation-induced neuropathies, lipoic acid has been able to reverse damage to nerve cells.

N-Acetyl cysteine

Another naturally occurring amino acid is N-acetyl cysteine (NAC), a sulfur-containing amino acid, which acts as a precursor to the synthesis of glutathione (GSH) in the body. Dietary cystine converts into the more stable cysteine in the cells of the body. Both cysteine and L-cystine are important detoxifiers capable of converting back and forth as needed.

Cysteine is present as alpha-keratin and forms the primary protein of skin, hair and nails. It is also present in collagen and promotes skin elasticity. Being found as part of a number of proteins, it is a component of various digestive enzymes. Vitamin B6 has been shown to be important for the synthesis of cysteine. Again, because glutathione is poorly absorbed orally, the combination of NAC, lipoic acid and Vitamins C and E will raise glutathione more effectively than the use of oral glutathione alone.

NAC is anti-mutagenic, antioxidant and protects the DNA. It protects against extracellular mutagenic hits from both endogenous sources (physical and emotional stress) and exogenous sources (environmental and food), it neutralizes free radical damage and prevents the formation of oncogenes that lead to the development of cancer. As an immune modulator, NAC has been found to increase T-cell lymphocytes, making it useful for the treatment of AIDS. Because NAC has been found to offer a protective effect in the development of oral cancer, it is an important protective nutrient for those who smoke, chew tobacco or drink alcohol.

N-acetyl cysteine is effective in preventing the side effects of chemotherapy and radiation therapy. It increases glutathione in the lungs, kidneys, liver and bone marrow and has an anti-aging effect, as can be seen in its ability to reduce the accumulation of age spots. Like lipoic acid, it has also shown liver-protective effects and has been used as an antidote to acetaminophen overdose (Tylenol). A unique feature is its ability to thin mucus viscosity, making it useful for a number of other conditions involving mucus such as upper respiratory conditions, emphysema, bronchitis, tuberculosis, asthma, sinusitis and otitis media. When combined with lipoic acid, NAC is an even more potent detoxifier for other serious diseases including rheumatoid arthritis. The exception is diabetes because supplemental cysteine can inactivate insulin and individuals with cystinuria, a rare genetic kidney disease, causes cystine kidney stones.

Studies have shown that by increasing plasma glutathione, NAC is uniquely beneficial for the treatment, prevention and recurrence of cancers. Because of its ability to increase glutathione, NAC was found to increase the antitumor effects of IL (interleukin)-2 making it a useful antitumor adjunct.[30]

Glutamine

Being the most common and abundant blood amino acid, glutamine has many important functions, primary of which is maintaining the immune system, preventing muscle atrophy and healing gastrointestinal ulcers. It is an essential amino acid for people who are undergoing periods of stress and injury that may adversely affect stomach and intestinal function. Therefore it is prescribed to patients who are recovering from surgery or are experiencing severe weight loss and gastrointestinal and immunological side affects associated with chemo and radiation therapy.

Most remedies that are intended for digestion work better as a powder and it is no different with L-glutamine for which 1 to 2 teaspoons can be given daily. Many foods contain glutamine, such as spinach and parsley, but it is easily destroyed with cooking. Individuals with cirrhosis of the liver, kidney problems, Reye's syndrome or any condition indicating an accumulation of ammonia in the blood should not take glutamine as it can cause further damage.[31] Finally, one should be aware that there are a number of substances with similar names, such as glutamine, glutamic acid, glutathione, gluten and monosodium glutamate, but these are all very different substances.

Calcium D-glucarate (CDG)

Glucoronidation is part of the process that the body uses to detoxify estrogen, xenohormones from foods, fat-soluble toxins and other stress hormones through the liver. When these hormones enter the liver, they bind with glucuronic acid before being passed out through the bile into the stool. CDG is a calcium salt of D-glucaric acid, used as part of glucoronidation and is naturally found in many animals and plants. This supplement is valuable to help reduce serum estrogen which aids in the prevention and treatment of breast cancer and other cancers that are hormone driven. The recommended dose is 2-4 500 mg capsules, two or three times daily.

Taurine

Taurine is found in high concentrations in the heart muscle, white blood cells, skeletal muscles and the brain. It is a key component of all other amino acids as well as bile. As such, it is needed for the digestion of fats, the absorption of fat-soluble Vitamins and for the control of serum cholesterol. Taurine is also useful for hypertension and to reduce cholesterol levels in the blood. As a constituent of bile acids, it forms tauracholate, which helps eliminate cholesterol in the bile. This makes it a well-established supplement for cardiovascular disease that should be taken with Vitamin E, omega 3 fatty acids and Coenzyme Q-10. For hypertension one should also take magnesium as well. People with congestive heart failure are treated with 5-6g of taurine which are taken daily in three divided doses, while congestive heart disease has responded with as little as 2g daily.

Taurine can function as an inhibitory neurotransmitter and has a protective effect on the brain and is useful for anxiety, epilepsy, hyperactivity, impaired brain function and seizures. It may be of benefit to children with Down's syndrome and muscular dystrophy. Taken with magnesium, it helps reduce the side effects of Dilantin given to patients suffering from brain tumors. For this effect the dose is approximately 500 mg three times daily.

Taurine is also important in liver function, being a component of bile. Finally, Taurine helps regulate glycogen synthesis and maintain proper levels of blood glucose making it useful for diabetes.

Lower levels of Taurine are often associated with patients undergoing chemotherapy. Though not an amino acid, it plays a role in clearing free radicals by assisting the body's ability to produce glutathione.

Coenzyme Q10 (CoQ10)

Because of its ability to remove toxic material from the body at a rapid rate, CoQ10 has been shown in both human and animal studies to be very effective for aiding tumor regression. It is also extremely valuable for patients undergoing chemo and radiation therapy. Cancer patients who are on the drug Adriamycin should especially take Taurine with CoQ10, since the latter drug is known to cause heart damage.

The daily recommended dosage of CoQ10 is 30-400 mg. It is best absorbed when taken after meals with fat such as EPA rich Eskimo Oil made by Tyler Encapsulations.

Ellagic acid

Ellagic acid is a plant polyphenol derived from berries including strawberries, raspberries, grapes, black currants and walnuts. It has both antimutagenic and anticarcinogenic properties. Besides lycopene from tomatoes, researchers found that strawberries were also effective in inhibiting and preventing prostate cancer. Various studies on rodents have found it to be effective for cancer of the lung, liver, skin and esophagus. It inhibits certain enzymes that tend to liberate unstable elements from chemicals, which in turn promote cancer. It also stimulates glutathione and other detoxification enzymes. Ellagic acid is further understood to protect the DNA and prevent mutations.

Various studies, mostly on lab animals, has substantiated ellagic acid's ability to protect the liver and the body generally from exposure to carcinogenic chemicals, from tobacco smoke, carbon tetrachloride and aflatoxins from rancid peanuts and corn. Ellagic acid is one of the more promising newer antioxidants on the market. As a supplement, the dose will be dependent on the indications of the manufacturer.

Flavonoids

Some traditional herbal systems classify the properties of plants and vegetables by their color. In fact, flavonoids, one of the most common constituents of plants responsible for their brilliant coloring, have been found to possess potent therapeutic value. Flavonoids have been found to be anti-inflammatory, antiallergenic, antibacterial, antiviral, antifungal and anticarcinogenic. Flavonoids act as plant antioxidants and are found in a wide variety of fruits, vegetables and herbs. Some of the best-known sources of flavonoids include grapes, blueberries and other berries, cherries, buckwheat, rose hips, hawthorn berries, ligustrum berries, the white pulp of citrus fruit, apricots, peaches, plums, black currants, green tea, soya and other beans and legumes, and various types of peppers.

Various phytochemicals found in plants and herbs have many ways to offset cancer. First, they stimulate the vital processes of detoxification in the body that eliminate carcinogenic factors; secondly, they powerfully stimulate and strengthen the body's immune system which help it to inactivate, fight and destroy cancer cells; and thirdly, many herbs have free radical scavenging properties. There are literally thousands of herbs that are known to have therapeutic value, but less than 1% of them have been researched.

Flavonoids include the following:

- Anthocyanins – these account for the red-blue pigments of grapes, plums, cherries and berries.
- Anthochlors – these are yellow and found primarily in flowers such as calendula, dandelion flowers and chamomile.
- The minor flavonoids – these include catechin and epigallocatechin,

which are present in green tea and the pycnogenols found in grape seed and pine bark.

- Flavones and flavonols – these include quercetin, a flavone found in the onion family including garlic, the brassica family including arugula, broccoli, brussels sprouts, cabbage and blue green algae.

- Isoflavonoids – these are primarily found in legumes including genistein found in soya and other beans.

- Tannins – these include proanthocyanidins, anthocyanides and galic acid phenolics (which is responsible for the health benefits of red wine). PCO's or pycnogenol from white pine bark and grape seeds are also in this category.

Pycnogenol

One of the most powerful plant derived free radicals is pycnogenol (OPC's) derived in large amounts in both pine bark and to a lesser extent from grape seeds. Pycnogenols derived from pine bark and grape seeds are a primary anti-inflammatory nutritional treatment for a variety of conditions ranging from sports injuries to recovery from surgery. Yet, tests have found OPC's to be twenty times more effective than Vitamin C and fifty times more effective than Vitamin E as a free radical antioxidant scavenger.

It is recommended that for the prevention and treatment of cancer, grape seeds should be chewed and consumed whenever organic grapes are eaten. In addition, cancer patients should take a high daily dose of pycnogenol that contains 25 mg of pine bark (OPC 85) and 25 mg of grape seed (OPC 85+). In addition, the use of whole grain fiber and citrus pectin has beneficial effects in inhibiting and preventing cancer of the large intestine and prostate.

It certainly would not hurt to chew and eat some of the seeds when we eat organic grapes. In addition, I would recommend cancer patients take a daily high dose of pycnogenol that contains 25 mg of pine bark (OPC 85) and 25 mg of grape seed (OPC 85+).

Quercetin

Quercetin is a bioflavonoid that is found abundantly in the onion and brassica family, cayenne pepper, green tea and in blue-green algae. By lowering cholesterol levels in the blood and making the platelets less sticky quercetin, like pycnogenol, has not only a beneficial effect on the cardiovascular system but it also helps against metastasis by preventing the cancer cell's ability to stick to other tissues and form new tumors. It is valuable in preventing genetically caused cancers by inhibiting the tumor-suppressing gene p53. The mutation or defect in this gene is associated with better than half of all cancers including breast, ovarian and prostate cancers.

Quercetin, like genistein, is derived from the soybeans. It binds to estrogen receptor sites even more effectively than the anti-estrogen drug tamoxifen. These binding sites are present in a number of human cancers including the female reproductive organs and melanoma.[32] Because of these abilities, quercetin inhibits the growth and proliferation of several varieties of human cancers including breast cancer (estrogen-receptor (ER) positive and ER negative forms), ovarian, squamous cell, cervical, bladder, gastric cancers, leukemia and some lymphomas.

Once again, counteracting the misinformation that nutritional supplements and herbs should not be taken with conventional cancer treatment, quercetin enhances the efficacy of chemotherapeutic drugs by blocking the (HSF) factor produced within the cell as a response to various forms of stress such as chemo and radiation therapy. As such quercetin helps reduce the cytotoxic effects of many well-known chemotherapeutic drugs including Adriamycin and Cytoxan.[33,34]

Quercetin, more than any other antioxidant, is well absorbed orally. Donald Yance recommends for maximum assimilation that approximately 1 to 3g be taken with Vitamin C and bromelain in two or three divided doses. Quercetin is also effective as a sublingual powder.

Essential Fatty Acids (EFAs) and Other Fats

Good quality fats are essential for every living cell in the body. Fundamentally necessary for the absorption and utilization of protein, EFA's are essential in helping the manufacture and rebuilding of cells throughout the body. Designated as Omega-3 and Omega-6 fatty acids, these form an important balance with each other necessary for many important life sustaining processes including the production of prostaglandins, which serve as chemical messengers and regulators of various physiological processes. In the prevention and treatment of cancer, the proper balance of EFA's have potent anti-inflammatory properties, detoxify cellular waste associated with cancer and conventional cancer therapies and inhibit the formation of tumors through the immune system and assist the process of metastasis to other areas of the body.

A South African study compared the rate of colon cancer in people living in a small fishing village with that of similar people living in Cape Town. The Cape Town city folk consumed as much as twice the amount of fruit and vegetables that are high in nutrients known to prevent colon cancer – fiber, calcium and antioxidants. However, they had a six times greater incidence of colon cancers than those who lived in the fishing village. Laboratory analysis revealed that the villagers had 3 times more omega-3 fatty acids n their diet with considerably less omega-6 fatty acids. This came as a result of their substantially higher fish intake. In general, the ideal ratio for cancer prevention is a higher relationship of Omega-3's to Omega-6's EFA's, similar to the ratio of people living in Cape town.

In the Mediterranean and Northern European cultures people would normally consume foods such as anchovies, sardines and herring in various forms. In Japan, small dried fish are added to miso soup broth. Besides adding protein and flavor, these foods also contribute to the regular intake of omega-3 fatty acids.

In France, researchers monitored 120 breast cancer patients over a three-year period and found that women who maintained high levels of linolenic acid (LNA) (abundant in flaxseeds and the building blocks of omega-3 fatty-acids) in the tissues of their breasts were better able to prevent the spread of cancers to other tissues. Women with low-level LNA had five times greater propensity towards metastasis to other areas of the body.

One of their most important virtues lies in the ability to prevent the tendency of cancer patients towards cachexia, which is severe weight loss due to protein malabsorption. I routinely recommend cancer patients take the equivalent of 6 to 12g of Omega-3 oils,[7] have 3 or 4 servings of fish weekly. I also recommend that they use 3 tablespoons of freshly ground golden flaxseeds mixed with yogurt to aid in assimilation. Golden Flax seeds are superior in flavor, quality and content of EFA's and are available direct from the Heintzman Farms (1-800-333-5813).

Omega-6 fatty acids including linoleic and gamma-linolenic acids are primarily derived from plant sources such as nuts, seeds, legumes and vegetable oils like sesame and olive oil (actually classified as an Omega-9 fatty acid). Omega-3 fatty acids, including alpha-linolenic and eicosapentaenoic acid (EPA), are found in fresh deep water fish, fish oils and certain vegetable oils such as canola oil, walnut oil and flaxseed oil. In order to be of nutritional value, these oils must be consumed as food or in a liquid form that has not been had not been subjected to heat since heat destroys fatty acids and, worse yet, causes the dangerous creation of free radicals.

By far the best source of omega-3 fatty acids is fish oil. These are derived from salmon, mackerel, herring and sardines, to name a few sources. Flaxseeds are another rich source of Omega-3 fatty acids and, while lower in this respect than fish oils, possess other benefits including being a good source of protein, B Vitamins and zinc. Flaxseeds and flaxseed oil are very beneficial in lowering cholesterol and triglyceride levels in the blood. Because of their propensity towards rancidity, all cold pressed oils should ideally be kept refrigerated. The exceptions are sesame and olive oils that resist rancidity, even unrefrigerated, for a much longer period and therefore have earned a

---

[7] I use Eskimo Oil made by Tyler manufacturing company

place of high esteem in Asian and Mediterranean cultures.

Sources for Omega-6 EFA's are much more common and easily derived from the regular use of olive and sesame oils. Gamma-linolenic acid (GLA) is found in evening primrose and borage seed oils. Studies have substantiated that evening primrose oil is able to increase cellular fluidity and flexibility, which tends not only to prevent metastasis, but also at the same time it increases the efficacy of chemo and radiation therapies.

Both olive and shark liver oils are also rich in squalene, which is known to have potent anti-cancer properties.

Based on the findings of Dr. Johanna Budwig, the combination of any EFA supplement is greatly potentiated with the use of sulfur-rich foods such as low-fat cottage cheese. I also recommend taking these with a garlic supplement because garlic is also high in organic sulfur.

Squalene

Squalene, naturally found in the body primarily in the skin was originally derived from the liver of a rare species of shark. Through a simple chemical process, it has the ability to increase oxygen in the tissues and organs of the body, though it will not alleviate asthma or other upper respiratory conditions. By oxygenating the cells of the body, it is able to impair the development and proliferation of tumors. Another rich source of squalene is olive oil.

It is hypothesized that the heart protective and cancer inhibiting effects of olive oil consumption in Mediterranean countries that consume an otherwise high fat diet is due to the presence of high amounts of squalene naturally found in olive oil.[35] More than 30 percent tumor shrinkage was demonstrated in a laboratory study through the combination of squalene, vitamin E and aloe vera.[36]

Enzymes

Enzymes are substances that act as catalysts, causing and accelerating the innumerable biological reactions that are involved with all of life's processes. Each enzyme has a specific role to play exclusive to a particular function. Digestive enzymes break food down for storage in the liver and muscles. Other enzymes are then used to convert these nutrients as the body needs them. Enzymes are used to concentrate iron in the blood while others are used to coagulate the blood to stop bleeding. Other enzymes are used to assist the lungs, kidneys, liver, colon and skin in the process of detoxification and removal of metabolic wastes. There are also enzymes used to build new tissues such as bone, muscle, skin, nerve and glandular tissues in the body. Enzymes are used to convert phosphorus into bone and to oxidize glucose for the creation of cellular energy. In fact, there is no biological process that is not triggered by a unique enzyme.

Enzymes are of two types: digestive and metabolic. Some of the digestive enzymes include amylase, protease and lipase. Amylase is found in the saliva, pancreatic and intestinal juices for the break down of carbohydrates. Lactase is a specific enzyme which is lacking in some people, especially those of African descent, that is necessary for the digestion of dairy products. Maltase is used to break down malt sugar while sucrase is used for beet sugar. Protease found in the stomach and pancreas is used for protein. Lipase, also found in the stomach and pancreas, is used to break down fats.

Metabolic enzymes catalyze the various reactions within the cells such as the production of energy and the elimination of waste. They are the workers that run the functions of all the body's organs and tissues and each bodily tissue has its own unique enzymes to do the job.

Two enzymes in this chapter have also been previously described. Superoxide-dismutase (SOD) is used as an antioxidant to protect the cells from free radicals. Catalase is responsible for breaking down hydrogen peroxide and releasing oxygen for the body to use.

Food Enzymes

The body manufactures a supply of enzymes that extracts enzymes from living foods. There is a particular feeling of lightness associated with eating raw foods that many associate as an enzyme reaction. However, subjecting foods to temperatures of 118 degrees Fahrenheit or higher will destroy most food enzymes. Sprouts are the richest source of enzymes, but papaya and pineapple are specifically rich in proteolytic enzymes for the digestion of protein. It is these same enzymes that are used as a meat tenderizing salt.

Many foods contain their own enzymes, which allow them to naturally rot and breakdown. Even fat contains lipase that works with the lipase in the pancreas to help break down fat. As previously stated, superoxide dismutase naturally occurs in a variety of foods and is particularly rich in barley grass, wheat grass, the product known as chlorella, broccoli and other cabbage family vegetables.

All of this would suggest that possibly eating only raw foods is, as its adherents proclaim, a panacea for all diseases. This seems especially obvious in light of the claim that the body's innate enzymes diminish with age. To whatever extent this is true or not, there are many other problems associated with digestion and assimilation that occur as a result of overeating raw foods, not least of which is the lack of a specific enzyme for breaking down the cellulose bond that surrounds the cells of most vegetables. The problem is always one of balance. If we are not taking in and/or assimilating the proper balance of protein, carbohydrates, fats and other nutrients for whatever reason, it makes no difference whether a particular food has an abundance of enzymes. It is a particularly good idea to have some raw foods, such as seasonal fruits or a small raw salad, as part of our daily dietary intake of enzymes, yet eating all raw foods creates other metabolic deficiencies that may be more serious in the long run.

There is no question that as we grow older our digestion weakens. Eventually, we assimilate less nutrients from the food we consume, causing deficiencies, which contributes to diseases associated with aging. An alternative is to ensure that supplemental enzymes are part of the dietary protocol of all elderly persons. If untreated, cancer usually degenerates in to cachexia or protein malabsorption, and cancer treated with chemo and radiation therapy severely injures the digestive system causing loss of appetite and severe indigestion. Thus, proteolytic pancreatic enzymes are an extremely valuable protocol for the treatment of cancer.

A good alternative source is Wobenzym™, also called Wobe-Mucos in Germany, where it is manufactured. It is a proteolytic enzyme preparation designed to optimally interact with each other that includes bromelain, chymotrypsin, pancreatin, papain, rutosid, trypsin, serratio-peptase, SOD (superoxide dismutase), amylase, lipase and protease.

Similarly, fermented foods provide abundant enzymes and are easily digested. All traditional cultures include fermented foods as part of their diet. Besides containing beneficial flora to maintain healthy digestion and assimilation, these are the 'live' foods that are rich in enzymes and are known to optimize human longevity. In Japan we find the regular use of miso and other fermented vegetables and in Korea there is 'kim chee' consisting of various fermented vegetables and spices. In Northern Europe, Russia and Siberia there is the tradition of fermented dairy or yogurt. In middle European countries such as Germany fermented cabbage, or sauerkraut, is made. These are only a few of the world's traditions in the use of fermented foods.

Cancer cells produce an abundance of fibrin that they use to insulate themselves from breakdown and dissolution. This is called the glycoprotein shield. Besides assisting in digestion, proteolytic enzymes act like blood-moving herbs to breakdown fibrin, or the glycoprotein shield. Bromelain, derived from pineapple, has been found to break down the glycoprotein shield, and has potent anticancer properties as well.[37] Herbalist Donald Yance, AHG finds the combination of Bromelain (or Wobenzyme), quercetin (which also has an inhibitory effect on the glycoprotein shield) and turmeric to be highly beneficial. The recommended dose for Wobenzyme is 2-4 tablets 3 or 4 times daily and for Bromelain, 1,000 to 6,000 mg.

Glandular Supplements

Thymus Extract

Thymus extract is specifically used to strengthen the immune system by increasing the number and activity of the T-lymphocytes. It is useful for all cancer patients, but especially those whose immune systems have been compromised as a result of chemo and radiation therapy.

Spleen Extract

Spleen extract is often taken together with thymus extract to strengthen the immune system. It is specifically useful when there is a low white blood cell count, exposing one to opportunistic bacterial and/or viral infections.

Desiccated Liver

Beef liver is especially useful for building strong red blood cells, making it very useful for cancer patients who have associated anemia. The liver is the most important organ of detoxification in the body. Gerson therapy used to require patients to consume organic calf liver daily, which is taken uncooked and juiced. This is very hard to obtain and many patients find it difficult to consume. I would recommend anyone with anemia to have a serving of cooked organic calf or pork liver daily. Desiccated liver is dried liver extract and can be used as an alternative to fresh liver. Even more effective are liquid liver capsules. It is easily taken either in powder or tablet form. Only use organic liver products.

Green Drinks

There are a number of green drinks on the market which are important because they are high in Vitamins, minerals, amino acids, enzymes and chlorophyll in a balanced, easily assimilable form. They are usually available as a dried powder extract intended to be mixed with water.

Chlorella

I recommend chlorella to all cancer patients regardless of any other green drink they might use. Chlorella is a small, one-celled algae containing a nucleus and a large amount of chlorophyll. Its protein content is approximately 58% with the balance made up of carbohydrates, all the B Vitamins, Vitamin C and E, amino acids and valuable trace minerals. It has more B12 than liver and a substantial amount of beta-carotene. Because it has a strong cell wall, it requires processing in order to make all of its nutrients available. It is virtually a complete food in itself. It acts as both a powerful nutrient and a detoxifying food.

Green Magma

Green Magma consists of the pure juice of young organically grown barley leaves. Brown rice is added to supply Vitamin B1, nicotinic and linoleic acids. Barley is used therapeutically for all conditions associated with dampness and contains potent anticancer properties. It is also used for other degenerative conditions including arthritis and rheumatic conditions. In this form it is rich in thousands of enzymes along with superoxide dismutase (SOD) that have potent and immediate antioxidant properties.

Probiotics

Lactobacillus Acidophilus

Affirming that the digestive system is the most important function to support in the treatment of cancer, lactobacillus acidophilus is an essential supplement for all cancer patients. Acidophilus bacteria is important to assist in the digestion of proteins, which involve a process in which lactic acid, hydrogen peroxide, enzymes, B Vitamins and antibiotic substances are manufactured. Together these form the basis for healthy digestion, assimilation, elimination, detoxification and for maintaining the immune system. Acidophilus is indicated to reduce high blood lipids, gas, bloating, intestinal and systemic toxicity, constipation and malabsorption. Because acidophilus helps to normalize the intestinal flora, it is an essential supplement for cancer patients and patients undergoing chemo and radiation therapies.

There are a number of good acidophilus products on the market but one with a basic bacterial count of 1 billion acidophilus organisms per gram should be used. Acidophilus will die at high temperatures and should be kept refrigerated and dried. Acidophilus should be taken first thing in the morning and approximately one hour before each meal. Alternatively, fermented foods, mentioned under enzymes, also provide plentiful favorable bacteria.

Lactobacillus Bifidus

This is another 'friendly' intestinal bacteria that has a particular benefit for the assimilation of B Vitamins and liver detoxification. L. Bifidus is considered preferable for children and adults with liver problems.

Miscellaneous Nutritional Supplements

Modified Citrus Pectin

Modified Citrus Pectin (MCP) is made from the peels of citrus. There is considerable research that substantiates its benefit in all stages of cancer by inhibiting metastasis. Carbohydrate lectins are found along the walls of the blood vessels and assist a cancer cell's growth, providing sites on which to adhere. Modified Citrus Pectin specifically binds to these sites and thereby helps keep cancer cells in circulation until they either die or are eliminated.

A 1995 study on mice found that MCP was able to inhibit the spread of prostate cancer to the point where eventually the cancer was eliminated by the immune system altogether.[38] As a result of this and other studies, MCP has deservedly become an established supplement for prostate cancer. However, based on its ability to inhibit the growth and proliferation of cancer cells, it is undoubtedly useful for many other types of cancers as well. The recommended dose is 1 tablespoon mixed with water, vegetable juice or a green drink, three times daily between meals.

Low Temperature Whey Protein

In one sense, cancer can be considered a disease of protein malnutrition. Because the assimilation of protein is a major issue for cancer patients, especially in the advanced stages, whey protein supplementation is of great value. Low temperature whey protein provides high quality, easily assimilated protein rich in immune patenting properties similar to colostrum. Whey is also very beneficial in enhancing the growth of L. acidophilus and L. Bifidus in the intestinal tract while concurrently having antipathogenic properties. Whey protein offers a safe alternative (not substitution) for the use of soya and other legumes as a non-animal source of protein. Like soya and other legumes, whey also possesses potent anticancer properties.

The whey protein powder I use is called Probioplex, made by Metagenics. It consists of lactalbumin, eighteen amino acids, calcium iron-binding protein, various cellular components and other nutrients.

Melatonin

Melatonin is a hormone that is naturally produced by the pineal gland located within the brain. As with other anti-aging hormones, such as human growth hormone (HGH) and dehydroepiandrosterone (DHEA), the body's natural production of melatonin tends to diminish with age. Melatonin is one of the most powerful of all antioxidants, more effective than Vitamin C, Vitamin E or beta-carotene. Because of this, it may play a role in many age-related conditions, including insomnia in the aged, hypertension, cardiovascular problems and cancer. Research seems to indicate that diminishing levels of melatonin may leave the body more vulnerable to the production of free radicals and oxidative damage that is associated with these conditions. Melatonin seems to play a major role in the production of other hormones, including estrogen and testosterone, and at least slows the growth of malignancies. Interestingly, if melatonin is taken in the morning it may speed the growth of tumors while if it is taken at night, it slows them.

The most common understanding of the use of melatonin is that it helps the body keep in sync with the circadian biorhythms, which allow sleep to occur at night. Thus, melatonin is commonly used to help restore the biorhythmic clocks of travelers and to help those who are prone to insomnia.

Sleep serves as a general restorative and is ultimately the way our body repairs itself. Lack of sleep sets up a cascade of deficiencies that ultimately compromises the immune system. This will obviously further the development and proliferation of cancer.

Melatonin, being a hormone, should only be used if there is a sleep related problem. I recommend Source Naturals melatonin, in 3 mg size tablets. Begin with ½ tablet before retiring and slowly increase to 6 mg (two tablets) as needed. Never take melatonin during the day.

DMSO

Dimethylsulfoxide (DMSO) is a by-product of wood pulp used for making paper. It appears as a clear liquid with a mild garlicky odor. It has been shown to be an excellent solvent and degreaser for paint and antifreeze. It is widely used in veterinary medicine externally for the healing of fractures, sprained ankles, pulled muscles, dislocated joints and arthritis where it provides remarkably fast-acting pain relief. It also promotes the immune system.

DMSO is quickly absorbed by osmosis through the capillary walls of the skin. This makes it very useful for a wide variety of conditions, including the treatment of brain and spinal cord damage, arthritis, Down's syndrome, sciatica, keloids, acne, burns, muscular skeletal problems, sports injuries, sinusitis, headaches, skin ulcers, herpes, cataracts and cancer.

Use DMSO in treating cancer whenever it is desirable to carry the properties of herbs and essential oils directly into the skin or blood. For this use, DMSO is mixed with the herbal poultice, fomentation or ointment for the treatment of cancer.

DMSO is usually available from veterinary supply houses.

Hydrazine Sulfate

In the early 1930's Nobel laureate Otto Warburg proposed a theory that cancer lived on anaerobic glycolysis (i.e. fermented sugar) and that chemicals could be used to control their growth. Drawing on Warburg's theories, during the late 1960's and early 1970's Dr. Joseph Gold, M.D., of the Syracuse Cancer Research Institute found that hydrazine sulfate, an ingredient in rocket fuel used during the Second World War, inhibited the growth of leukemia, lymphoma, melanoma and other cancers in rats. This occurred as a process of starving the tumor by cutting off its supply of glucose from the liver. By so doing, it would slow or stop the cancer from consuming the body's innate resources. This in turn would at least slow or stop the relentless progression of wasting known as cachexia, which is variously estimated to be responsible for 40 to 80% of the deaths of all cancer patients.

Cachexia occurs as a result of cancer cell metabolism where cancer cells greedily use glucose as fuel of which the concomitant waste becomes lactic acid. Normally an enzyme in the liver is responsible for breaking down the lactic acid and reconverting it back to glucose. When a patient has cancer, this becomes a vicious auto consumptive cycle where the newly created glucose is in turn taken up and used as fuel for the proliferating cancer cells.

Dr. Gold discovered that hydrazine sulfate was able to block the liver enzyme that converts lactic acid back into glucose. Besides its powerful effects against cachexia, hydrazine sulfate increased appetite, decreased pain, lessened anorexia, inhibited tumor growth and enhanced the cytotoxic effects of chemotherapeutic drugs, including, ironically, various chemotherapeutic drugs[39] with few or no side effects.

Double blind studies conducted in both the US and in Russia substantiated that there is no bone marrow depression and that the side effects of hydrazine sulfate were indeed few and far between and ranged from a mild tingling in the fingers and toes to mild nausea, itching and drowsiness. These were easily remedied when the dosage was lessened and were further obviated by allowing short periodic brakes between courses of treatment.

For maximum effectiveness, treatment protocol using hydrazine sulfate is of great importance. Dr. Gold recommended the following protocol for people who weigh more than 100 lbs.

Begin with one 60 mg capsule once daily for three days taken before breakfast. For the 4th to the 6th days increase the dose by taking 60 mg before breakfast and 60 mg before dinner. From the 7th day on take one 60 mg capsule three times daily before breakfast, lunch and dinner.

For those under 100 lbs. reduce the dosage to 30 mg each time. The effects of hydrazine sulfate are accumulative. Prolonged and sustained treatment without periodic breaks may induce peripheral neuritis, though I have neither seen nor heard of this. To prevent side effects, treatment with hydrazine sulfate should be maintained for 45 days after which a break of one to two weeks is advised before resuming.

Hydrazine sulfate is a very useful adjunct for cancer and according to Dr. Ross Pelton, "very effective against solid tumors,"[8] but it is not a natural

---

[8] Hess, David J., Ph.D, *Evaluating Alternative Cancer Therapies*, pub by Rutgers University Press, 1999, p. 148.

substance. To achieve any benefit, Dr gold found that individuals who use it should avoid drugs such as alcohol, barbiturates, tranquilizers and anti-depressants. Pain medication may be safely used without interfering with the positive actions of hydrazine sulfate but one prominent practitioner, Dr. Michael B. Schachter, M.D., feels that doses of more than 25 mg of Vitamin B6 and more than 3gms of Vitamin C may interfere with its positive effects.[40] Studies that purport to debunk the effectiveness of hydrazine sulfate were flawed because approximately 94% of the patients were taking one or a number of these drugs.

Finally, because hydrazine sulfate is a controlled substance, preparations manufactured by companies must bypass the FDA requirements by not labeling it at all or by labeling it as "not for human consumption." As a result, one must scrutinize the purity of the quality of any hydrazine sulfate sold in such an unregulated manner.

Soybean Extract: Special Nutrition for Cancer Patients

One of the most valuable anticancer food agents I have found is a special fermented soybean extract that was first developed in a cancer hospital in China. It is made by concentrating approximately 25 to 27 pounds of organic soybeans down to 8 ounces of liquid. This is then fermented for several days to form and release thousands of bioactive phytochemicals that have anti-inflammatory, antibacterial, antiviral, anti-osteoporotic, anti-mutagenic and anti-carcinogenic properties. The phytochemicals generated from the concentrated fermented soybean extract are able to prevent cancer by capturing free radicals and prevent them from damaging DNA. In animal studies they have been found to be effective in the prevention and treatment of most cancers including breast, colorectal and prostate cancer. They assist in detoxifying the liver and lowering the number of histamines in the blood that helps clear various allergic reactions, including bronchitis and nasal congestion. They also help relieve pain, lower cholesterol, heal stomach ulcers and stop menstrual cramps.

Research has shown that soybean products contain five cancer preventive or reversal chemical agents: 1) protease inhibitors, which hold off activation of the specific oncogenes that cause cancer, 2) phytates, which bind iron in the intestines to prevent it from generating free radicals resulting in cancer, 3) phytosterols, which neutralize the breakdown of cholesterol and reduce the development of colon tumors and skin cancer, 4) saponins, which stop cellular mutations that could inevitably lead to cancer, and 5) isoflavones, which are plant estrogens with strong inhibiting effects in hormone-related malignancies such as prostate, ovarian, cervical and breast cancers.[41]

The isoflavones are a group of phytochemicals that include genistein. Genistein is an estrogen precursor that binds to receptor sites and either blocks estrogen uptake, if there is too much, or supplies it, if there is too little. This is thought to be why Asian women who eat a traditional diet including soy foods have a noticeable lack of gynecological problems associated with menopause, fibroids and of breast cancer (more than a 45% lower incidence). The assortment of other isoflavones found in soy are effective against a wide variety of cancers including lung, brain, breast, colon, prostate, skin and even blood dyscrasias, including leukemia and Hodgkin's disease.

Fermented soya extract is very expensive but as a special food for cancer patients it is worthwhile for those who can afford it and is especially recommended to counteract cachexia. It is recommended that one 8-ounce bottle a day is taken for the first month. For the second month and subsequent months thereafter, especially if price is a factor, this can be cut back to a half bottle, or 4 ounces daily. Because the flavor leaves much to be desired, I have been able to increase its palatability by teaching patients to add a few drops of tangerine oil or vanilla extract and liquid stevia extract as a sweetening agent, all to taste. Fermented soya extract, the richest source of cancer-blocking genistein and phytoestrogens is available from Haelen as Haelen-851 and –951 (see resources).

Urea

Urine has been used since ancient times for the diagnosis, prevention and treatment of disease. Today a number of useful drugs are derived from it, including anticoagulant urokinase (Abbokinase), the sex hormone Premarin (originally from pregnant mare's urine) and the experimental anticancer treatment of Stanislaw R. Burzynski, M.D., Ph.D. using antineoplastons.

Drinking one's own urine is, needless to say, a highly controversial topic. However, it has a long tradition of use claimed by its adherents to be capable of both preventing and treating a wide range of both acute and chronic conditions. Urea in the body functions as a diuretic and it has been used in conventional medicine for various skin disorders.

During the Second World War in England there was a controversy over a urine-based product called "H11." An English research laboratory produced it and it was based on a growth-retarding ingredient found in the parathyroid gland of animals. It was found that urine was a much cheaper and more accessible source of the same constituent.

E. Cronin Lowe, the pathologist of Southport Infirmary, published a report from an obscure laboratory based on a review of 243 cancer patients. He found that there was a 40% partial or complete response in 96 cancer patients tested. In another 69 patients there was a 28% temporary reduction of tumor size. Finally, of the remaining 78 there were 32% who exhibited no effect on tumor growth. This substantiated the claim that H11 offers a significant "growth inhibiting factor" on tumors.

In the 1960's, Evangelos D. Danopoulos, M.D. of Athens, Greece wrote of his extensive use of urea for the treatment of cancer. His articles were peer-reviewed in a number of the prestigious Lancet medical journals. Danopoulos, an ophthalmologist and professor at the Medical School of Athens was also a member of the board of the Hellenic Anti-Cancer Institute. In practice, his special was eye cancer.

He said that the "smaller the tumor, the shorter the duration of treatment. Small lesions can be cured within one to two years, whereas in cases of more extensive tumors, the treatment has to be continued for longer periods, or even for life" (*Townsend Letter for Doctors,* Feb.- March, 1988). Danopoulos reported numerous cures of eye cancers and various other cancers from both topical application and internal ingestion of urea.

Urea was the first chemical to be synthesized and has been used in medicine for over a century. Danopoulos used it with Heat therapy and described how urea breaks through the "structured water system" that surrounds tumors. He claims that it has absolutely no toxicity. Urea taken orally, according to Danopoulos, goes to the liver and provides a powerful anticancer effect. However, if the liver is more than 30% involved with cancer, the urea will have no effect.

For a more in depth guide to this therapy I recommend *The Golden Fountain, The Complete Guide to Urine Therapy* by Coen van der Kroon, published by Amethyst Books, distributed in the UK by Gateway Books, The Hollies, Wellow, Bath BA2 8Qj, telephone 01225 835127

General Nutritional Supplements Protocol for Cancer Patients

The following 21 supplements form a basic set of nutrients, which I modify according to the individual patient. Because many of these have overlap in benefits, it may not be necessary to take all of them.

- *Multivitamin/mineral formula* –Take the "optimal" recommended dosage stated on the bottle. Some good varieties are Rainbow Light and Source Naturals.

- *Vitamin E* –Take 1000 IU's as mixed tocopherols from a natural source. Since this is never sufficient in a multivitamin, one needs to supplement it either individually or as part of an antioxidant supplement.

- *Mixed carotenes* –Take 100,000 IU's as mixed carotenes. Obtain a portion from the multivitamin and the remainder from another antioxidant supplement. I recommend Beta-Plex made by Scientific Botanicals.

- *Vitamin C* – Most multivitamins never carry enough Vitamin C. I would suggest supplementing the minimum daily dose from 500 to 2,000 mg.

- *Antioxidant formula* – This should contain Vitamin C, Vitamin E, beta-carotene and mixed carotenes, and selenium. A comprehensive antioxidant formula that I recommend is Cyto-Redoxin made by Tyler Encapsulations. This formula includes Vitamins C, E, A, selenium, N-acetyl cysteine, zinc, grape seed extract, and green tea extract.

- *Coenzyme Q10* – This is an important antioxidant and detoxifying agent. It has potent anticancer properties, protects the heart and is specific for patients given Adriamycin. Dose: 100 to 600 mg daily.

- *Fish oil (EPA)* – Omega–3 fatty acids have anticancer properties, inhibit metastasis, are anti-inflammatory and counteract cachexia. Take 1000 to 1600 milligrams EPA as fish oil. The amount per capsule and gram of fish oil differs depending on the source. Check the bottle for EPA levels. I recommend Eskimo Oil made by Tyler Encapsulations. *Warning:* When supplementing any fat-soluble Vitamin or oil, you must also take a Vitamin E supplement to protect against oxidation.

- *Wobenzyme* – Maintains digestion and assimilation, activates the immune system and inhibits metastasis. Dose: 2-4 tablets 3-4 times daily a half-hour before meals.

- *Lactobacillus Acidophilus* – Important to maintain digestion, assimilation and elimination and general intestinal health. It is also necessary for immune strength. Dose: For better assimilation take once or twice daily with whey protein before meals.

- *Chlorella* – Nutrient-dense green algae that is rich in easily assimilable protein, Vitamins and minerals. It supports the immune system of patients undergoing chemo and radiation therapy, increases phagocytes, T-cells and cancer killing B cells. Take twice daily in doses ranging from 1 to 2 teaspoons or more at a time.

- *Inositol Hexaphosphate (IP6)* – Inhibits cancer development and metastasis. Dose: 4-16 capsules or more divided into two daily doses.

- *Kelp and other seaweeds* – Take supplementally if it is not a regular part of the diet. It supplies important cancer fighting nutrients including calcium potassium, all other minerals and iodine. Take several tablets two or three times daily.

In addition to the above, the following are added according to special needs and indications:

- *Selenium* – One of the most important antioxidant minerals against cancer, it is needed in the manufacture and utilization of glutathione. Dose: 100-800 mg

- *Modified Citrus Pectin* – Inhibits cancer cell proliferation and metastasis. It is especially good for prostate cancer. Take with chlorella or a green drink such as Green Magma.

- *Thymus extract* – Strengthens the immune system by increasing the activity and number of T-lymphocytes.

- *Spleen Extract* – Regulates white blood cells as needed and has a generally beneficial effect on the immune system. It is a useful adjunct for patients undergoing chemo and radiation therapies. I recommend SP500. Dose: 2-6 tablets twice daily.

- *Glutathione* – The most powerful antioxidant self generated by the body. It deactivates free radicals of cells of the liver, lungs, heart and blood, promotes DNA repair and activates T-lymphocytes and Natural Killer cells in the fight against cancer. Presence in the body declines with age and it is poorly absorbed orally. A combination of N-acetylcysteine (NAC), lipoic acid, selenium, Vitamins C, E and selenium together will effectively raise glutathione levels. Counteracts the toxicity of the chemotherapeutic drugs, cisplatin and cyclosphamide and may even improve therapeutic results. Dose: 2,500 mg

- *Lipoic Acid* – This antioxidant has detoxifying properties, especially to the liver and kidneys and is an immune tonic protective from the effects of chemo and radiation therapy and increases glutathione levels. Dose: 200-600 mg

- *N-acetyl cysteine* – Helps to synthesize glutathione, inhibit cancer and protect DNA damage. Dose: 500-3,000 mg

- *Quercetin* – Has anticancer properties, is anti-inflammatory, inhibits breast, ovarian and prostate cancers and works synergistically with many chemotherapeutic drugs. Dose: 1,000-6,000 mg

- *Folic Acid and B 12* – The combination is anticancer and improves general well being. Dose: 400-2,000 mg

- *Vitamin K* – Take this Vitamin as part of a multivitamin supplement. Large doses of Vitamin E require extra Vitamin K. Be sure to take a total of 5-20 mg daily.

- *Molybdenum* – This is especially useful for esophageal cancer. Dose: 200-400 mg

- *Zinc* – Antioxidant mineral useful for the prevention and treatment of cancer and the prevention of DNA damage. Used for prostate cancer, to accelerate healing after surgery, improve appetite and maintain taste sensation. Dose: 10-50 mg

- *Taurine* – Detoxifies heavy metals and inhibits seizures associated with brain tumors. Dose: 1,000-6,000 mg.

- *Glutamine* – Useful for protein synthesis, removes ammonia from the urine and heals gastrointestinal ulcers. Dose: 2,000-6,000 mg

- *Calcium D-glucarate* – Aids detoxification and neutralizes excess estrogen and other hormonal driven cancers. Dose: 1,000-6,000 mg.

- *Bromelain* – Use instead of wobenzyme when treating breast and ovarian cancers. Dose: 1,000-6,000 mg.

- *Whey Protein* – Use freely as a nutrient to maintain protein levels, counteract cancer, prevent or treat cachexia.

- *Fermented Soya Extract* – Use as an anticancer nutrient as indicated.

- *Lactoferrin* – Use for deficient red blood cell anemia and to stimulate the immune system against cancer. Dose: 4 capsules before going to bed.

- *Melatonin* – Use only if there is a sleep problem. Stimulates the immune system against cancer. Take 5 to 10 mg before retiring at night. Discontinue if it is not working and never take during the day.

In his book *Antioxidants Against Cancer* (published by Equinox), Dr. Ralph Moss offers a good general daily supplement program that may be useful for the prevention of cancer and other health problems (such as heart disease). Once again, it may offer a good starting point, which should then be adjusted to suit one's individual requirements.

- A good multivitamin (without iron)
- Vitamin A – 10-20,000 IU
- Vitamin C – 500 to 2,000 mgs
- Vitamin E – 200 to 1,200 IU
- Coen`zyme Q10 – 30 to 300 mgs
- Lipoic acid – 50 to 200 mgs
- Zinc – 15 to 30 mgs
- Selenium – 200 mcg
- Pycnogenol, grape seeds – 50 to 300 mgs.
- Mixed carotenoids – 10,000 to 25,000 IU

We increasingly find oncologists specifically telling their patients that antioxidants should not be taken during chemo or radiation therapy. If it isn't already evident from the many citations associated with the description of individual antioxidants and other supplements, such precautions seem contrary to existing research. In fact, in can be argued that since the body naturally manufactures antioxidants such as glutathione and the fact that they are found in most wholesome, organic foods it defies reason to specifically deny the body's need for them especially at a time when, through depletion as a result of surgery, chemo and radiation therapy, the body is most in need. This is especially true in view of the numerous citations that prove the value of antioxidants against cancer and even their ability to enhance the cytotoxic effects of radiation and chemotherapy.

Nutritional Support During Radiation Therapy [9]

1. Increasing oxygen to the area of the tumor makes the cancer cells more vulnerable to radiation. [42]

2. Whey powder: (2 tsp, 3X daily, with meals) selectively deprives antioxidants from the tumor, making it more sensitive to radiation as well as chemo-therapy. Whey is also beneficial for raising oxygen supply by increasing hemoglobin. From a study conducted in 1994-95,[43] it was found that whey selectively depleted glutathione from tumor cells, without adversely affecting the healthy cells. This in turn enhances the effects of radiation and chemotherapy by increasing the vulnerability of the cancer cells. Specifically one should use an undenatured whey product, which is cold-pressed and not centrifuged. For best effect this should not be processed in a blender but stirred by hand making a significant difference in raising hemoglobin levels.

3. Alkylglycerols: (2 capsules, 2X daily with meals). This product is made from shark liver oil purified of excess vitamins A and D, pesticides and heavy metals. Good research on alkylglycerols shows that they minimize radiation damage to healthy tissues, supporting the immune system while actually enhancing the effect of radiation on tumor cells. It is contrain-dicated for individuals with elevated platelet levels. Companies are now making both 250 and 500 mg caps of alkylglycerols. This 2-cap dose is based on using the 250 mg caps. So perhaps it would be better if the dose reads 500 mg, 2x/day with meals. Best results are obtained by a loading period of 7-10 days period prior to starting radiation therapy.

4. Antioxidants: Vitamin C 1-3g/day, enhances the effect of radiation while protecting healthy cells. It also supports the immune system.

   Vitamin E 400-800 IU daily; it sensitizes tumor cells to the destructive effects of radiation while protecting the healthy cells. Higher doses may be inappropriate for individuals who are taking blood-thinning drugs.

---

[9] "A Database of Nutritional and Botanical Agents as Adjuncts in Oncology" (self-pub; hope-fully due out early 2002)

5. Glutamine: (1 tsp, 3X daily). Dissolve the powder in chilled water and sip throughout the day. It helps to protect against the destruction of gastrointestinal cells. This is especially true if the gastrointestinal tract is affected by radiation. Glutamine is also required for a healthy functioning immune system, reducing the lowering of white blood cells.

6. Ashwagandha (Withania somnifera): take one teaspoon of the powder mixed with honey three times daily. It is well known to enhance the effects of radiation while affording some protection against adverse reactions. (Partially adapted from the notes of Jeanne M. Wallace, Ph.D., CNC)

7. Essential Fatty Acids (EFA's): research has shown that at 3g a day, fish oil with combined EPA/DHA reduced long-term side effects, e.g., necrosis, from radiation therapy. This study initiated supplementation 2 weeks post-treatment.

8. Possible contraindications: Some animal studies seem to suggest that both soy and ginseng may interfere with Radiation Therapy via DNA repair capacities.

9. According to nutritionist Jeanne Wallace, many practitioners recommend seaweed baths for internal detoxification during and after radiation with the intention of attempting to protect thyroid function from the adverse effects of radiation. In light of newer research and my own and Jeanne's personal experience, it seems that while low thyroid seems to be a risk factor for developing cancer, once one has cancer it seems to offer a significant survival advantage. Instead of seaweed, one should consider using alginate or pectin to help removal of radioactive isotopes following treatment.

Nutritional Support During Chemotherapy [10]

1. Increase protein, especially in the form of whey, soy and coldwater fish. This is important to protect against weight loss and rebuilding destroyed tissues. Because digestion is seriously impaired after chemotherapy, food should be well cooked for chemotherapy patients. Ideally, one would use glutinous rice congee cooked with mung beans and shiitake mushrooms. Dilute with 7 to 10 parts water and slow cook over 12 hours. Other foods that can be added to the congee is fish. Whey powder, undenatured as described above is another ideal food for patients undergoing chemotherapy. In general it is a good idea to not eat anything that you normally really enjoy because food eaten immediately after chemotherapy is often associated with a sick feeling so that cancer patients may lose their predilection for them in the future.

---

[10] ibid

2. Take EPA (Eicosapentaenoic Acid)/DHA (Docosahexaenoic Acid) which are essential fatty acids that are known to enhance the uptake of chemo-therapeutic drugs into tumor cells, prevent chemo resistance and weight loss. (6 to 9 capsules or more daily). It is important to ensure the product is good quality and not rancid. It should not have a fishy smell/taste or bitter taste.

3. Take acidophilus bifidus (a tablespoon of the powder two or three times daily). It helps replenish beneficial intestinal bacteria, reduce gastrointestinal side effects and raise the immune system. Because white blood cell count often lowers after chemotherapy, one should be very careful about exposure to harmful bacteria. For this reason, one may need to be careful about the quality/purity of certain products such as probiotics. In general we have found that Metagenics probiotics to be of exceptional quality.

4. Glutamine to chemo section: (1 tsp. 3X daily). This decreases the side effects of chemotherapy such as: peripheral neuropathy, diarrhea/constipation, low white blood cell count, and mucositis. It can be used as "swish and swallow" for mouth sores. Research shows that glutamine can increase the concentration of chemo drugs delivered inside the tumor cells!

5. Medicinal Mushrooms: Especially maitake, reishi, shiitake and turkey tail mushrooms. Maitake D- fraction has been shown to enhance the effects of chemotherapy as well as having anticancer and immune strengthening properties. New research shows maitake D-fraction also has apoptosis (cancer cell death) inducing properties. Planetary formulas Maitake Mushroom and Reishi Mushroom Supreme have shown themselves to be very efficacious.

6. Astragalus: Boil 9g in 2 cups of boiling water and take with food. This can be cooked with glutinous white rice using 9g of astragalus root, 1 cup of glutinous white rice and 7 to 10 cups of water – slow cook for 8 to 12 hours.

7. Take the Chinese formula Six Gentleman Combination or Planetary Formula's Ginseng Classic combination. Both are traditional Chinese formulas well known to support the immune system and counteract the negative effects of chemotherapy by supporting the immune system and enhancing digestion and assimilation (With permission, partially adapted from the notes of Jeanne M. Wallace, Ph.D., CNC)

Despite the substantial evidence in support of the use of vitamins and antioxidants during chemo and radiation therapy, one alternative strategy to prevent any possible interaction is to suspend, with the exception of those previously mentioned, all other antioxidants two days before each chemotherapy session and resume them again two days after the session ends.

However, one should always consider telling their doctor what supplements and herbs they are taking regardless of whether they understand or believe in their efficacy. At the same time it would be good to enlist expert professional guidance in their use. There are only a few contraindications that may be worth considering. Dr. Ralph Moss embodies these in his ten cautionary statements on the use of specific supplements.[8]

1. Do not take very high doses of Vitamins A, D or E, except under a doctor's direction.
2. Do not take synthetic beta-carotene, especially if you smoke.
3. Do not take high-dose Vitamin C as a single agent while taking either Methotrexate or DTIC.
4. Do not take high-dose Vitamin C supplements if you have a hereditary tendency to accumulate iron (hemochromatosis).
5. Do not take N-acetyl cysteine while you are taking cisplatin or Adriamycin.
6. Do not take high-dose Tangeratin, especially with tamoxifen.
7. Do not take zinc while you are taking cisplatin or carboplatin.
8. Do not take melatonin if you have leukemia or any other proliferative disease of the blood or lymph.
9. Do not take folic acid while you are taking Methodrexate.
10. Have your progress checked periodically by a qualified alternative health practitioner.

In conclusion, nutritional supplements including vitamins, minerals and other supplements that serve as antioxidants are for the most part contained in whole, organic foods. A selective supplementation may be beneficial for the prevention and treatment of cancer but their use is not a substitute for a life supporting diet. With few minor exceptions, there are no dangers in their use when accompanying chemotherapy or radiation and, in fact, research seems to demonstrate that many of them enhance the effects of conventional medicine.

Because digestion is the foundation to healing cancer and all disease, there is a danger of injuring digestion associated with taking so many supplements at once. For this reason, they should be ingested at different times throughout the day, some before and some after meals. Further, because many of them overlap in benefits, it is possible to derive many of these from special foods therefore one should learn to integrate those that may be most relevant to one's particular needs.

Endnotes

[1] Associated Press release March 27, 2000, "Doctors warn against big doses of Vitamin C during cancer treatment."

[2] Reported in *Nutrition and Cancer*, 1999.

[3] Moss, Ralph W., *Antioxidants Against Cancer,* pub by Equinox Press, 2000, pages 14-19

[4] Atkins, Robert, Dr., *Dr. Atkins' Vita-Nutrient Solution*, p66, publ 1998 by Simon and Schuster.

[5] Rohan, Jain; Howe, Miller, "Dietary Folate Consumption and Breast Cancer Risk," *J. of the National C. Intst*, Vol 92, No. 3, February 2, 2000.

[6] Carmel, Ralph, M.D., "Subtle and Atypical Deficiency States," *American Journal of Hematology*, 1990; 34:108-14

[7] "Cerebral Manifestations of Vitamin B12 Deficiency," Damien Downing, M.B., B.S., *Journal of Nutritional Medicine* 1991; 2, 89-90.

[8] "Vitamin C and Cancer Prevention: The Epidemiologic Evidence," Gladys Block, *American Journal of Clinical Nutrition*, 1991;53:2,701-282S.

[9] "Glutathione Blood Levels and Other Oxidant Defense Indexes in Men Fed Diets Low in Vitamin C," S. Henning, et al, *Journal of Nutrition*, 1991; 121:169-75

[10] "A Major Symposium on Vitamin C sponsored by the National cancer institute," Morton A. Klein, Linus Pauling Institute of Science and Medicine, December 1990:7

[11] "Vitamin C and Reduced Mortality," Gladys Block, Epidemiology, May 1992; 3(3): 189-91

[12] Marshall, James, Dr., editorial in the *Journal of the National Cancer inst*. Vol. 92, No.12, June 21, 2000

[13] Teicher, B.A., et al. "In vivo modulation of several anticancer agents by beta-carotene." *Cancer Chemother Pharmacol.* 1994;34(3):235-41

[14] Schwartz, J.L., et al. "Beta-carotene and/or Vitamin E as modulators of Alkylating agents in SCC-25 human squamous carcinoma cells." *Cancer Chemother Pharmacol.* 1992;29(3):207-13

[15] Park, J.S., et al. "Dietary lutein from marigold extract inhibits mammary tumor development BALB.c mice." *J. Nutr.* 1998 Oct; 128 (10):1650-6.

[16] Narisawa, T., et al. "Inhibitory effects of natural carotenoids, alpha-carotene, beta-carotene, lycopene and lutein, on colonic aberrant crypt foci formation in rats." *Cancer Lett.* 1996 Oct 1;107(1):137- 42.

[17] "Vitamin E Protects Nerve Cells from Amyloid B Protein Toxicity," Christian Behl, et al, *Biochemical and Biophysical Research Communications*, July 31, 1992; 186 (2) 944-50.

[18] Bendich, Adrienne Ph.D., "Vitamin E Status of U.S. Children." *Journal of the American College of Nutrition*, 1992; 11: (4) 441-44

[19] Nesaretnam, K., Stephen, R., Dils, R., Darbre, P., "Tocotrienols inhibit the growth of human breast cancer cells irrespective of estrogen receptor status." *Lipids* 1998 May; 33(5): 461-9

[20] Yance, Donald, A.H.G., *Herbal Medicine Healing & Cancer*, pub.1999, Keats publishing

[21] Clark, L.C., M.D. et al., "Effects of Selenium Supplementation for Cancer Prevention in Patients with Carcinoma of the Skin. A Randomized Controlled Trial," *Journal of the American Medical Association* 276 (24): 1957-63 (1996).

[22] Hehr, T., et al., "Role of sodium selenite as an adjuvant in radiotherapy of rectal carcinoma" Med Klin., 1997 Sep 15-92 Suppl 3:48-49

[23] Xu, Z.L., et al. "The effect of lisheng-se (selenium) on cisplatin and its relation to metallationein indiction, " Chung Hua Chung Liu Txa Chih. 1994 Jul; 16(4):280-3

[24] Luo, X.M. et al., "Inhibitory Effects of Molybdenum on Esophageal and forestomach Carcinogenesis in rats," *Journal of the National Cancer Institute* 71: 75-80 (1983)

[25] Moss, Ralph W. *Antioxidants Against Cancer*, pub by Equinox Press, 2000

[26] B. Donnerstag et al., "Reduced Gluthione and S-acetylglutathione as Selective Apopto-sis-Inducing Agents in Cancer Therapy," Cancer Letters 110 (102):63-70 (1996)

[27] Locatelli, M.C., et al. "A phase II study of combination chemotherapy in advanced ovarian carcinoma with cisplatin and cyclosphosphamide plus reduced glutathione as potential protective agent against cisplatin toxicity." *Tumori*. 1993 Feb. 28:791):37-30

[28] M. Tedeschi et al., "Glutathione and Detoxification," *Cancer Treatment Review* 17 (2-3): 203-8 (1990)

[29] A. Bauer et al., "Alpha-Lipoic Acid Is an Effective Inhibitor of Human Immuno-deficiency Virus (HIV-1) Replication," Klin wochenshr 69 (15): 722-74 (1991).

[30] V. Bongers et al., "Antioxidant-Related Parameters in Patients Treated for Cancer Chemoprevention with N-acetyl cysteine," *European Journal of Cancer* 31A (6): 921-23 (1995).

[31] Teran, J.C., et al., *American Journal of Clinical Nutrition*, 1995; 163(7): 385-388.

[32] M. Piantelli et al., "Tamoxifen and Quercetin Interact with Type II Estrogen Binding Sites and Inhibit the Growth of Human Melanoma Cells," *Journal of Investigative Dermatology* 105 (2):248-53 (1995)

[33] N. Kioka et al., "Quercetin, a Bioflavonoid, Inhibits the increase of Human Multidrug Resistance Gene (MDRI) Expression Caused by Arsenite," *Febs Letters* 301 (3):307-9 (1992)

[34] G. Elia and M.G. Santoro, "Regulation of Heat Shock Protein Synthesis by Quercetin in Human Erytroleukemia Cells," *Biochemical Journal* 300 (Pt. 1): 201-9 (1994)

[35] Newmark, H.L., "Squalene, olive oil, and cancer risk. Review and hypothesis." Strang Cancer Research Laboratory, The Rockefeller University, New York, New York 10021, USA (1999)

[36] *Cancer Letters*, 1996; 101 (1):936

[37] S. Barkin et al., "Antimetastatic Effect of Bromelain With or Without Its Proteolytic and Anticoagulant Activity," *Journal of Cancer Research and Clinical Oncology* 114 (5): 507-8 (1988)

[38] K.J. Pienta et al., "Inhibition of Spontaneous Metastasis in a Rat Prostate Cancer Model by Oral Administration of Modified Citrus Pectin," *Journal of the National Cancer Institute* 87 (5): 348-53 (1995).

[39] Moss, R., *The Cancer Industry* (New York: Equinox Press, 1996), 192-93

[40] Goldberg, Burton, *Alternative Medicine Definitive Guide to Cancer*, p. 386-387, publ 1997 by *Future Medicine*.

[41] St Clair, W.H.; Billings, P.C.; Kennedy, A.R., "The effects of the Bowman-Birk protease inhibitor on C = MYC expression and cell proliferation in unirradiated and irradiated mouse color." *Cancer Letters* 52-145-152, 1990

[42] Crawford & Gabrilove, 2000

[43] Kennedy et al 1994, 1995

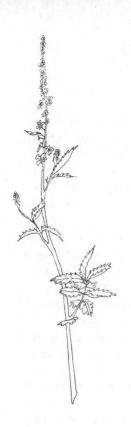

CHAPTER TEN

EXTERNAL CANCER TREATMENTS

T here are many important external treatments that may be appropriate for different types and stages of cancer. There is some controversy as to how systemic a disease cancer is. Repeatedly when we are discussing the treatment of cancer, cause is always an issue. This is because there are probably many causes for cancer depending on individual circumstances. Without metastasis most cancers remain a local phenomenon perhaps, but not always, induced by a generally unhealthy condition of the body. Without metastasis, most cancers are curable.

It is a principle of herbal medicine that the closer to an affected site one can deliver the healing properties of an herb, the quicker and faster the result. This may involve the use of medicated enemas, boluses, poultices, fomentations, ointments and the combination of herbals with DMSO as a carrier. Other issues such as metabolic detoxification are also greatly assisted by certain external treatments. These also involve enemas, dry skin brushing, enzyme implants and Epsom salt baths.

Enemas

Coffee Enemas

Coffee enemas during the initial stages of treatment are important to maintain regular detoxification from the overburdened liver. As tumors breakdown, whether as a result of conventional treatment or through the use of herbs, they cause an added toxic burden. First associated with the Gerson anticancer method, coffee specifically draws toxins from the liver through the mesentery of the small intestine, promoting a general sense of well-being and pain relief as a result of detoxification. While a small amount of caffeine may be absorbed, the detoxification is of far greater benefit.

Depending on the individual case, coffee enemas taken once or more daily are useful throughout all stages of treatment. If possible, a coffee enema once daily is highly beneficial. Many promote them as much as three times a day during the initial stage. These should be supplemented with weekly colonics if at all possible. If the process is neither convenient or the patient is too week to undergo them, one may consider forgoing this aspect of treatment.

Dissolve 3 tablespoonsful of ground organic coffee in one quart of water. Boil for three minutes and then simmer for another fifteen minutes. Strain and allow cooling to body temperature. Place in an enema bag, which can be purchased from a pharmacy. Be sure the stopper on the enema bag hose is closed. Apply oil to the enema tip and the anus. Position a place in the bathroom with towels and blankets as necessary. Hang the bag no higher than 3 feet above the area where you will be laying on the floor. Lay on your back and gently insert the oiled enema tip into the anus. Try to have your feet slightly elevated, perhaps against the wall near where enema bag is hanging. Allow the coffee to flow gently into the bowel slowly so as not to cause cramping. Gentle pressure on the bag will encourage the flow. At the same time massage upwards on the left side of the abdomen from the descending colon to the transverse colon just under the ribs and then down to the ascending colon on the right side of the abdomen. Retain for 4 or 5 minutes and expel. Often within 20-30 minutes the patient will expel up to a gallon of fluid. Initially this will take an hour or so but with practice it is possible to get the entire process down to 20 or 30 minutes.

Coffee enemas are best taken once or more times daily for several days in succession, later tapering down to once or twice a week or on an 'as needed' basis. They should be considered anytime added detoxification is needed or when the cancer patient feels bogged down, tired or is in pain.

While coffee enemas do help to detoxify the liver, there are some valid criticisms of coffee enemas. One is the issue of getting people hooked on caffeine. While this may be true to some extent, most consider that the benefits of coffee enemas outweigh its disadvantages.

Other Types of Nutritive and Herbal Enemas

Besides coffee enemas, an herbalist may prefer to use other herbs such as bayberry bark, agrimony, marshmallow root and garlic tea as an enema. Here the astringent and soothing action of the herbs combined with the stimulating and detoxifying properties of the garlic will assist general detoxification.

A retentive, nutritive enema is useful when a patient is unable to efficiently absorb nutrients by mouth. Typically these may involve the use of a meat soup, perhaps cooked into a broth with tonic herbs such as shiitake mushrooms and astragalus root.

High Colonic Enemas

A colonic therapist usually administers high colonic enemas. It is possible with practice that one achieves a high enema by eventually taking in as much as two quarts of enema solution at one time. However, through a system of repeatedly discharging and irrigating the bowel mechanically, a colonic therapist can affect detoxification of the entire colon. Again, convenience, cost and time are the limiting factors but having a high colonic enema at least once weekly during the initial stages of treatment would be appropriate.

Oil After Taking an Enema

Whenever one adds water and voids fluid from the intestines, there is a drying action that ensues that can mildly aggravate nervous energy. In Ayurveda, the use of a small amount of sesame added and an entire oil enema is used to relieve nervous affections including irritability, pain and even insomnia. Injecting from a quarter to a full cup of sesame oil using a bulb syringe, following every enema or colonic treatment, is very beneficial and balancing to the enema procedure.

Enzyme Enemas

Cancer cells are highly susceptible to lysis (dissolution) when exposed to proteolytic and lipolytic enzymes. The theory is that rapid process of cell division of cancer cells causes cancer cells to generally have weaker outer membranes, making them highly susceptible to destruction with enzymes.

Proteolytic enzymes as found in papain from papaya and bromelain from pineapple are used in extract form as meat tenderizers. When the more vulnerable membranes of cancer cells are exposed to these enzymes they also tend to soften and dissolve.

We have already recommended the use of oral enzymes for cancer patients. However, in many instances, proteolytic enzymes are found to be more effective when taken rectally. I dissolve three Wobe Mugos wafers (Retenzymes may also be used) in a cup of warm water (not hot) for this. Again this is intended to be a retentive enema and the cup of enzyme water can be injected along with a quarter cup of sesame oil once daily, separately or following other types of enemas or colonics. Place 3 enzyme wafers in a single enema once a day for 3 days, then 2 wafers in a single enema 2 times daily for 3 days and finally a single wafer dissolved in a cup of warm water and oil taken consecutively for 5 or more days as needed.

A syringe and enema tip accompanies the Wobe Mugos enema wafers. Place the number of wafers in the syringe and draw from 15 to 200 cc of distilled water into the syringe (body temperature). Shake a few times until the wafer dissolves and attach the plastic tube to the syringe. Lubricate the tube syringe and insert into the rectum. Slowly allow the fluid to enter the rectum. This usually does not stimulate bowel movement. The whole process should be performed in 5-6 minutes or the enzyme will be deactivated. The enzyme is rapidly absorbed within a few minutes by the large intestine and enters the blood stream to the site of its action.

Baths and External Applications

Medicated Epsom Salts Bath

The medicated Epsom salts bath should be taken at least twice a week before retiring to bed. It neutralizes toxins, relieves pain and calms the nerves. Simply dissolve 6 tablespoons of Epsom salts in warm water in the bathtub. One can add a few drops of various essential oils such as a few drops of lavender, tea tree, rosemary, rose or eucalyptus oil to the bath water. The patient should soak in this bath for 15 to 20 minutes. The salts will open the pores and draw toxins from the body. This can be taken just before bedtime. Eli Jones recommends that the Epsom salts bath be taken as often as twice a week. While in the tub, one can vigorously rub all parts of the skin with a natural bristle brush or luffa sponge to help remove the dead skin and other material. Another benefit from using Epsom salts is that the magnesium in Epsom salts helps to neutralize the toxins throughout the body and will help soothe the nerves and induce a much-needed sound sleep.

If there is no bathtub, dissolve one ounce of Epsom salts in a pint of warm water and bathe the body all over with the mixture. For cancer, the bath should never be omitted.

Skin Brushing

The skin is the largest organ of detoxification for the entire body and is capable of discharging through its pores up to two pounds of toxins daily as well as sloughing off dead skin. Because of this, it is sometimes called the "third kidney" or the "third lung."

In sickness, the fact that the pores of our skin may be clogged thus hampering proper elimination, becomes a negative factor in our recovery especially from a disease such as cancer.

Each day before showering, the skin should be vigorously dry brushed with a natural fiber brush or luffa sponge. Then a warm bath or shower can be taken which should always be followed by a cool rinse to invigorate blood circulation and stimulate surface warmth.

Castor Oil Fomentation

The remarkable mystic-healer Edgar Cayce first popularized castor oil fomentations. Castor oil in Ayurveda is the ultimate nutritive nerve-soothing agent. Of course, internally, it is a surefire purgative, guaranteeing evacuation within 8 to 12 hours after ingesting it. The plant and seeds are toxic but the oil is an age-old purgative. It is extremely viscous and when applied over an area, it penetrates and helps dissolve congestion and stagnation. As a fomentation, castor oil is applied topically for purposes of detoxification and pain relief.

To administer a castor oil fomentation assemble the following:

A large bottle of food grade castor oil

A cotton or flannel cloth

Plastic to cover the application

Hot water bottle

A towel

First saturate the cotton or flannel cloth with castor oil. Next apply over the affected area and cover with plastic. This is then followed with a towel and a hot water bottle. The entire treatment should take about 45 minutes. This should be repeated consecutively for at least three days in a row. There are no contraindications so it can be used as often as convenient.

Castor oil packs are often applied over the liver to aid detoxification and as such it is a very good daily application at least periodically for all types of cancers. They can also be applied over areas of pain and non-suppurating tumors. Applying diluted DMSO topically first will make the treatment even more effective since the DMSO will assist the penetrating action of the castor oil.

Dimethylsulphoxide (DMSO)

DMSO is derived as a product of the wood pulp industry. There are literally hundreds of acknowledged research papers attesting both to its efficacy and safety. The major advocate and researcher of DMSO is Dr. Stanley Jacobs, called 'the DMSO guru' who resides in Oregon. Through his efforts he was able to attain FDA approval for the injected use of DMSO for the treatment of interstitial cystitis (a very painful and difficult disease).

DMSO was first synthesized in 1865. It is 'officially' sold as a highly effective degreasing solvent but unofficially it has been used for decades by veterinarians for a wide variety of inflammatory ailments of domestic animals. Most commonly it is topically massaged on horses to relieve painful joint, legs and tendonitis. It is also widely used, again unofficially, by athletes to speed recovery from contact sport injuries.

It has a wide range of applications including being used as a topical liniment for tendinitis, arthritis, rheumatic disease, retarded children, cancer, skin conditions, shingles and the list could go on. DMSO has been hailed as one of the most important medical discoveries of the 20th century, along with aspirin.

One of the peculiarities and the basis of caution for its use is that DMSO acts as a carrier through the skin for anything with which it is combined. This can be of great value for herbalists using a liniment with, for example, 20% DMSO added as a carrier. I add DMSO to a liniment made from alcoholic extracts of lobelia, myrrh, goldenseal and cayenne. DMSO can also be mixed into an herbal poultice to further assist in carrying the constituents of the herbs into the body. I also combine 20% DMSO with poke root oil to be rubbed directly over breast lumps and various other masses and tumors that are close to the body's surface.

As a solvent, DMSO is very effective for a wide range of chemicals. One should be very cautious in handling DMSO in conjunction with any chemical solvent such as industrial cleaning solvents, for instance. Practitioners and patients who handle DMSO should be warned about using these at least two hours before or after handling such solvents.

When applied by hand, it should be kept in mind that DMSO will go through one's hands as well as the patient. It is helpful to either use laboratory gloves or to at least wash one's hands immediately after handling DMSO to diminish and prevent a clammy taste in the mouth that occurs later after handling DMSO.

For cancer DMSO has the following benefits:

1. It is a powerful antioxidant.
2. It increases circulation and has been found to revert cells to normal.
3. It relieves pain.
4. It can be used as a carrier when applying herbs topically over the site of various cancers and tumors.

5. It potentiates the intended effects and mitigates the side effects of chemotherapy and radiation.

DMSO has the property to increase circulation and normalize cells. Dr. Jacob described twelve tumor-cell types in vitro that DMSO was able to stimulate to change to a more normal non-cancerous cell.[1] In another study conducted in New York on leukemic mice, Charlotte Friend M.D. of New York's Mt. Sinai hospital found that when injected with DMSO, cancer cells reverted to normal function including the ability to make their own hemoglobin, which leukemic cells are unable to do.[2] The ability of DMSO to convert neoplastic cells to benign tissue offers a novel approach, called maturational-agent therapy, in place of the slash, poison and burn approach used most.[3]

In 1981 DMSO was given concurrently in a 5% intravenous solution along with 1500 mg Cyclophosphamide (CYC), a highly toxic chemotherapeutic drug, over a period of three days to 14 patients with squamous cell lung cancer. This was repeated in four week intervals. While there was no noticeable effect directly on the tumor from the DMSO the urinary excretion of harmful CYC was much lower.[4]

This makes it very efficacious adjunctively in the treatment of cancer both for helping to treat the cancer and to relieve pain. Similarly, DMSO can be used for topically lipomas (fatty growths), warts, toenail fungus, and other growths and excrescences.

DMSO potentiates the intended effects of chemotherapy while lessening its harmful side effects. At the oncological depart of a military hospital in Santiago, Chile, 65 patients with various localized incurable cancers were given DMSO along with conventional chemotherapeutic drugs. It was found that DMSO, in combination with the drugs, strengthened antiblastic activity (cancer destroying) as a result of its circulating and penetrating properties. It also reduced the side effects of these drugs, especially of Cyclophosphamide, the chemotherapeutic drug that is usually prescribed long term.[5] From this study it was found that DMSO greatly benefited anemia and relieved pain to the degree that in many cases morphine was not necessary. It was also found that patients who were intolerant of cyclophosphamide in saline solution had good tolerance with DMSO. It was also found that DMSO had its best results for the treatment of lymphomas.

DMSO, when topically applied over the area, is able to protect against burns and mutagenic damage from x-rays and other forms of radiation therapy. This has been demonstrated in numerous animal experiments and one Russian study.[6]

Besides the clammy mouth taste, too much DMSO can cause minor temporary reactions of heat, flushing, dizziness, gastrointestinal reactions and in sensitive individuals a temporary heat rash. These are all relatively mild and temporary. It will also dry the oils of the skin, therefore, after applying DMSO topically it is a good idea to apply a lubricating substance such as aloe vera. One should use the purist high grade pharmaceutical DMSO, beginning with a 70% concentration. After patient sensitivity has been determined, the 90% grade DMSO can be used with even faster results.

Basic topical application for inflammatory as well as various musculoskeleton conditions is simply to lightly dab DMSO over the affected area one to three times daily.

To attest to its safety, Dr. Jacobs has personally ingested a teaspoon of full strength DMSO for over 30 years and claims no adverse reaction except that he has never gotten a cold or flu throughout the entire time.

As a more stable source of sulfur and a spin off from the research on DMSO, Dr. Jacobs and colleagues has developed a metabolite made from DMSO called MSM (methylsufonylmethane). MSM has most of the benefits of DMSO without the negative aspects of its odor and resultant clammy mouth taste. MSM would be good to use for long-term treatment of all forms of arthritis including rheumatoid arthritis and also has penetrating properties. Unlike DMSO, however, it does not have the same ability to carry other substances with which it may be combined into the body. Further, it may not have the potent cell normalizing properties of DMSO that is useful for cancer. In all of this it seems that it is not so much whether it lacks these properties but that little research has been done to evaluate this. I suspect that because Jacobs and company have developed MSM as a popular health supplement, the last thing they want to do is show that it has qualities for which the FDA previously rejected DMSO. Both DMSO and MSM would be classified in TCM with warming, blood moving properties. If only for the mouth taste and odor alone, MSM is generally better for long term use by arthritic and rheumatic sufferers.[1]

Escharotic Pastes

Escharotic pastes are salves or ointments that are applied topically to the skin to destroy and remove various types of cancers, tumors and other excrescences.

---

[1] DMSO can be purchased from DMSO marketing 1-800-367-6975. Whoever you purchase it from, remember that it is not legally approved in the US for anything other than medical treatment of interstitial cystitis so don't ask the sales person about therapeutic usage. You can also look up DMSO on the Internet and even find Stanley Jacobs' own DMSO website. Interestingly in the UK it is only approved for shingles while in Germany it is only approved for arthritic and rheumatic problems. Because of this issue no distributor of DMSO is allowed to discuss any of its therapeutic applications with their customers in the US. I also recommend Dr. Morton Walker's book *DMSO, Nature's Healer*, published by Avery, 1993.

In general they work by eroding the surface layers of the skin, dislodging or drawing out whatever material that lies below.

Since ancient times, along with surgery, various caustics (substances that burn) in the form of herbs or minerals have been used to directly remove tumors, cancers, warts and various other excrescences. Such methods were described in the *Ramayana*, an Indian Hindu epic where a paste of arsenic is mentioned. In Greece, Hippocrates used various caustics as well as direct burning or cauterization similar to that practiced in Tibet on tumors and cancers. The treatment of breast cancer, particularly through the use of dandelion latex, was described as a folk remedy by the Chinese, and the use of taro potato made into a mash and applied topically was part of the standard Japanese macrobiotic treatment of breast and surface cancers. There are numerous references to the topical application of the latex or juice of a wide number of herbs including chelidonium, the common buttercup (ranunculous) and the seeds of brucea javonica (used in TCM) for the removal of warts and other skin excrescences of which some must have been cancerous.

Prior to, and during the early part of the 19th century in Europe, various compounds, some of which utilized zinc chloride, were topically applied as a paste to burn off topical cancers. Without the benefit of modern analgesics, reports of the time describe the excruciating pain suffered by those who underwent such treatment.

Samuel Thomson (1769-1843), an iconoclastic herbalist-medical reformer is reported to have successfully treated a woman with a breast tumor by the topical application of a thickened paste made from boiling down kettle's full of fresh red clover blossoms.

One of the most important North American herbs used in escharotic salves is Bloodroot, *Sanguinarea canadensis*, a beautiful eastern woodland herb. One of the active constituents of bloodroot is an alkaloid, sanguinarine, which is known to have powerful anti-cancer properties. Based on Indian lore, Dr. J.W. Fell, working at Middlesex Hospital in London in the 1850's, developed a paste made of bloodroot, zinc chloride, flour, and water. It was directly applied to a malignant growth and the paste generally destroyed the tumor within two to four weeks. He would spread the bloodroot paste onto a cotton cloth, which was then applied directly over the tumor. A fresh application was made and reapplied daily. For deep tumors, he would use nitric acid to break through the healthy tissue. The necrotized cells would eventually form a scab-like slough with a greenish and yellowish color. At this stage, the slough is painless and Fell would cut incisions into it and put the paste into the cuts to be sure that it penetrated deeply enough to destroy all of the cancerous cells. Eventually the mass would separate from the healthy, untreated flesh and literally fall off, leaving perfectly clear uninfected tissue that would subsequently granulate and heal over. Considering how badly the entire process appeared, it is remarkable that the open cavity that is left behind after the tumor falls off seems to never get infected and relatively quickly heals over with a minimum of scarring.

Following the example of Samuel Thompson and Fell, the mid-19th century North American Eclectic Medical doctors continued the use of Fell's escharotic paste. One of a number of medical doctors of the time, Dr. John Pattison attempted, evidently with some success to effect a less painful process though of considerably longer duration, through the use of an escharotic compound substituting goldenseal (hydrastis canadensis) rather than bloodroot in the process.

Another Eclectic medical doctor, Eli Jones, published in 1905 and 1911 his protocol for the treatment of cancer. Jones emphasized internal treatment with herbs, diet and other methods including the Epsom salt bath described earlier. While he did not consider escharotic salves a cure for anything but the most superficial cancers, he did employ a salve consisting of bloodroot, galangal, sandalwood, zinc chloride, flour and water.

His book, *Cancer, Its Causes and Symptoms* (first published around 1911 and reprinted in India by Jain) gives a detailed account of how to apply the escharotic salves as well as several recipes. Cancer being a systemic disease, he cautions against the overuse of escharotics and favors internal treatment with herbs, diet and lifestyle modification.

Despite controversy over its effectiveness and use, the basic escharotic salve formula which consits of equal parts bloodroot, galangal, flour and zinc chloride with water continues to circulate throughout the underground by exponents throughout the world. It was used as a part of the Harry Hoxsey (1901-1974) cancer treatment along with his famous Hoxsey herbal formula based on the earlier Eclectic Trifolium Compound.

Throughout the early part of the 20th century up to the beginning of the 1940's Dr. Perry Nichols, M.D. and his successors operated a sanatorium in Savannah, Missouri specializing in the use of the escharotic paste. He treated approximately 19,000 selected patients over the course of thirty years. The sanatorium published a nicely bound yearly publication entitled *The Value of Escharotics - Medicines That Will Destroy Any Living or Fungous Growth in the Treatment of Cancer - Lupus - Sarcoma*. These journals seem to not describe the use of the salves as much as they presented thousands of names with addresses, photographs and testimonials of patients who underwent successful treatment for a variety of cancers. Looking over a couple of these journals, it seems that by far the majority of cancers, if not all, were close to the surface and included cancers of the lip, breast, jaw, arm, hand, tongue, nose, ear, cheek, leg, etc. There are no cases of internal cancers such as cancers of the pancreas, liver, brain, lungs or internal reproductive organs. I mention this because Nichols prided himself in making a stronger escharotic with two to three times the amount of zinc chloride as the most active caustic. His goal was to burn a perimeter of healthy flesh around the tumor along with the tumor itself ideally in one day. He claimed that the patient hardly suffered any discomfort since he would adjunctively prescribe strong pain medication for the course of one or two days.

Escharotics received modern medical sanction through the work of Dr. Frederic E. Mohs, M.D. Without a mention of at least a century of previous use of bloodroot-based escharotics Mohs called his method "chemosurgery," because he offered it as an alternative to surgery for many types of cancers that were located closer to the surface of the body. For very large tumors, he would favor partial removal of as much of the mass as possible before applying the escharotic to remove the deeper portions.

Mohs' escharotic compound consisted of the following:

Bloodroot - 10.0g

Zinc chloride saturated solution - 34.5 ml

Stibnite (an antimony-based substance) - 40.0g

Mohs' textbook, Chemosurgery (published 1978 by Thomas Books) is well known by contemporary oncologists. In it, he describes with graphic photographs the successful treatment of a wide variety of external cancers, achieving 99 percent success for all basal cell carcinomas. The effectiveness of Mohs' treatment is borne up by decades of medical study and scrutiny and remains today the preferred treatment for a number of skin cancers.

Caution

I must strongly caution against anyone trying this on their own since one can easily find one'self in circumstances that are over one's head. One southwestern naturopath treated a tumor that was on the carotid artery of a patient's neck. The salves 'going for' the cancer cells actually penetrated the carotid artery, creating a medical emergency that required heroic surgery to correct.

What can happen with the escharotic salves is that they can affect an area larger than the intended site. Again this is conjectured to be based on the presence of a wider area of the cancer than one might have suspected. Application to large breast tumors or other areas of the body may result in unintended disfigurement. If after experiencing some discomfort with the escharotic salves, aggravated by fear and trepidation, there may be an inoculation to stop the process. Unfortunately this may not be possible since in many cases even after an application of 24 hours, most of the process of necrotization, with subsequent sloughing of dead tissue, will occur. Considering this, one may as well go forward with the complete treatment.

This having been said, following is the protocol for the formulation and application of escharotic pastes based on the formulas and procedures of Dr. Eli Jones' work and others:

Dr. Eli Jones' escharotic pastes:

Paste No. 1

Saturated solution chloride chromium

Saturated solution of zinc chloride

Solid extract sanguinaria

Pulverized sanguinaria

Glycerin

Prepare as needed since the paste tends to harden. Dr. Jones regards this as the least painful of the pastes but states that it does not always go deep enough. He recommends using it on any repeated procedures or if the tissue is healing too quickly or reactions are too slow. He suggests wetting a camel's hairbrush with the solution and dabbing it over the site two or three times to stimulate the process to continue.

Paste No. 2 (used for small skin cancers on the nose or forehead)

Pulverized galangal root

Zinc chloride

Starch

Enough water to make a paste

Paste No. 3

4 parts solid extract (alcoholic) sanguinaria

12 parts zinc chloride

1 part starch (this could be flour)

2 parts Red Saunders (sandalwood powder)

This salve is recommended in cases of breast cancer, cancer of the lip, hand, foot, arm, back or wherever there is a need for deeper penetration. He said to use the soft sanguinaria, not the dry solid extract. More water can be added to soften it or more powdered sanguinaria to thicken it.

Paste No. 4

To paste No. 3 add equal parts of the saturated solution of zinc chloride and 25% solution of carbolic acid. This paste is used where the condition is ulcerated and it is necessary to penetrate more deeply to the bottom of the tumor mass. This is often indicated for more advanced breast cancers.

Most salves in circulation today consist of the following combination:

Bloodroot powder

Galangal powder

Zinc chloride

Flour and water to form a paste

Some may add various herbs with the bloodroot; however, in general this seems to not be necessary. There is much speculation as to the value of adding 20% DMSO to the cancer salves and poultices to relieve pain and promote deeper penetration.

Three stages to escharotic treatment:

1) The application of the black escharotic paste,

2) the application of either the poultice or the yellow salve, and

3) sloughing off of the dead necrotized tissue and subsequent healing of the shallow open cavity that is formed.

First Stage

Dr. Jones attempted to protect the healthy tissue by first encircling the area where the paste is to be applied with an easily removed adhesive. One may also apply a thick layer of Vaseline around the periphery of the intended site to confine the action of the salve to the affected area. The salve itself is applied fairly thick to a density of approximately 1/4 inch on clean cotton or linen cloth. This is then placed over the intended site to cover the apex of the palpable tumor. Adhesive is applied around the edges to fasten the application to the body and to seal in the moisture of the salve. The application is renewed once daily so progress can be assessed.

The dressing is changed every 24 hours with the previous salve removed as carefully as possible to alleviate any discomfort. The affected area is cleaned with a solution of hydrogen peroxide, followed with witch hazel extract. There may be minor bleeding but this is not generally a cause for alarm. Except for the removal of the bandage, none of this is uncomfortable. A new application of the escharotic patch is then reapplied.

This first stage is completed in usually three to seven days depending on the amount of zinc chloride in the formula when the treated area exhibits a whitish, yellowish to greenish appearance of necrotized (dead) tissue covering at least 85% of the treated area.

During this process the patient may experience moderate discomfort to severe, though not unbearable, pain. The patient may be given a suitable analgesic herbal formula or over the counter pain reliever such as Tylenol to take the edge off the pain if necessary.

Second Stage

After the first stage has reached completion Eli Jones then switched to the following poultice:

Poultice Powder

Combine equal parts powdered slippery elm, flaxseed, lobelia seed and bayberry bark. Put 1 to 2 teaspoons of the powder in a ¼ cup of boiling water. Stir it to a smooth, non-lumpy consistency. Spread onto a white cloth large enough to cover the area and apply. This is changed every two hours. The skin around the growth is bathed with witch hazel tea. When the growth breaks loose and drops onto the poultice, examine the area to see if it appears healthy. If so, apply the Yellow salve. If not, continue applying the poultice.

Yellow Healing Salve

Burgundy pitch (pine tree pitch)

White pine turpentine

Beeswax

Mutton tallow

Olive oil

Melt, stir and cool. Then add Cosmoline, which is a special grease applied to prevent rust. Spread onto a soft white cloth and apply three times daily. It will draw out the unhealthy pus. If it draws too hard it may cause smarting and pain. If so, dilute it by adding one part Vaseline to three parts salve and apply as described.

Dr. Jones comments that "The above Yellow healing salve I have used in all the years of my practice and I have never found anything to equal it."

As with the escharotic salve, there are many variations for the Yellow Healing Salve. Proportions of ingredients should be varied until the desired consistency is achieved, which is fairly hard and thick so that it will not melt and run. The amount of pine tree resin one uses can be approximately the size of a walnut to a pound of mutton tallow. If one using a pound of tallow (lard), about half as much olive oil and a quarter cup of white pine turpentine. The bee's wax is melted into the heated mixture, cooled and spoon tested to determine its consistency. If it is too soft, melt more beeswax. If it is too hard add more olive oil or turpentine.

Third Stage

The most passive stage is when the eschar actually sloughs off. This process should be allowed to happen of its own accord and should not be forced.

One may be surprised to find a perfectly clean crater of exposed flesh formed at the site of treatment. Neither I, nor any of my colleagues, have ever seen this become infected. Nevertheless, this can be treated with an application of echinacea and calendula salve or some other suitable healing ointment such as plantain and comfrey salve. It can also be left loosely bandaged, with the bandage changed once daily following a rinsing off with hydrogen peroxide and witch hazel. One may be amazed at how such a crater can heal over, sometimes with only a minor scar.

Perry Nichols and others may examine the area after the second or third stage and decide that cancer remains and further application of the black salve of stage one is repeated to remove the cancer from the deeper levels. This is another area where it can become dangerous and proper professional assistance is strongly recommended.

This brings us up to the present. While I have interviewed and spoken with a number of practitioners and patients who claimed success in removing their cancer through the use of escharotics, long term, critical studies need to be made concerning the efficacy of escharotics especially for deeper, internal cancers. It is obvious that escharotics are effective for some cancers, especially those that are closer to the surface of the body. While it is a debatable issue, one of the touted claims of proponents of escharotic salves is in their ability, at least to some extent, to be selective in destroying the more vulnerable cancer cells, leaving the non-cancerous tissue intact.

In my own practice I have had 100 percent success in successfully treating a variety of small basal cell carcinomas as well as the routine removal of warts, excrescences and small skin cancers. The value in the use of the salve for these as opposed to the use of other medical procedures such as cryosurgery or surgery, is my sense that the salve does to more specifically target cancer cells, while other procedures are non-selective.

My personal use for breast cancer (one of the types of cancers that are widely self treated by desperate women, often with disastrous results), internal cancers such as lung and liver cancer (the only ones that I have escharotics to date) is difficult to evaluate. One of the problems is that patients who come to me are often too far advanced and one needs to exercise maximum prudence as to who might be a likely candidate for the application of escharotics. One patient with small cell lung cancer, after having an escharotic applied to her back over the approximate site of the tumor, seemed to exhibit by X-ray a shrinkage of the primary tumor. I think this worked not so much by removing the tumor but by topically affecting a strong counterirritant effect that ultimately stimulated a favorable immune response internally.

Another case was a woman in her late 50's with advanced liver cancer. The escharotic patch was applied on the front of her chest directly over the approximate location of the largest tumors on her liver based on x-rays that were previously taken. Before undergoing this process she was experiencing severe pain and fatigue which, except for the fatigue, did not worsen after the application of the patch. Different people have widely varying responses to the escharotic patch while it is on. This can range from a mild sense of discomfort and heaviness over the site to severe discomfort. There seems to be no way of predicting how one individual will react as opposed to another. It so happened that for this woman, there was hardly any added discomfort, just the characteristic feeling of mild irritation and heaviness. In any case, it certainly didn't interfere with her daily activities, nor did it prevent her from her usual sound sleep over the course of 4 days or so while it was applied.

From the day the eschar sloughed off, the woman claimed greater freedom from pain, and more energy than before. From being given only two or three months to live, she went on to live another year and a half. It was felt by her daughter that if she would have removed herself from a stressful relationship with her husband and continued taking her anticancer supplements, she might have continued to live on.

Oncologists have come to measure success by many standards and criteria. They often consider chemotherapy or radiation therapy successful even if it only increased expected longevity by a few months. Of course this is at the expense of the patient's overall immune system and subsequent quality of life. In this sense, the woman's expected longevity and quality of life seemed to improve as a result of escharotic and internal herb treatment up to the last couple of months until her final demise. She and her family agreed that from this perspective, the treatment was successful.

Afterthoughts

My own personal opinions as to how the escharotic pastes work are as follows:

Counterstimulation

This is a process where a strong topical irritant is applied on the skin over an affected area to relieve underlying pain and inflammation by breaking up deeper congestion. Traditionally, herbalists have used various ointments and liniments for this purpose such as an ointment or plaster of cayenne pepper or a mentholated application. Acupuncturists use moxabustion, which is the topical burning of an herb (Artemisia vulgaris), on or near the skin. This can result, depending on the method used, in the formation of a reddening of the surface area or a blistering. The effect of moxabustion is profoundly healing for a wide variety of diseases and is regarded as the 'left hand' of an effective acupuncture practice.

No one has fully explained how moxabustion may work but I believe that many of the effects of the topical application of the escharotic pastes are similar. One of the ways they may work is to create a minor crisis on the surface of the body near a diseased site. This in turn provides a strong neurological and immunological response that increases the circulation of blood and nutrients to and through the area, optimizing and carrying with them a concentration of immune potentiating antibodies along with an increase of natural killer cells and other immune potentiating agents. It may be one of the ways that escharotics work towards stimulating the removal of deeper cancers and tumors.

Removal of surface tumors and cancers

This is the most obvious claim that somehow escharotics draw out and destroy tumors and cancers from the body that then simply fall off.

The issues surrounding the use of escharotic salves seems to focus around issues as to whether it is only useful for those cancers that are closer to the surface and can be directly exposed to the surface influence of the escharotic paste during stage one. One clinic I visited claims success in treating large numbers of patients using the salve to purportively "draw out tumors" from the deeper internal organs and even the brain. I have personally spent a short time at this clinic and interviewed extensively both the practitioners and their patients. They all claimed success, however, in retrospect, without careful scrutiny of before and after x-rays, biopsies, etc., it is difficult to substantiate these claims.

Unfortunately, one patient I referred was treated for breast cancer over the course of three months. Treatment included a barrage of colonics and daily coffee enemas, supplements, juices, herbs (not very specific in this way) and escharotic application directly on the breast to remove the tumor. The patient happened to complain over the severity of pain from the escharotic but nevertheless followed through to completion. The eschar, which was called the "tumor," fell off leaving a cavity and breast disfigurement to which she did not object so long as the tumor was gone. Unfortunately, after the area healed over, a lump remained deeper in her breast, which has continued to grow and suppurate over time.

I have met other women who claimed to successfully use the escharotic to remove their breast tumors; however, there have been no long-term follow-up studies to substantiate any of these claims. This is not the fault of the method and may not even be a reason to not use it. Rather it is a failure of our medical system that is unable to designate time, money and energy to investigate the validity of the use of escharotics and other alternative cancer methods.

Perry Nichols claimed with sufficient proof and validity to treat some

19,000 patients over 30 years with 90% long term cure rate. From his published annual journals, this included a large number of breast cancer patients. We also have the compelling results of Harry Hoxsey, who through the middle of the 20th century operated several cancer clinics throughout North America. Despite repeated legal harassment by the AMA and law enforcement agencies, his claims of success in curing cancer through the use of internal herbs and an escharotic paste have never been refuted. In fact, in one informal study by a number of doctors they were substantiated.

Escharotics continue to be made and sold on the Internet and by individuals throughout North America and Europe. They literally cost pennies to make but bear a heavy cost of responsibility to the one who uses or sells them. One individual I met makes it up in large batches and gives it away to anyone who wants some. He then dedicates around-the-clock hours of his personal time to guiding people by telephone through the fear, discomfort and pain they may be experiencing as they go through the first and second stages of their use. He has literally given the salve to hundreds of people, mostly women with breast cancer and claims no serious negative reactions from their use.

Personally, despite the drastic and extreme reactions to the escharotic pastes, I think that when used with a generous dose of reasonable common sense they are remarkably safe. I treated one woman with a very large breast tumor whom I advised to not use the escharotic paste because it was too large an area and it would probably require repeated applications accompanied by considerable agony and ultimate complete breast disfigurement. I advised her to resort to conventional means first to shrink or remove as much of the tumor as possible through surgery or radiation before considering the use of escharotics. Unfortunately, at the time she did not want to do that and insisted that I use the escharotic. I refused her, as I do many, because I don't think they should be considered a panacea for all types of cancers and situations.

They are one important weapon, however, that can be considered for certain types of cancers. Those who are interested in reading more about the use of escharotics might refer to a book called *Cancer salves: A Botanical Approach To Treatment* by Ingrid Naiman, published by North Atlantic Books (1999).

As stated, escharotic pastes have been used for at least 200 years and they continue to be unofficially manufactured and distributed by individuals throughout the world. One area where escharotics continue to be passed on is in the mid to southwestern states of North America. At one point when I was actively searching out anyone who had experience I found that one of my older students, a quiet older gentleman that had been studying herbal remedies with me for several months, was involved in one of the most interesting ventures with the escharotic salves. It almost resulted in research and FDA approval for the salves in the treatment of cancer. It did however lead to the development of a popular anti-gingivitis toothpaste. One of the interesting facts with Clark's story is the use of the paste internally. Following Clarks' recommendation, I feel comfortable and have seen no serious adverse reaction when patients take only the recommended small bean sized amount of the salve internally. They can put this in a capsule but it should be only taken after food since solo, it can be irritating.

With the combination of Dr. Moh's medically recognized use of escharotics and the following story I feel that there is enough legitimate evidence for further scientific examination of the efficacy of escharotics in the use of the salves.

Following is Clark Bingham's interview about his use, discovery and experiences with the sanguinaria paste:

Contemporary History of the Escharotic Black Salve

Narrated by Clark Bigham to Dr. Michael Tierra

Twenty-Eight years ago my son was diagnosed with glomurulonephritis. Since conventional western medicine has nothing to offer for this condition except palliative treatment with cortical steroids, I was looking for any other viable alternative that was available. It was during that time, in the middle of Wyoming, that a friend told me about a cowboy named Howard McCreary. He said that Howard had a mysterious black salve that could be used either externally or internally to treat and cure a wide variety of problems and that it could be possibly effective for my son's glomurulonephritis.

Howard was indeed literally a cowboy, famous at the time for winning numerous awards in rodeos throughout the country including Madison Square Garden in New York. He received two silver buckles and was named world champion for two years in a row. At the time that I met him, he weighed around 275 pounds, mostly muscle. It seemed that Howard's father passed down a secret anti-cancer formula in the form of a paste comprised of Sanguinaria, commonly known as "bloodroot", Galangal, Zinc Chloride and distilled water. Through a dream, Howard further developed a modification of this formula, including a proprietary method of preparation that increased its efficaciousness not only for cancer but a broad spectrum of other diseases, simple and acute, as well as chronic.

I spent the better part of an entire day speaking with Howard about my son and the various uses for which he had successfully employed the salve. He had an album of photographs showing the many successfull treatments he had accumulated over the years. The pictures were very similar to those found in Dr. Moh's book, *Chemosurgery* (published by Charles C. Thomas, 1978). Throughout all of this, he was very open and gracious with me in every way, bought me lunch and even invited me to stay at his home overnight. Upon leaving, he gifted me a half-pint of the salve to bring home. Because this was all given freely with no hooks attached, I was predisposed to trust and believe him.

Among the many wondrous uses of this seemingly miraculous salve, Howard told me of using it as an eyewash, diluted one part to a thousand parts water. One way he had to determine whether anyone was with him or 'agin em' was to ask them to put it in their eyes. This I did, putting a drop in each eye. At first it stung for about 30 seconds and caused my eye to become mildly irritated. Within a short while, however, the mild irritating condition completely cleared up, leaving my vision clearer and brighter than before. You might consider this my initiation to it.

As a result of Howard's eyewash trial I have personally recommended it to a number of people with glaucoma and macular degeneration. It seems to be highly effective for one type of glaucoma and in about five cases of macular degeneration it proved to be 100% effective.

My wife used the salve topically on a mole. It developed the characteristic minor inflammation with accompanying pain and discomfort.[2] Generally it takes about 8 hours for the area over which the salve is applied to blow up with the characteristic inflammation and whitening on the surface of the skin. Following this, from 7 to 11 days later, the core (eschar) drops off, leaving a shallow hollow core in the skin. Rarely would this be accompanied with bleeding and never with infection. This is simply kept clean with an antiseptic solution such as hydrogen peroxide, and covered. Usually it heals within a month with barely a scar. The fresh skin that healed over it was tender, like a new baby's skin. In the case of my wife's mole, it was completely eliminated. I have never found the salve to damage unaffected tissues. Since my wife had a hair mole, when the tissue healed over, the hair came back. This attests to the fact that the salve didn't even disturb the underlying hair follicle.

Now with over 28 years experience in using the Black Salve it is my belief that, applied topically or taken internally, it has the ability

---

[2] This method uses only the Black salve and does not use the either the herbal poultice or the yellow salve. It seems to be effective in this way as described.

to seek out problem areas throughout the body. It is not a universal panacea for all ills but at least offers a window of opportunity for the individual to make other changes that may be necessary for lasting healing to occur.

Despite all of this, influenced by the negative opinions of the doctors who were overseeing the care of my son, I remained reluctant to give it to him. For the next two years my son was in and out of the hospital almost weekly. Finally, out of desperation, I decided to give him the salve internally. It was interesting because after taking the salve he did not go into the hospital again for over six months. Without any recent checkup, and based only on prior history, the doctors decided that it was time for him to have a kidney transplant. We trusted the doctors and we stopped giving the salve to my son because of the fear that it would stimulate the immune system and result in his body rejecting the transplanted kidney.

In fact, despite the fact that my son had not been taking the salve for some time, he rejected the transplant and a subsequent second transplant later. Later, however, he developed peritonitis and I gave him the salve to take internally and it worked very well.

I learned from the cowboy that the salve generally works very well with all infections, perhaps with the exception of gastrointestinal ulcers for which it can be irritating. I gave the salve to one person with colitis and told him that it may cause a temporary aggravation. This it did for about three or four days, after which the colitis was completely cleared up with no recurrence.

This same man, however, told me that while he had no further colitis symptoms, his ankle developed an unusual pain. I asked him if he ever had an injury to his ankle. He said that when he was much younger, he jumped off the end of a bridge and broke his ankle. I asked if it was the same foot. He said "Yes." "Was it the same place?" "Yes." About a week later he called me again and said "yep, the ankle seems fine now."

The Development of
Vipont Chemical Pharmaceutical Company

Vipont Pharmaceutical Company was located in Fort Collins, Colorado. Howard McCreary and a friend specifically developed the company over 30 years ago to research and develop the salve pending eventual FDA approval. Vipont had a very sophisticated laboratory and was able to raise between one and one and a half million dollars to fund their research. I served as chairman of the board over a period of three years.

My first intention for getting involved with the company was the prospect of financial reward from developing the salve. Eventually, after seeing all the good it was doing and could do for so many people with otherwise incurable diseases such as cancer, I personally invested over $500,000 of my personal funds in the venture.

At that time the FDA may not have been as rigid as they are today and the salve was classified "IND" meaning "Investigational New Drug." 'Officially' its first intended purpose was for the treatment of periodontal disease for which it had been extensively used on animals in veterinary practice. Of course, it was also used extensively and successfully on animals for various types of cancer. While our primary aim was to have the salve approved for the treatment of cancer in humans, at one point we realized that we needed more money to continue our research and to go through the complicated and expensive approval process. As a result we petitioned its use for periodontal disease. In general the FDA has had problems approving a substance for as diverse a usage as periodontal disease and cancer. Because of this, the FDA eventually shut us down.

At one point we sent a sample to be tested at the Mayo clinic. I still have the letter from the investigating researcher stating that the black salve exhibited the highest in vitro (a test tube) reaction against cancer that he had ever seen.

Eventually Vipont was bought out by Viadent (a division of Colgate) and remains an ingredient in one of their toothpastes to this day. Because Viadent chose to use it as an extracted ingredient and leave out the galangal, claiming that it had no therapeutic value in the formulation, it never worked as well for cancer as it did previously. To this day, I make the Black Salve toothpaste and give it away to friends, adding about a 5% ratio to Tom's toothpaste, not other commercial brands. It is highly efficacious with even casual brushing in clearing up periodontal disease.

Since the Black Salve was taken internally, Vipont funded an LD50 toxicity test.[3] It turns out to be quite safe with an LD50 of 700 mg. per kilogram of body weight. The recommended daily internal dose for an average person is only around 150 to 250 mg, taken once daily. This is well within the safe, non-toxic range. In fact I had a man who misunderstood my instructions and took one teaspoon a day for three days. He said he felt nothing but a slight gastric discomfort.

In general, for internal use, I recommend that it not be taken on

---

[3] LD 50 is how much of a given substance is necessary to kill 50% of the test animals (usually mice).

an empty stomach and that the salve be put into a small gelatin capsule.

While the ingredients in the salve are simple, consisting of zinc chloride, powdered sanguinaria and galangal and distilled water, the sequence and conditions of how these are put together are also important. In general, we have found that the Black Salve does not work as well when a lot of things are added to it. It may also be that the preparation lessens and alters the caustic principle of the zinc chloride.

I have given it to numerous people for a wide variety of problems ranging from moles, skin cancers, other cancers, influenza, colds, eye problems, gastrointestinal inflammations, skin diseases including psoriasis and other conditions too numerous to list. My inclination, since the Black Salve seems to seek out diseased areas of the body, is to try it for just about any known condition. More often than not, I have been astounded with the results.

Cosmetically, I have added a 5 to 10% solution to a cream (not moisturizing) to be put directly on fingernails. This seems to make them grow stronger and faster. At one time I added a 15 to 20% solution to shampoos and hair conditioners and the result was that it stopped dandruff and other scalp diseases and brought life back into the hair, making it grow fuller and more lustrous. I have never used it to stimulate hair growth. Now I only use a 5% solution for the scalp for fear that it may unintentionally remove a cherished mole.

Regarding claims of others that the Black Salve is dangerous, I have never seen any serious adverse reaction in over 28 years of its use. I have personally found that while other formulas advocate up to 50% zinc chloride, the version that I use and that was extensively tested by Vipont Chemical Company, only uses about a third and this seems enough to produce its therapeutic effects.

* * *

Moxabustion and Cancer

As previously described, moxabustion is a well known technique associated with the art of acupuncture involving burning the dried herb called mugwort, *artemisia vulgaris*, on or near the skin. There are broadly two techniques for applying moxa, direct and indirect. Direct moxabustion is where, after applying a little oil to the surface for adhesion, the cotton-like dried herb is rolled into small cones about the size of a mung bean and placed on specific acupoints on the skin. These are then lit with a stick of incense and allowed to burn down to the skin. Usually there are repeated applications ranging anywhere from 5 or more which are performed on the same point. Obviously this will leave a small blister, which is allowed to run its course perhaps only with a topical anti-infection salve, but only if it is absolutely needed.

Indirect moxabustion is the more common method preferred in the West for obvious reasons. This is done with commercially available cigar-like moxabustion sticks, although if one is determined, it is certainly possible to role the moxa into a stick using thin tissue paper. The stick is lit at one end and held or passed back and forth over a specific area or acupuncture point. The patient is instructed to say "hot" when they desire that the stick be lifted away momentarily. This process is applied repeatedly until there is a reddening of the area.

Moxabustion is particularly indicated for conditions associated with coldness, but in fact it is effective for a wide range of conditions including cancer. It has the ability to powerfully stimulate a local immune response by increasing the circulation of blood and qi. It is very effective for pain, which while not its only use, makes it particularly useful for cancer.

There has been some controversy even within the acupuncture community, about whether moxabustion is appropriate in the treatment of cancer. In fact, the Chinese have performed research on induced cancers of mice using moxabustion. They found that the direct application of moxabustion on a specific well-known acupoint had powerful antitumor effects by stimulating immunomodulators (IMC), which inhibited the DNA reproducing effects of tumor cells.[4]

I have used moxabustion widely in my practice for a variety of conditions including cancer and I find it to be an invaluable aid in treatment that tonifies the immune system, especially when used on specific points including the following: Back – Bladder points 13, 43, 18, 20, 23 bilaterally and Governor 14 and 4 on the spine. Front – on Conception points 4, 6 and 12

---

[4] Zhao Cuiying, Chen Yunfei, Zhao Jiazeng, Chen Hanping, Zhang Yingying, and Hong Xian (Shanghai Research Institute of Acupuncture and Meridian, Shanghai 200030, China)

Abstract: In the study, the antitumor effect was observed by employing HAC-tumor-bearing mice treated with direct moxibustion on point Guanyuan (CV 4) (Group M), subcutaneous administration of liposome encapsulated immunomodulators called IMC(Group IMC), and combination of these two methods (Group M + IMC). Parameters reflecting biological characteristics of tumor cells, including 5 kinds of lectins, mitotic cycle, expression of C-erbB-2 oncogene and counts of AgNORs were further investigated. The results showed that treatment with a combination of moxibustion and IMC could significantly lower three lectins (ConA, LCA, RCA) among these five lectins (BSL, ConA, LCA,RCA, WGA), significantly reduce the expression of C-erbB-2 oncogene, the counts of AgNORs and the percentage of phase S in HAC tumor cells (compared with Group IMC). Moxibustion or IMC alone did render a certain degree of influence on the above-mentioned parameters, although most of the changes were not statistically significant. The above-mentioned results indicated that the antitumor efficacy achieved by treatment with combination of moxibustion and IMC was mainly through its influence on biological characteristics of the tumor cells, namely, its reducing effect on DNA synthesis or on the proliferating rate of tumor cells and its influence on other biological characteristics of tumor cells.

as well as indirect moxabustion directly over the navel. Stomach 36 on the anterior lateral side of the tibia about 3 inches down from lower border of the kneecap. In addition I would do indirect moxabustion directly over the tumor and instruct the patient and their helpers how to administer this on themselves at home.

Because a treatment is generally done when the area being treated takes on a reddened blush, the moxabustion sticks are seldom consumed in one treatment and can be used repeatedly. When a session is completed it is a good idea to wrap the burnt tip of the moxabustion cigar in tinfoil and lay it down on a wide plate. The procedure is very easily done but it is probably a good idea to have it shown and demonstrated at least once before attempting it.

Magnet Therapy for the Treatment of Cancer

Much less heroic than escharotic salves is the topical application of permanent magnets for the treatment of cancer. Magnets are highly effective for a wide variety of conditions involving the regulation of blood and energy circulation through an affected area. This is their domain of effect and as such they can prove to be a powerful asset for many conditions. I have written a small book[5] on magnet therapy drawn from my personal experience, to which anyone who is interested in their wider therapeutic application may refer. I also recommend the books and work of Dr. William Philpott, M.D., who published the most books on the use of magnets in the treatment of cancer.[6]

The earth upon which we live, including all of life down to the smallest cells of our body, possesses magnetic energy. All magnets have two poles, the positive being the power of attraction and the negative being the power of repulsion. For most types of magnetic healing, magnet therapists the world over agree that it is the negative pole (sometimes misleadingly called the "north" polarity) that is needed, as it is the one that promotes movement and circulation. The positive pole (called the "south" polarity) is more static and will coalesce or stagnate an area to which it is applied.

For healing two types of magnets are used. One is from an electromagnetic field generated by a machine and the other is the use of permanent magnets made of various metallic ores capable of maintaining a magnetic charge. Magnetic properties occur when all of the atomic molecules are aligned to move in the same direction on a piece of metal. Magnets are approximately measured and sold according to their strength measured in 'gauss' units and beyond the direct sense that one magnet is stronger than another; it is

---

[5] Tierra, Michael, *Biomagnetic and Herbal Therapy*, published Lotus Press 1997

[6] Philpott, William H. 17171 SE 29 St. Choctaw, Oklahoma 73020, (405) 390-3009 or fax (405)390-2968

difficult to standardize gauss strength. The strength of a magnet is based on its attraction-repulsion power plus its size. So a small magnet that is claimed to be 9,000 gauss is weaker than the earth, for instance, which is only a half gauss.

The magnets I use for the treatment of cancer are primarily called Neodymium, which are a combination of various metallic ores capable of holding the highest magnetic charge. Sources are provided in the footnotes below. It is posited that all diseased cells, including cancerous cells, have a weaker magnetic charge than a healthy cell. By applying the negative polarity of a stronger magnet over an area where such weaker, compromised cells are located, such as the site of a cancer or tumor, the weaker cells take on the magnetic charge of the stronger cell. This tends to effect a number of very positive organic processes namely 1) imparting great strength and normalcy to the weaker cells, 2) relieving oxidative stress (antioxidant) over the area, 3) promoting circulation and thereby breaking up stagnation while inhibiting the formation of vascular supply to tumor (angiogenesis), 4) relieving inflammation and pain, and 5) shrinking tumors.

To accomplish these powerful effects with a magnet, only the negative polarity should be applied over the site of a cancer or tumor and it should be left on the body as long as possible (ideally 24 hours).

For cancer, one needs to fasten (usually by taping them on) one or more small neodymion magnets, with the negative polarity against the body, over the site of any known cancer. A single neodymion magnet can be taped over the thymus gland, using the positive polarity against the skin, for two hours daily. This is to strengthen the immune system while the negative polarity magnets are to dissolve the tumors. It is also beneficial for anyone with a chronic disease to sleep on a magnetic bed pad on which are placed a large number of 3,950 gauss magnetic (again negative polarity facing the body) spaced approximately on and one half inches apart to conform to the shape of a person's body.

The magnetic field generated by a topically applied magnet must be larger than the area intended for treatment. If the area of the body to be treated is raised one can use a foot corn pad so as not to have continuous pressure against the affected site. For larger areas one can use a multi-magnet mat or apply a flexible disk mat over the site to which is topically applied one or a number of strong neodymium or ceramic disc magnets. In the case of a metastasized cancer, every lesion must be individually treated.

I have seen magnets shrink a variety of tumors when the therapy is properly administered. They offer a relatively inexpensive and effective topical treatment for most solid type cancers. For non-solid lymphatic or leukemic cancers, one may only be able to use the positive facing neodymium magnet over the thymus gland for two hours daily. Some also claim a benefit from the use of negatively charged water. This is made by exposing a glass of water (or herb tea) to the strong negative polarities of a magnet. There are special magnetic cups that one can purchase for this or one could easily fasten two negative magnets to the sides of a special cup or glass or simply place a glass of water on top of a negative pole facing neodymium magnet. It is difficult to substantiate the benefits of the magnetically charged water however, for the topical application of magnets over tumors, the results are easily perceived.

For some reason, they may not work all of the time. This could be for a variety of reasons since the patient has to wear these magnets on the affected site continuously to achieve benefits against cancer. Magnets afford a wonderful ongoing external treatment in conjunction with other external and internal therapies.

Cases

A *38-year-old male* patient diagnosed with a slow growing glioblastoma (brain cancer) was treated for six months with a neodymium magnet sewed into a special pocket on a cap situated over the site of the tumor determined by x-ray and brain other visioning methods. He wore this cap continuously, including at night in bed. After a period of 6 months he returned to his native country in France and had another examination and they found that the tumor had shrunk to a third of its original size.

A *43-year-old woman* with metastatic breast cancer suddenly developed a metastatic tumor lump just above her forehead. It was quite large, about half the size of a golf ball. She was also experiencing some balance and visual impairment. I fastened a small neodymium magnet to the top of the lesion. The same evening, upon driving home, she experienced a remarkably sudden restoration of her mental and visual faculties. The next morning the lesion was reduced to half its original size. She continues to use the magnet topically while pursuing other internal approaches to managing her cancer. This woman is a survivor. While her condition was too advanced to cure, she has continued to survive for at least 4 years using herbs, diet and magnets without any further medical intervention.

A *55-year-old man* dying with advanced liver cancer was able to completely control his pain with the topical application of magnets and without requiring the use of morphine to control the pain.

Other magnet practitioners in the Caribbean and Central America use magnets extensively for the treatment of cancer, evidently, in many cases, with good success. In my experience, while not always effective except for relieving pain, they are an inexpensive and sometimes highly effective modality that can be incorporated into a comprehensive natural cancer treatment.

Meditation

Meditation is a process where one gradually learns to clear the mind of all thought. Easier said than done but to whatever extent it is possible, there is profound and lasting benefit. The best times to meditate are first thing upon arising in the morning and just before going to sleep at night.

There are countless ways to meditate but the goal of clearing the mind is ultimately the same for all.

Find a comfortable place to sit with your spine in as comfortable and upright position as possible. Ideally this is by raising one's buttocks slightly on a pillow on the floor. Meditation begins with concentration. To aid in this, one can create a small altar space, with a candle and a picture of one's chosen form of deity.

Take a few deep abdominal breaths and lightly close your eyes. Sit at first for five minutes, and gradually increase to 10 and eventually more minutes each time. Focus on the non-forced inner and outward expulsion of breath.

At first one's mind will try to resist any attempts to subdue its tyrannical hold on our consciousness. It may have a painful tendency to stray to various thoughts and concerns. When this occurs, keep returning to focusing on the breath. Above all, do not allow yourself to chase after your thoughts. Gradually, by not attributing any significance to them, they will with practice come to relative submission. Perfect suspension of thought is hardly achieved by most and you will find that, like the weather, some days will be better than others.

Remember that whatever uncontrolled thoughts are happening to us each day has a powerful effect on everything we do. Healing others, or ourselves, requires as much calm, focused attention as possible so that daily meditation is one of the most powerful of all healing methods.

Some of the other methods to still the thoughts is through prayer, repeating a sacred name of a deity such as "Jesus, Son of God, have mercy on us." or the Hindu name for God which may be "Rama," "Shiva" or "Krishna." A Mantra such as the syllable "Om" repeated at first aloud several times and then inward. A Buddhist mantra is "Gate, Gate, Para Gate, Para Sam Gate, Bodhisattva." This basically signifies our journey inward and roughly translates as "Gone, Gone, Gone Beyond, Hail the Goer."

Sleep

Sleep is not simply something we do but it is a form of deep nourishment. It is surprising how many have trouble achieving a deep restful sleep. We speak of nourishing our yin or essence with certain herbs and foods, but nothing nourishes yin essence more than sound, restful sleep.

In today's world, it seems that everything around us is antithetical to a calm relaxed state and sound sleep. Ever increasing excitement and stimulation is like a drug, the more we get, the more we crave. Eventually, this takes a negative toll on our nervous system and we are unable to sufficiently relax or sleep as well as we should for optimal health.

It is impossible to live a life completely without stress. For a patient with cancer, this may be even more of an issue, which is one reason why it is so important to focus on this aspect of our life.

Begin by limiting the amount of stressful activity and entertainment. Deliberately avoid the news, TV, the Internet, violent movies and other forms of excessive stimulation to our nervous system. Set aside time out periods of each day, or an entire day each week where one remains as much as possible deliberately silent throughout the designated part of the day, or an entire day, specifically letting people know that at a designated time, you are simply not available. This is a good time to take quiet walks in nature, listen to gentle music, read poetry, do hand crafts, practice journal writing, do qi gong or meditate.

One can use herbs such as camomile, passionflower and valerian taken a half hour before bed to promote a more restful sleep.

Without proper sleep and relaxation, the body-mind will be unable to heal and repair itself. Therefore, this aspect of treatment is extremely important for cancer treatment.

Exercise

It has been found that people who exercise have lower death rates from cancer than do people who do not exercise. Further, by reducing a person's fat ratio exercise generally improves immune system function. Through maintaining healthy circulation, some studies have shown how exercise may prevent malignant cells from spreading.

Too little and too much exercise is debilitating. One should begin with a regular program according to one's capacity. In general, a brisk daily 20-minute walk first thing each morning is ideal. Other forms of exercise that have been shown to be powerful for both the prevention and even the cure of cancer include yoga, tai chi and qi gong (discussed in another chapter). These combine movement with mental focus to optimize the circulation of vital energy and blood throughout the body.

Endnotes

[1] Walker, Morton, *DMSO, Nature's Healer*, p. 60-61, published by Avery, 1993

[2] Friend, C., and W. Scher, "Stimulation by dimethyl sulfoxide and hemoglobin synthesis in murine virus-induced leukemic cells," *Ann. N.Y. Acad. Sci.* 243:155-163, 1975

[3] Spremulli, E.N., and D.L. Dexter, "Polar solvents: a novel class of antineoplastic agents," *Journal of Clinical Oncology*, 2(3):227-241, March, 1984.

[4] Ostrow, S.S.; M.E. Klein; N.R. Bachur; M. Colvin; and P. H. Wiernik. "Cyclophosphamide and dimethylsulfoxide in the treatment of squamous carcinoma of the lung. Therapeutic efficacy, toxicity, and pharmacokinetics," *Cancer Chemotherapy and Pharmacology*, 6(2):117-120, 1981

[5] ibid

[6] ibid p. 53-54

Part Four

FINDING THE
QUIET CENTER
OF THE CYCLONE

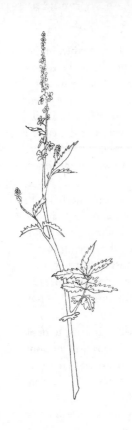

CHAPTER ELEVEN

EMOTIONAL, SPIRITUAL & OTHER ASPECTS RELEVANT TO CANCER

After the initial shock associated with a highly stressful experience of a cancer diagnosis fear, often followed by anger, are the most dominant emotions. Unfortunately while preparing us for an immediate physical threat, these same emotions can be an obstacle to the treatment and healing of a protracted life-threatening disease. This would be true if for no other reason than the fact that these emotions can cloud our judgment at a time when we are most in need of clear inner guidance. Further, the adverse effect on the immune system by these emotions has been shown repeatedly to be an obstacle to healing.

Some of the many outer, emotional and spiritual changes include a radical shift of lifestyle that includes seemingly endless doctors and other therapist's appointments, dietary changes, increasing discomfort and altered relationships with friends and family all imbued with a sense of fear and urgency. The fears can be many and include amongst others, concerns for oneself as well as the fate of those loved ones, who in the event of our passing, would be left behind. However, the root of all our fears emanate from the primal fear of death.

To whatever extent we are able to diminish this penultimate fear, there will be a degree of clarity and space that will serve us to better confront and deal with the inevitable decisions and choices one who has had a cancer diagnosis must make. It would be foolish optimism to categorically state that by overcoming fear one would automatically survive cancer but to the extent that we are able to lessen fear's impact it would most assuredly increase the quality of our lives and perhaps even its longevity as well. For the cancer patient it is even more imperative that they do whatever it takes to be able to approach each day with hope and the openness to receive whatever support or assistance is available at each moment.

Whether it be the loss of some cherished object, position, another with whom we are close, or our own life, such loss is an expression of death in one form or another and it is death that is at the basis of all of our fears. Thus, when we say that someone is in denial of having cancer, they are ultimately in denial of death. However reasonable this may be, just as fear beyond a reasonable limit impairs our ability to act effectively, it is stress-inducing fear that can impair our much-needed natural immunity that is of vital importance in fighting cancer.

Because death is an inevitable part of life, in one sense at least, to deny death is ultimately to deny life itself. Embracing death is certainly not our natural impulse but ironically many have found that to the extent that we are able to accept death positively as a part of life, we are able to live life more fully even to the extent of lessening in some measure life's attendant pains and the physical pains of life's final days. This is why to whatever extent we are able to see beyond the paralyzing influence of our immediate pain and fear we are able to live life more fully. In this same way, I have known courageous cancer patients who have found a life of greater purpose and meaning in the days after a cancer diagnosis than in all of their preceding life.

From the ancient drawings on the walls of caves up to the present, we witness how our need to memorialize a moment of our experience is in one sense to deny its death and it is this same impulse that is at the basis of all of our religious and spiritual beliefs. The attempt to find meaning in life, which is also at the basis of human artistic expression, is another way that we attempt to reach beyond the anxieties, frustrations and fear of death. Thus to lose our creative potential, the ability to see a common thing or anything in an uncommon way is the very essence of death. It is common to witness death but to view death, as a transformative process as all religions tend is to employ not only our ability to believe but also an even more fundamental creative impulse that is at the basis of our being. Thus we see how through the ages art and religion are so often entwined. To live well is to some extent the ability to live artfully, which includes the interweaving of our personal spiritual and religious beliefs into our life in the from of prayer and ritual as well as the adoption of artful life-sustaining activities such as yoga, qi gong, meditation and so forth that can serve us especially at such times in our lives.

For some, meaning and peace is found in surrender to a higher power. Still for many, this is either not possible or not enough so that another way is yet possible. This is in service to a cause greater than their individual life or service to others.

Not only people with cancer but all people, and especially those with cancer or some other deemed terminal disease, should feel encouraged to seek out a positive creative activity or endeavor based on their innate inclination and proclivity. For some this may be in the form of religion, prayer and other spiritual practices but for others activities that involve spending time in nature, completing a yearned for unfinished goal, journal writing, painting, music and yoga are all valuable useful ways to reach beyond our fears to some extent. Not to be overlooked is sharing our feelings, thoughts and experiences with others either one on one or in some organized group experience. To this purpose, there are many cancer support groups available that one may participate in or one may feel called upon to start their own.

There are many methods one can use to gain a measure of clarity in the hopes of achieving some measure of personal clarity and direction. One mind game that I have used with cancer patients is to have patients close their eyes and relax as much as possible and then imagine a radio blaring F-E-A-R louder and louder until it seems completely overwhelming. I then suggest that they reach out with one hand, imagining themselves turning the fear dial louder or softer until it is as faint as possible. For most it is impossible to completely eliminate all fear and in fact a certain amount of fear helps to foster preparedness. With the ever present input from physicians, friends and family, the goal is for the cancer patient to assume as much control over their destiny and fate as possible. To do this they need to recognize when their inclinations and goals are becoming overrun by crippling fear and to be able to turn those fears down as much as possible whenever needed.

Full cooperation between the doctor, various caregivers and the cancer patient

Attitude is of tremendous importance in the treatment of cancer. The most difficult thing for many is the realization that the first and most important step is for the patient to assume full responsibility for his or her own treatment. Overly solicitous family members, doctors, herbalists, acupuncturists and friends should be seen as resources and extensions that can offer suggestions, choices and vitally important assistance, but in the end the choices one makes, whether to undergo conventional medical treatment or not, whether to take herbs, supplements and so forth, rests entirely with the patient. Patients often find themselves intimidated by their oncologists, family or friends and this creates a great amount of confusion.

Since most medical oncologists are not trained in herbal medicine, they often represent a very limited perspective and theoretical assumptions that often do not represent empirical facts. Nevertheless, these assumptions put forth by recognized authorities can prove very intimidating.

It takes at least as many years to become a qualified herbalist as it does to become a qualified medical doctor. Things are very different in the West where herbal medicine is barely recognized as a valid healing system of its own, as opposed to countries such as China and India, where it is esteemed based on centuries of traditional usage, along with contemporary Western medicine.

Seeking the advice and guidance of a qualified professional clinical herbalist is not easy at this time but they do exist in growing numbers throughout the West. One place to go for such guidance is the American Herbalists Guild (AHG).

It cannot be emphasized enough that cancer patients need to take as full responsibility for their treatment as possible. This means that they should not hesitate to question their oncologists, herbalists or alternative practitioners about their experience, qualifications, and whether the practitioner is willing to provide as much information as possible and then support them in whatever choices they make.

One of the most essential prerequisites for every cancer patient is to have a personal lay caregiver who will assist them in their various day-to-day needs. Cancer patients typically go through many emotional changes through the course of their treatment. These range from fear, anger, sadness, irritability, worry and depression to the point where it becomes very difficult to carry on with the tedious daily ritual of herbs, supplements, doctor's appointments, etc. They may develop a lack of appetite or insomnia, which can be very debilitating in itself and requires preferential treatment. Besides physical assistance, cancer patients need to be encouraged to take their herbs and supplements, do their enemas, go for their chemo or radiation treatments and so on. Included in all this, it is probably very wise to have regular "days off" from everything but the barest essentials. I recommend one day a week when no supplements or therapies are undergone and the patient is encouraged to think about other things that will refresh their spirit for when they begin the routine anew.

Having said this, the intimidation and pressure that patients have to endure, not only from arrogant medical doctors but also from close family and friends, can be frustrating and exhausting in the extreme. I would direct the reader at this point to Catherine's story immediately following where she specifically told all her family and friends that she no longer wanted their opinions but she did want their support.

There is no doubt in my experience that those cancer patients who manifest as optimistic an attitude as possible do the best. They are also likely to receive the best care from those they employ.

Following are some actual cases from my files reported by myself or directly in the words of the patients of their experience while undergoing various treatments for their particular cancers. These are not all intended to be success stories in terms of all the patients being cured of their cancer, but they are success stories in terms of the way these patients found inner emotional resources that allowed them to carry on in the most optimal way possible.

Case Studies

Catherine G. – Breast Cancer

Catherine is a close friend who after undergoing a few lumpectomies disdained all further conventional medical intervention and has been subsequently engaged in a valiant battle with breast cancer for over seven years. Like many, she found that the preoccupation with fear was an obstacle to life itself. She soon learned that her task was "to create a space in her life where she didn't feel the compulsion to be always reacting from a place of fear."

For her, healing was coming into right relationship with all that exists: people, plants, animals, the earth and all of nature. Her stand against conventional medicine was based on a basic philosophical difference of having no faith in the American Medical Association and a refusal to align with what she felt were their negative aspects. Because of this, she has lived with breast cancer far beyond the normal expectations, and we are quite certain that the intervention of chemo or radiation therapy after a certain period would probably have compromised her survival more than enhanced it.

Besides being confronted with her own personal concerns and fears, Catherine had to deal with the pressure from family and friends who themselves were caught up in their fears by association. Catherine is a particularly bold individual who had no trouble eventually telling all of her family and friends that while she wanted them to have their own feelings, she wanted no more of their opinions towards her since she felt she had her hands full dealing with her own feelings. What she wanted from them, on the other hand, was their support for whatever decisions she made. Fortunately, all her family and friends rallied to support the decisions that Catherine made in treating her cancer and learning to live with her cancer.

According to Catherine, the greatest relief and support came from an intense daily commitment to hatha yoga. She maintained this for several years until the situation of her breast prevented it. After her cancer diagnosis, Catherine undertook a completely new and more creative livelihood, selling handcrafted objects to friends at various fairs and other occasions. Then she wrote a self-help book for other women with breast cancer. She also explored various alternatives including acupuncture, herbal medicine and most recently she is working as a student-assistant of a shamanic plant healer.

Indeed we can see how Catherine's ongoing experience with cancer has fully changed her life to creative adventure, carrying her to dimensions and places that are far beyond the scope of conventional medicine. Most important, as of this writing, Catherine still lives and remains intensely and creatively engaged and satisfied with her life.

Joan M. age 45 – Cancer?

I have come to suspect anyone who claims a 100% or even a high cure rate for treating cancer. In many cases, curing is not an option while healing in the sense of relieving the suffering of another to improve their life quality is always possible. However, there are experiences that have happened in my career that by typifying a powerful healing principle, stand out as extraordinary.

Following is an extract from a letter from one of my patients who seemed to present with a variety of serious symptoms. After following a vegetarian, macrobiotic diet and a detoxifying herbal regime for a few weeks she experienced dramatic relief from all of her symptoms:

> A little note to say 'thanks' for the wonderful new life you have led me to. Last year I was under treatment for severe rheumatoid arthritis. The pain was severe and constant. Most of the time I could hardly walk and I was unable to use my hands. I had also been 30 pounds overweight for years. I was given numerous drugs, all with very dangerous side effects. These resulted in a deepening depression and feeling I just wanted to die.
>
> I am a very rigid and conservative Christian and have really been praying for a healing or to be led to someone who could help me. One day someone mentioned your book "The Way of Herbs." I read it and was very impressed. I made an appointment. I had to wait 2 weeks. The same morning I had the appointment with you I had a biopsy report telling me I had cancer. The doctor had me all set up for various treatments. I was in a state of shock. I left his office and went directly to your office. You talked to me about diet, attitudes and things no medical doctor ever bothered to mention. At that point I really felt that the Lord spoke to me and I made the decision to abandon all medical treatment and go for what you suggested – and that was the beginning of many miracles in my life.
>
> I immediately started with the herbs, weekly acupuncture and the macrobiotic diet. The first miracle was that within a week the arthritis

was much better. In 5 months it was gone along with 30 pounds of fat. As far as I know the cancer is gone too.

The most important changes were those within. As my body healed so also did my spirit. I will never be the same (thank God!). I have not arrived nor will I ever, these changes and new things come to me every day – this is a lifetime journey, not a destination, nor a place I will arrive at. My walk with the Lord is closer than ever.

During the early days of treatment many times I was discouraged and fearful. In those times you gave me the gentle guidance that I needed and when necessary you reminded me how I was responsible for my own healing. With much love and gratitude, Joan M.

My approach to treating Joan was to promote circulation and detoxification. She was instructed to remove all refined sugar and denatured foods from her diet along with dairy and red meat. I recommended the grain based diet of kicharee for 10 days which consists of mung beans and rice with specific spices. She was then instructed to take five herbal formulas.[1]

Frank Y. age 74 – Prostate and Colon Cancer

Frank had been diagnosed some years previously with prostate and colon cancer. This resulted in a prostectomy with removal of nearby lymph glands. Later it was found that it had metastasized to his colon, liver and lungs. A port-a-catheter was inserted into his abdomen. By now his entire abdomen, extending from the right side over the liver to the right over the spleen was a hard tumorous mass. He had stomach and digestive problems alternating with constipation or diarrhea. When there was a blockage, he had liver and intestinal pains. He was unable to digest solid foods and was given "Insure," a sugar based liquid nutritional food prescribed by his medical doctor. He consequently had a very poor appetite and appeared very thin (cachexic, having lost 20 pounds over the course of 2½ months. He complained of

---

[1] The first was an herbal formula that consisted of a powder of the following herbs: equal parts chaparral and red clover taken as two 'OO' sized gelatin capsules 6 times daily for the first month, then 3 or 4 times daily thereafter. Her second formula was Triphala about two capsules three times daily. Her third combination was for the kidney and urinary system and consisted of a combination of the powders of uva ursi, parsley root, cleavers, a quarter part ginger and a half part marshmallow root. Again two 'OO' sized capsules were to be taken three times daily. The fourth formula was to promote circulation and consisted of a powder of equal parts cayenne and ginger. Two OO sized capsules were to be taken three times daily. The fifth formula was an herbal tea that consisted of Burdock root, dandelion root, sarsaparilla and a half part licorice. This was made by simmering three tablespoons of the herbs in three cups of water. One cup was to be taken three times daily. She could take all the herbs together with a cup of the tea before meals except for the Triphala, which was to be taken after meals.

feeling very tired and weak. Previously he was treated with chemotherapy but no radiation therapy. [2]

He was completely free of pain within three days. I saw him again two months later and he was greatly improved, had more energy, no pain and his tumor had even shrunk somewhat. As much as anything, the success of his treatment was due to the dedication of his wife who prepared everything for him and saw to it that he took them as indicated. They both were very grateful and said that I was the only one to offer them something to do and some hope of recovery.

The lesson in this case demonstrates a complex daily regime and the necessity of an advanced cancer patient to have a dedicated helper to see to it that they have the encouragement and ongoing support to take their supplements.

Mary, age 89 – Breast Cancer

Healing does not always mean to completely cure a disease such as cancer. For many, the best approach is through coping and management. Sometimes medical intervention may be needed and useful, but too often its slash, burn and poison approach adds little, if anything, and may actually compromise one's life quality and hasten one's demise.

I have not been able to find any studies thus far comparing the survival rate of patients who, after a cancer diagnosis, opt to do nothing compared

---

[2] Following is the program I put him on:

1. Planetary Formula's Red Clover Cleanser and the Complete Pau d' Arco Formula, six tablets of each four times daily.
2. Reishi mushroom, three tablets three times daily.
3. Wheat grass, one ounce added to 8 ounces of fresh squeezed carrot juice twice daily.
4. Bio-Radiance chlorophyll-rich green drink, one tablespoon in 4 ounces of liquid or added to the carrot juice twice daily.
5. Metagenics Health Gain, 2 scoops with 8 ounces of water, soy or rice milk three times daily.
6. Slippery elm powder, 8 level tablespoons (1/2 cup) each time to which warm, pure water is mixed to form a porridge consistency. Honey, cinnamon and ginger is added to taste. This was gradually reduced to 3 tablespoons.
7. Tea consisting of a combination of 2 parts each of Red clover blossoms, chaparral, dandelion root, 3 parts each of burdock root, stillingia, sarsaparilla, Oregon Grape and prickly ash, 1 part buckthorne and one part licorice root. All these herbs were mixed together. One handful of the mixture was simmered in a quart of distilled water for 20 minutes. It was then allowed to cool. He was instructed to consume the entire quart throughout regular intervals each day.
8. He was also given a daily warm castor oil fomentation over the liver. Various vitamins were recommended including a multivitamin pill, a dessivated liver pill three times a day with the protein drink, Vitamin E 1000 IU's, Beta-carotene 25,000 IU's daily, Vitamin C 2,000 mg daily, selenium and lipoic acid.

to those who undergo conventional therapies. The problem is that if no one sees these patients in a medical context they are not likely to figure into the dire cancer survival statistics that cause oncologists and patients to over-react in favor of the most heroic, desperate treatment protocol.

Again, I think that there are some instances, especially with fast growing tumors where a combined approach is optimal. There is at least a suggestion that any heroic attempt to quickly rid the body of a tumor might indeed promote its recurrence and metastasis elsewhere.

Mary is a case that demonstrates a woman who was never part of a statistic. She was the mother of one of my patients. When her daughter took me out into the waiting room to meet her mother, the spry 89-year-old crone jumped up enthusiastically to shake my hand vociferously, exclaiming how happy she was to meet me and how she had read my books for years. She told how she has had undiagnosed breast cancer for 25 years and everytime the tumors would form, she would prepare strong burdock root tea and drink a quart a day until they went away, usually within two weeks to a month.

Whether she actually had breast cancer or not is irrelevant in view of the fact that something positive was happening for her and to have enough faith and confidence from what she read in one of my books to drink a full quart of strong burdock root tea every day until her lumps disappeared is no small achievement.

This led to my asking at the beginning of every lecture on cancer how many people in the audience either themselves, or someone they know who after receiving a cancer diagnosis, chose to do nothing and survived past the designated 5 year cure time. Usually from 40 to 60 percent of every large group of people raised their hands. In some cases, doing nothing might mean to only take herbs or follow a special diet.

I don't know if it is still the case, but in China it used to be that someone diagnosed with cancer was treated, but not told that they had cancer. Studies there seemed to show that those who knew they had cancer died more quickly than those who didn't.

This case shows that sometimes it is better to not know of the severity of one's condition and to encourage the pursuit of avenues of self-healing, perhaps with the guidance of an experienced practitioner or even a credible book. It also shows that one needn't know a wide number of exotic herbs and formulas and that there is a power for some, in taking concentrated daily amounts of a relatively safe, mild herb in the treatment of a serious disease.

Richard B. – Brain Cancer (astrocytoma)

Richard was of French origin and he was recommended and brought to me by a former client who took on the task of directly assisting cancer patients in their healing for which he received room and board and a financial stipend. Richard had a slow growing astrocytoma brain tumor, which was first diagnosed in France.

He came for weekly acupuncture and herbal appointments for a period of three months. After this time, he needed to relocate to another area but he continued the dietary, acupuncture, herbal and magnet therapy I recommended to him.

I put him on a mostly macrobiotic dietary regime, allowing some fish two or three times a week as the only source of animal protein. He began with a Kichari fast for 10 days. He was also given several herbal formulas, including Planetary Formula's Reishi Mushroom Supreme, Red Clover Cleanser and the Complete Pau D'Arco Formulas. He was given a specific TCM formula that included powdered 5 to 1 extracts of scorpion, centipede, silkworm, tienchi ginseng, andrographis and scutellaria Barbat. He was also directed to drink three cups of tea made of burdock root, dandelion root, red clover blossoms and a half part of licorice root. The tea was prepared by slowly simmering an ounce of the herbal combination in four cups of water down to three cups. He was directed to have one cup of this tea (sweetened or not with honey), three times daily. He could take this with the other herbal formulas.

I decided to use the strongest neodymium magnet to reduce the tumor size. In order for this to be effective it needed to be on most of the 24 hours a day, situated approximately over the area of the head where the apex of the tumor was thought to be. An x-ray determined this. In order to fasten the magnet over the tumor, Richard devised a baseball cap with a small pocket sewn inside the cap over the appropriate area. The neodymium magnet was placed inside the pocket of the cap, with the north-seeking side face down against the body. Richard literally wore this cap continuously day and night for approximately three months, after which time he returned to France. Upon his return he went for another MRI and the French doctors who originally diagnosed the tumor were amazed to find that it had reduced to nearly half its original size over the interim.

Melissa H. – Brain Cancer (astrocytoma)

(In her own words)

> "Why don't you give it a name?" my friend suggested. Of course, I thought, this tumor has come to me as a teacher and we'll get along better as partners than as adversaries. From that day on, the tumor in my brain became Maud. Maud caught my attention through blind spots in my vision. At its worst, the entire right side of my sight was gone. I was passed along from my optometrist to an opthalmologist to a radiologist and finally a neurosurgeon who ordered an MRI

(Magnetic Resonance Imaging) scan.

The results showed the tumor clearly resting on the optic track deep in the left lobe of my brain. My doctor labeled her an astrocytoma and his only solution was radiation. But I clearly felt that attack only leads to stronger defenses, and this tumor was not something to battle with or wage war against. I had no desire for my brain and body to be under siege.

I chose the different, less-traveled path, and my world expanded as I turned the singular focus from my tumor to the broader view of my life. I saw illness not as a punishment or sinister plot against me, but simply an attention getter. Illness is a voice calling out "Stop, something is out of sync and changes need to be made." I had ignored earlier hints and nudges to take stock of my life, but now my attention was riveted, and I thought it prudent to listen carefully.

Yes, I was scared and confused. With supportive family and friends I cried and screamed, punched pillows, and asked "why me?" I let my fears run wild with gruesome scenarios. I knew that these feelings had to be expressed and released. The flood of energy and calm that followed these sessions was magnificently soothing. With these emotions more or less out of the way, Maud's guiding voice became stronger, and I learned to trust it.

The next step was to reclaim my power and take responsibility for my own healing. I had grown up on the coast of Maine, the youngest of a hard working family that placed emphasis on accomplishment and putting others first. To avoid confrontation or conflict, either within the family or workplace, I accommodated as necessary to keep things smooth. The idea of standing up for myself or saying "No" or "I'll do it my way" was an alien concept. Also, our society has cultivated a dependency upon authority figures. We look for someone else to take care of us and to fix us right now so we won't be late for our next appointment. To say "No, I don't want radiation and I want to pursue alternative methods," to my doctor was a difficult but key step. When I hung up the phone, my body was shaking, but a new strength was surging through.

My job was next. Realizing that I was not indispensable, nor responsible for the make or break of the entire organization, I quit a stressful and emotionally draining job. Healing became my full time occupation, and now macrobiotics took the stage.

I had a better than average dietary rearing with awareness of "healthy" foods with homemade whole grain bread and lots of fresh vegetables from our garden, but the consciousness still revolved around meat and dairy with a hefty sweet-tooth to top it off. After leaving my parents' home, I evolved easily toward a vegetarian diet, but the amount of cheese, butter, eggs and yogurt I consumed was astounding. My roommate once remarked that I was a bovine delight. I used to tease with a friend that we could cook up anything with butter and love. We had half of the equation right!

I had known of macrobiotics for several years and now the time was ripe. Here was a very tangible arena for me to work in – and I loved it! The idea of letting my body heal itself by getting out of my own way appealed to me immensely. I had always loved to cook, and now the concept of food and healing fascinated me. I had an interview with a macrobiotic counselor and with a direction to go in, I easily spent 75 percent of my time dealing with food-planning, preparing, and chewing.

It became easier for me to chew (once my jaw muscles got in shape)[3] when I acknowledged that once I sat down at the table I knew I would be there for the next hour. It became part of my routine and released me from a sense of urgency and impatience that eating was taking so long. I really enjoyed just settling in and chewing.

The other aspect that made a tremendous difference was attending a weekly cooking class. The support, information, and inspiration received from human contact was so much more valuable than trying to memorize from a book. My Wednesday nights became sacred – and still are!

For the first three months on the healing diet I was exhausted, often constipated and lost 20 pounds, looking emaciated and frightening to my family and friends who bravely continued to support me.

Prior to understanding the all-encompassing effect of food in my life I watched my emotions shift with confusion. I had very little patience, became easily frustrated and intolerant of others. With tears of frustration I complained, "I don't know what's happening to me." My husband gently said, "I think it's your diet." Wow, the notion of food affecting my feelings was staggering. I had become 'tight!'

Yoga was an important aspect of my life, and I found that the movement and meditation was very soothing and relaxing to my body and wound-up emotions.

As I learned more and felt comfortable working with the food, to stop and really think about activities that made me happy was new. I needed to stop taking care of the rest of the world and neglecting myself. I had to figure out how to take care of myself, and I had to

---

[3] Macrobiotics recommends chewing every mouthful 100 times for serious diseases.

allow others to take care of me. This last aspect continues to be the hardest as it flies in the face of all my "It's OK. I can do it myself" upbringing, which is terribly isolating and not very helpful.

The autumn progressed, and my stamina slowly returned and then surpassed previous levels. I was still painfully thin (literally taking a pillow everywhere I went to sit on), but I felt great!

I wanted to give myself time before I had another (my fourth) MRI scan for feedback. My counselor had said that I could possibly go through a period of tumor enlargement as it attracted all the toxins my body was releasing. But in December 1990, six months after starting my healing macrobiotic diet, my doctor, my husband, and I were pouring over the picture of my brain taken that morning, and no one said a word. I finally broke the silence, "I don't see anything." After a pause and with sincere confusion my doctor said, "I don't either. Just where had the tumor been?" Maud was gone.

Now, two years later, I know that the essence of Maud has never left me. Her voice continues to guide me to doors that keep opening deeper into the worlds of macrobiotics, of yoga, and of self-reflection. Trusting this inner voice is the greatest gift Maud has given me and I am eternally grateful.

There are many lessons we learn from this courageous woman's approach. First we see how Melissa developed a creative approach in making her cancer an ally or teacher rather than an adversary by personifying her with a name. Second, we learn the ways she had to come to terms with her fears and confusions and then to eventually rise above them to arrive at a single clear choice for her treatment, which in this case was not to include conventional medicine. Thirdly, we see the power of diet, especially a macrobiotic diet, in helping her to overcome the years of fatty foods that she had been consuming that were probably at least a contributing factor for her brain tumor.

Characteristically, macrobiotics is a protein-lean diet rich in natural anti-cancer phytotherapeutic compounds that not only do not feed the cancer (as would sugar and fat), but it also provides sources of anticancer plant-based compounds that will inhibit cancer. Here the patient had to go through dangerous periods of weight loss but obviously she had enough nutritional reserves that eventually such a diet literally starved out the tumor before the patient.

Again, this case would not figure as part of the statistical averages that are often quoted when doctors offer their prognosis. It is also noted that in this case, this woman did not undergo a regime of supplements and herbs, but was able to accomplish her goals completely with diet.

Gary S., age 40 – Prostate Cancer

Following is a letter from one of my patients with prostate cancer. This is the case of a very intelligent man whose will allowed him to make a sudden complete change in diet and lifestyle but also able to consciously empower the guidance and treatment he was given for his own benefit. I asked him for a letter describing his ongoing journey which I enclose here in its entirety:

First of all, I'd like to make it quite clear that I'm not a doctor, or involved in the health care field in any way. I'm a commercial real estate broker in Downtown San Jose. I'm not promoting any products or special interests, and everything I talk about is based solely on my own personal experiences over the past year as a cancer patient.

My goal today is threefold:

First, I want to talk about the necessity of **taking control of your own treatment options** when faced with a life threatening disease such as cancer. A person is so frightened at the exact moment that they find out about their cancer, that they can be pressured into making premature decisions that are irreversible. It's easy to ignore the morbid side effects of the **"big three"** of surgery, radiation and chemotherapy when you believe your life is on the line and you have no choice. Well, you do have a choice.

Second, I want to stress the importance of strengthening the immune system through a strict regimen of **diet, exercise and attitude** to assist in the healing process. I believe that cancer starts because of a weakened immune system, which is the result of a lifetime of poor nutritional and lifestyle habits. As such, I believe strengthening the immune system can contribute to the reversal of cancer. It is also my belief that cancer is a systemic disease, and not a local one, and should be treated accordingly.

Third, I want to point out **how much better** my life has become since finding out I had cancer. **This is not a death sentence—it is a life sentence**. Since dropping all of my old "bad habits", and adopting a new and healthy lifestyle, I've never felt better. I've dropped thirty pounds and achieved a new level of fitness. My friends tell me I look ten years younger, and I've become a much better person because of it. There are some definite advantages to healthy living!

My particular wake up call to health came **last November** when I was diagnosed with what the doctor termed an **"aggressive and advanced"** stage of prostate cancer. I had recently turned fifty, and went for a standard PSA test. I felt well enough at the time, and was flabbergasted to find that the disease had spread so far without any warning signs. I spent the entire month of December in a blur of eating and drinking and doing whatever else I could to deal with the trauma of my pending death.

But as I began working through the haze of fear, and through the mountains of conflicting opinions and information, **I slowly came to realize that this really could be a blessing in disguise.** This was the opportunity I had been waiting for to really turn my life around health wise, and to become a more aware and compassionate human being in the process. With that thought in mind, I set January 1, 2000 as a new beginning.

The first step was to **gather as much information** as humanly possible on my disease. There are so many sources to go to for information. Western doctors are well versed in their particular field of bias, but offer little else in terms of treatment. **A urologist will recommend surgery, a radiologist radiation, and an oncologist chemotherapy. But when asked about treatments outside their particular field, they get vague all of a sudden.** But bookstores are filled with cancer books of every persuasion, the internet has endless sites to explore, and local cancer support groups offer another invaluable source of the most current information, as well as giving an opportunity to interact with other survivors. It is only by accessing every possible means of gathering knowledge that one can get their arms around this thing. This is when you need to assemble a health care team. My immediate team presently consists of a urologist, an oncologist, an herbologist, an acupuncturist, a chiropractor and a massage therapist. Add to this family and friends who will love and support you, and all of a sudden you are not alone anymore. It is not just you against the cancer. Each member of this health care team will have something important to contribute, and the sum of the parts is definitely much greater than the whole, or especially the opinion of just one team member.

Prior to the discovery I thought I was doing a well enough job of taking care of myself. I exercised once or twice a week, but drank too much, ate too many of the wrong things, and worked too many hours. I skipped breakfast each morning thinking there was no time, and my idea of a good lunch was a beer and a sandwich. My wife always cooked healthy dinners, but my overeating kind of defeated the purpose. I basically thought that as long as I looked good on the outside, everything on the inside should be OK too. I was basically walking around in a daze and a state of denial, planning on someday doing something about my health. Everything changed the day I met with my doctor at Kaiser to get the results of the biopsy. As my wife and I walked out of the office in total shock, **I could feel the hours**

and minutes of my life just slipping away.

You know, this is really the darkest hour for cancer patients, and this is when you are the most vulnerable. The **Western medical view addresses the symptoms more often than the causes,** and you are immediately offered one of the "big Three" in cancer treatment (surgery, radiation or chemotherapy) along with powerful hormone blocking drugs. At the time you are willing to do anything to "get well", and one of the saddest things I have seen is patients who jumped into a major procedure too soon without gauging the side effects and quality of life issues that will certainly arise. I had actually **signed my release** form with a clinic in Palo Also **to begin radiation treatments the next day,** but fortunately a conversation with my herbologist Michael Tierra persuaded me to postpone that procedure, and that was the pivotal point in my recovery process. Once you are cut, burned or poisoned, the immediate symptoms may be gone, but the cancer may still be there microscopically in your body. That is why it is so important to treat it as a systemic disease, and not rely on just one quick fix to solve the problem. **Every case is so different from the next,** depending on the type and severity of the cancer, and the lifestyle and overall health of the patient. **The many options and opinions are tremendously confusing,** and I can't emphasize enough the value of educating yourself to your specific disease.

The first thing to change was lifestyle, so on January 1 of this year I stopped alcohol, meat, caffeine, dairy products, fats, sugar, and processed foods in general. I concentrated on live foods. Eating "dead" foods is so hard on the body. The body must create enzymes to digest this food, and in the case of a cancer patient, you need those very enzymes to kill the cancer cells. Fruits and vegetables carry their own enzymes, and basically self-digest once they are in the body. I now start each day with a smoothy, and a handful of vitamins and herbal supplements, and burst out the door each morning with a tremendous burst of energy.

Added to this is a daily exercise regimen consisting of stretching, aerobics and strength training. This is followed by another round of stretching, and then I get cleaned up and in the office. I'm a morning person, and still the first one in. But after such a good start to the day, it is hard not to show up in a great mood, and keep that mood going through the day. On weekends I'll hike in the mountains (there are so many beautiful places close by), or walk on the beach. Just getting outdoors for any kind of activity

The final ingredient is attitude. All the knowledge in the world is useless unless you truly believe in the choices you have made, and commit to follow whatever path it is you have chosen. It is knowledge that gives us confidence, and empowers us to make our own decisions, but it is our belief in the wisdom of our choices that allows us to take it to the next level and actually make definitive changes that will improve our health.

It's been nearly eleven months and I can't begin to describe how much better a person I've become. In spite of the cancer I've never felt better. My PSA levels are presently undetectable, and my attitude and health are unstoppable. My life is calmer, and I feel so much in touch with both myself and those around me. I'm trying to squeeze out every minute of every day, and each day feel like I'm seeing the beauty of life around me for the first time. More than anything, I've become fearless. Of course we're all going to die, but why not concentrate on life instead of death? This thought right here can set you free, and on the road to healthy and happy living.

Vitamins and Herbal Supplements
Smoothie:
1 cup orange juice
1 banana
1 tablespoon "Green Magma" (powdered barley grass juice)
1 tablespoon of soy protein powder
3 powdered green tea capsules
Lemon or orange zest

Blend for thirty seconds and drink with daily vitamins and supplements. I have given this recipe to friends who have reported feeling a major energy burst. There's nothing better than eating live food (fruit) in the morning. It goes straight into the system and begins to digest itself because it is carrying it's own enzymes.

In Morning:
- *PC Spes* (author's formulation without drugs), containing eight different herbs and specific to prostate cancer
- *PectaGen*, containing saw palmetto and grape seed extract, among others
- *MycoCeutics*, containing ten mushroom formula
- *Eskimo 3* fish oil supplement with vitamin E
- *Bupleurum Liver Cleanse*, containing about sixteen different herbs

- *Cellular Forte* to promote healthy cell growth
- Vitamin C
- Vitamin E
- Multi Vitamin
- Calcium, Magnesium, Zinc
- Selenium
- Iron
- Aspirin

In Afternoon:
- First six again.

Unlike prescription drugs, herbal supplements come in pretty gentle doses, and rely on continued use to reap the greatest benefits. Only an herbologist can prescribe the right combination for any individual. Typically, after a lengthy interview, certain herbs and supplements will be given, and monitored on a regular basis. Everyone has a different set of health issues to deal with, and this approach can offer a much more tailored approach to therapy, rather than a "one drug for everyone" approach.

- TEA, taken before and after meals, made of red clover, burdock root and dandelion root.

The Team:

Herbology and Acupuncture: Michael Tierra at the East West Herb and Acupuncture Clinic in Santa Cruz 831-429-8066.

Chiropractic: Dr. Andre Chevalier at TEAM Clinic in Santa Clara 408 241-8326.

Massage: Tammy Puthof, Massage Therapy in Morgan Hill 408 683-0428.

Western Medicine: Dr. Harris, Kaiser Urology and Dr. Fischetti, Kaiser Oncology in Santa Clara. Dr. Eric Small, Urology, UCSF.

Spiritual Healing: My wife, family and friends who constantly surround me with love, and allow me to look beyond the immediate.

PC Spes: Mike Cook, Vivacity, 800 251-6315

San Jose Prostate Cancer Support Group. Over a hundred people at monthly meetings with speakers and lots of information.

Barnes and Noble: There is so much helpful information available both in bookstores and on the Internet.

Books:

A *Cancer Battle Plan* by Anne Frahm. This is an easy read, written by a "lost cause" survivor, who has covered all the bases in terms of treatment and recovery. A great little book.

Definitive Guide to Cancer by Burton Goldberg. This is the bible of alternative treatments, with over 1100 pages including recommendations of 37 leading cancer physicians and 55 documented patient cases, covering all types of cancer. Incredible in the amount and variety of information available.

Herbal Remedy for Prostate Cancer by James Lewis, Jr. Talks about various herbal treatments, with lots of information on PC Spes.

An Unfinished Cancer Story:

When you first hear the words "You have prostate cancer" you really only have two choices. You can roll over and wait for what you might think is the inevitable, in the meantime drowning in whatever temporary escapes (drugs, alcohol, self pity) you may find, or you can embrace the "cure", and go on the attack. There are so many weapons at your disposal, including the most powerful of all, attitude. Your attitude will dictate where you go in the fight, and can carry you through the toughest of obstacles, not the least of which will be fatalistic and preconceived notions from your doctors, friends and loved ones as to your early demise.

The first few weeks after receiving the news are undoubtedly the hardest, after hearing from a somber doctor who has recited various facts and figures about how long you are expected to live, given you treatment options of which none are very attractive (castration, radical prostectomy, radiation). You walk around numb, and fully convinced that it is just a matter of time. You forget that it is just a matter of time for each of us on this earth anyway, and become consumed with the thought of your own mortality. If you're even able to discuss it with other people, they may ask if they have "caught it in time". Well that's easy. They have always caught it in time if you're not dead yet! Look how close Lance Armstrong came to death, with tumors in his brain and lungs, and look how far he came back to win the Tour de France twice. There are many Lance Armstrongs in this world. Become one.

It is my firm belief that a balanced and all-encompassing approach to cure must be taken as quickly as possible. Don't mourn your own death too long, for it will start to become a reality. Spend just a little time, if you can, enjoying your "old" life. Remember those double martinis, rare steaks, triple espressos, or whatever else that was so much a part of who you were, and that unfortunately was probably in some way responsible for where you are today. Then drop them like a bad habit. It is time for a change. And if you can embrace this change, you will see that the knowledge of your cancer can actually become a blessing. It will change your life in some very positive and unexpected ways.

The first step is to fully understand the extent of your disease, so you can fully embrace the cure. Assemble a team of experts in their respective fields. Read books, get second opinions, go to support groups for information. The Internet is an invaluable resource. Get to the point where you know more about your specific cancer than even your own doctor does. Because when you have this knowledge, you are empowered to choose your own treatments and understand their benefits, as well as their side effects. Make no major decisions (surgery, radiation, etc.) until you have your arms around this thing. This is hard at first, because everything seems so confusing, but soon enough the fog will clear and you will find your right path. Through a combination of both eastern and western medicine, diet, exercise and mental attitude I have found my path to the cure. This is based on my firm belief that cancer is a systemic disease, and should be approached accordingly. This is what has worked for me...

At age 50 I knew it was time for a random PSA test, and after three years of asking my doctor at Kaiser for one, he finally consented. After a surprising initial PSA of 15.9 (which was alarming, but not too bad), I had a biopsy, and found a Gleason score of 9 (which was really bad). Although a bone scan and subsequent MRI revealed no metastasis, it was assumed that the disease had already spread microscopically through my system. I had no outward symptoms, so the news came as quite a surprise. I used to consider myself in fairly good health, although I had several "bad habits" I had been trying to ignore for years. Little did I realize at the time that everything in my life was about to change in a very rapid and a very exciting way.

The very first choice my urologist at Kaiser offered was a radical orchiectomy, or removal of the testicles (medical castration). Since prostate cancer is a hormone driven disease, this procedure would stop my body from producing testosterone, and slow the spread. This was absolutely out of the question, so then we moved on to plan B, which was implementing a hormone blocking therapy consisting of four month lupron shots and daily casodex (clinical castration). He took great care in describing the side effects, which included everything from hot flashes, short temper and loss of strength to impotence, incontinence, and even growing breasts. I immediately assumed the worst, and went home feeling like my normal life was over. This was right around Thanksgiving, 1999, and I spent the month of December eating, drinking and being as merry as possible under the circumstances, all the while contemplating my fate. Starting January 3, I took the first four month lupron shot, and began daily doses of casodex.

The next decision to be made was whether or not to start radiation treatments. Although it was assumed the cancer had already spread beyond the prostate, a second opinion at Stanford strongly recommended radiation treatment, just in case the disease had not gone that far. Side effects to be expected were the possibility of permanent impotence and incontinence. The decision to start radiation was especially difficult, because of the lasting side effects. In my confusion, I had actually decided to start, and had even signed the release form for the treatments to begin the next day, and at the last possible minute, I was dissuaded by Michael Tierra at the East West Clinic in Santa Cruz. Although I had wasted the time of a few of my western doctors, this proved to be the pivotal decision in my treatment program, and set in motion everything else I am doing today to maintain my health.

Michael Tierra had already counseled me in choosing a new diet, and incorporating herbal supplements into my daily routine. Even more importantly, he told me what to eliminate (alcohol, red meat, caffeine, dairy products, fats and sugars), which was most of the stuff I had been consuming for the past fifty years. I had been rather bored with certain parts of my lifestyle over the past several years, and this was just the jumpstart I needed to begin completely reinventing myself.

As the weeks went by, and as I began following this strict program of diet, exercise and attitude, I immediately began to see results. And the more results I saw, the more excited and committed I became to turn this thing around. In the first six months of my new program, I had lost thirty pounds, and looked years younger. My energy level shot up, and I found I could get by on an hour's less sleep each night. It was especially satisfying going to the tailor to get my clothes taken in... My PSA dropped from 15.9 to 3.5 to 0 (thanks to the lupron and casodex), and I was experiencing virtually no side effects from the medication. After eight months of the double hormone therapy, I decided to stop taking the drugs, and my doctors did not contest my decision. Where I've gotten to now is such a better place, physically, emotionally and spiritually, it really has been a blessing in disguise to find out about the cancer.

Here are some random thoughts on the quality of life after the knowledge of cancer...

Power of the Universe. Every day presents an opportunity to improve oneself, and to tap into what I call the Power of the Universe. Many people call this God. Pray, meditate, or just stare into the stars for inspiration and strength. Walk in the forest or on the beach. See yourself as a very small part of a very big plan. Wake up and see the world as a more immediate and urgent place to be in. Do good deeds, because it feels good and because karma is truly an underrated force in this world. Become spiritual in whatever way you choose, and pay attention to the big picture. Here you will find peace.

Love. Love truly does make the world go round. To get it, you must give it. The love and support of my wife, friends and loved ones throughout this past nine months has been truly incredible. So many have given me so much support, even though it took me quite a while to tell them. Remember it is always hardest for those closest to you, because they feel helpless. You must keep them pumped up, and let them know you are giving it your best, and it will come back tenfold.

Options. There are so many options, but you must search them out. Find out all you can about the disease, and the various treatment options, and then decide. And stick with that decision. Don't ever give up, not for a single day, not for a single minute. You must embrace your cure. You must live it and breathe it, and you will become it.

Form a team. I have consulted with three urologists, an oncologist, a radiologist, internist, chiropractor, herbologist, massage therapist, acupuncturist, personal trainer, and several cancer survivors. Each had a different take on things, based on their field of expertise. All have something valuable to add, but it is up to you to pick and choose what parts of the individual disciplines you want to incorporate into your personal program.

Attitude. This is what drives everything. All the knowledge in the world is useless until you truly believe in the choices you have made, and commit to follow whatever path you have chosen, at all costs. The amazing thing about attitude is that it is contagious.

Opinions. Don't ever settle for just one. Each doctor has his own bias, his own field of expertise. An oncologist will recommend chemotherapy, a urologist will suggest castration or radical prostectomy, a radiologist will prefer radiation. While there may be a time and place for these radical treatments, it is not within the first few weeks after receiving the knowledge. I've heard so many stories of patients who were pressured into making a quick decision that they later regretted.

Nutrition. This is the foundation for the cure. Stop putting processed foods in your body and get natural. Raw foods carry their own enzymes – save your body's natural enzymes to fight the cancer. Keep your immune system strong, because it is this that has allowed the cancer to grow, just as it is this that will keep it from spreading. Remember that your liver is the most important organ for eliminating toxins from your body. It must remain healthy and functioning, or all the poisons just get recycled and help create more cancer. Read books, and change your diet accordingly. It can be fun, and you will definitely see the results.

Alternative treatments. Explore acupuncture, massage, yoga, chiropractic, meditation and prayer as alternative and supplemental healing strategies. Your western doctors will not spend much time telling you about these. It is contrary to everything they have learned in and out of medical school. Yet there are so many alternative treatments based on years and years of cumulative human knowledge from around the world. Include these in your arsenal as well.

Routine. It is important to maintain a routine. To include a daily regimen of nutrition, exercise, work and spirituality, we all need a framework to function in. There is so much that needs to be incorporated into a plan of attack. If you get accustomed to doing each of these things every day, nothing will slip through the cracks. My routine starts early every morning with a hot tub under the stars, pondering the nature of the universe. Taking a blended drink of fresh juice and fruits, and all of the vitamins, minerals and supplements that I am supposed to be taking follows this. After that, I have a workout at the gym, and then to the office. And I'm still the first one in. I have some quiet time, and then work begins. By the time the office fills up I have already had a great day, and a tremendous feeling of accomplishment.

Cancer responsibility. I believe it is every survivor's duty to help others with the disease, whether it is through direct encouragement, passing of knowledge, or even financial support of the various cancer resource and support groups. Once you've come to terms with your own disease, find those new patients who are still in shock, or let them find you. They need the most support. Find those who have given up. They need hope, and an example from those who have not given up. It will truly make you feel better to help others in whatever way you can.

Be thankful. Spend every day in a state of thankfulness. It will help you to remember to enjoy all the wonderful things in life, and will translate into good actions and deeds that you spread around. It will boost up your attitude, and you will find even more things to be thankful for. Don't whine, don't complain, and don't feel sorry for yourself. There is no benefit in this at all.

Be fearless. We are all going to die. Humans are the only species on earth that is aware of this, which probably has a lot to do with the popularity of religions. Twenty years ago I had the privilege to briefly "die" in a diving accident. I saw the soul separate from the body, I went toward the white light, and I felt a great feeling of peace. It wasn't my time, and I came back, but that brief glimpse of the other side showed me that there is another place we all go, and in those last few moments of our earthly existence, there is nothing to fear. It is just a journey to the next place. So why be fearful of death? Embrace life instead, and you will never fear death.

In conclusion, I must emphasize again that each prostate cancer patient must find his own path to a cure. For some it will be through the Western methods of the big three (surgery, radiation and chemotherapy), for others it will be a combination of alternative therapies, eschewing the cutting, burning and poisoning. Whatever the path, it is up to you and only you to first acquire the knowledge you need to make up your own mind. This is the most important thing. Understand your enemy so you can fight the good fight. Once you have done that, you can follow your path with the full conviction that you are doing the right thing, and be confident of victory. You do have the power to heal yourself.

* * *

Lacking definitive scientific studies using alternative therapies, I can only offer my personal observation of hundreds of cancer patients who I have queried on this very topic. It would seem that there is at least a 50% improved survival and quality of life of patients who avoid conventional therapies altogether. This is based on my addressing large groups of people with the question "how many of you personally know or are one who was indisputably diagnosed with cancer over five years ago and chose to not undergo conventional medical treatment and are living past the 5 year survival rate established as the basis for cure by conventional medicine?" In every case the number of hands that would be raised numbered from 40 to 60% of everyone attending.

I know this does not prove anything but it does prove that there are a significant number of people who are not a part of the survival 'statistics' that doctors tell patients who inquire of their personal chances. That this number of survivors who refuse conventional treatment altogether could be a lot greater than is generally recognized can be troublesome because it is these very statistics that doctors use to convince patients to undergo their oftentimes-drastic treatments that also too often lead to a miserable and possibly untimely death. Again I am not saying that patients should discount the value of conventional medicine whenever it seems appropriate. However, given the poor prognostics associated with following a recommended protocol of chemo or radiation therapy, it would be wise to consider such an option carefully and to first give alternative methods including herbal therapy an opportunity.

Certainly the work of the Chinese with Qi Gong therapy and Dr. Carl Simonton on the mind-body relationship of therapy shows that there is indeed an important mind-body connection associated with cancer prognosis, but this probably varies according to each type of cancer and each patient.

What does it take for a cancer patient and his or her support group to evaluate such possibilities? For one thing, it takes courage and the willingness to look at a situation clearly. It may involve decisions such as, "if my chances of survival are minimal, how can I divert my attention profitably from complete survival and cure to quality of life?" Certainly too much treatment can in some instances be as bad or worse than the disease itself.

At this time there are very few assurances based on indisputable research that alternative medicine, herbs, diet, etc. can guarantee a reasonable survival percentage for most cancers. At the same time, there is no question of the efficacy of such treatment for those with cancer. When a patient dies after undergoing a protracted course of agonizing chemo or radiation treatments, I often wonder if they would have been better off avoiding these and using only diet and herbs. Given the dearth of credible research to date, one can only wonder and patients must make their own choices, hopefully after evaluating all the evidence pro and con involved with treatments for their condition.

For most cancer patients there comes a stage when the treatment seems to take over focus from the disease. After an initial 'loading' period, usually of around three months, the goal of therapy, whether one chooses conventional, alternative or a combination of both, is that treatment protocol be reduced from a plethora of daily tasks and supplement taking to the most effective ongoing maintenance program.

I love the music of Chopin. As I write this, I am listening to the middle section of his beautiful Fantasy impromptu in C sharp minor. The beauty of this soaring lyrical melody in the contrasting key of D flat major embodies the very essence of love and compassion and offers such a powerful contrast to the stormy opening and ending that might be seen to embody the dark fears of all those who have cancer. As the music returns to its stormy character, one may imagine how in the end they are about to become utterly consumed in the outer storm of their fears. Gradually the stormy music subsides in the upper register and we hear in the bass the reiteration of the one clear melody of peace and compassion sounding as a refrain in the bass like the reassurance of the cosmic mother. Instead of listening to loud blaring electronically generated popular music, I recommend cancer patients to purchase a recording of the beautiful piano music of Chopin that includes this short sublime piece and sit down in a quiet place and allow this music to imbue your essence with its shimmering beauty.

Music, for many, is a simple and powerful way to achieve a level of detachment from the nagging fears accompanying cancer. Another patient, who himself was an accomplished musician and both a classical and jazz pianist, was dying of a rare fast-progressing cancer. He sought refuge in composing some of the most beautiful music, which he would present to me in lieu of payment for the treatments I was giving to him. Being a pianist myself, I particularly appreciated these musical offerings far more than money and was honored to perform one of them for a concert given in his honor after his passing.

The point here is that this patient was able to find piece in his music and as the disease progressed and it was no longer possible to compose, he contented himself with listening to the music of the Papae Marcello mass of the 16th century Italian composer, Palestrina. This music had particular significance for him since in his youth he sang it in English cathedral choirs.

For Catherine, her most successful method of overcoming her fears was through hatha yoga. Until the discomfort of her breast cancer prevented the stretches of daily yoga, she would spend hours each day in strenuous hatha yoga practice. Besides helping her to overcome her fear, the yoga practice powerfully assisted her in maintaining optimum mental and physical health.

In conclusion, while it is impossible to predict how anyone, even ourselves, will react to a life-death crisis such as a cancer diagnosis, it is obvious that at least two perspectives are relevant. First is that one is likely to respond according to their prior orientation of how they have learned to deal with crisis throughout their previous life. Secondly, that it is possible for one to perceive in the midst of crisis an opportunity to discover potentials and resources that were previously not evident. In either case there is an important psycho-spiritual aspect to healing that is reflected at all levels, from our relationship with our friends, family, therapists and healers as well as the way we view and utilize the prescribed treatments, therapies and lifestyle changes.

In all cases there is a common thread of determination, faith and the will or inspiration to take personal responsibility for the direction of our healing. Witness, for instance the high minded determination of Catherine G. with breast cancer in contrast to the naïve and simple faith of Bernardo A. with pancreatic cancer. No two individuals could be more different and yet they have both succeeded in improving their life based on an inner principle.

So how do we energize the inner resources we need for healing? It is obvious that it is a personal choice. For some it is through religious or spiritual belief, for others it is part of a philosophical or sociological point of view. Still for many others the ability to positively utilize the fear that is inevitable under such conditions, especially with the realization that there is no way out from this one except finding the quiet center of the cyclone.

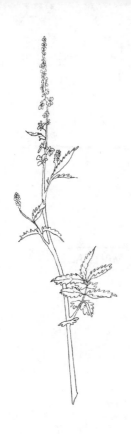

CHAPTER TWELVE

CANCER AND QIGONG
By Arnold Tayam, D.M.Q.

Introduction

T he ancient Chinese had a great reverence for the way of nature, or
"Tao," and viewed the entire universe as being composed of vital
energy, or "qi". This energy manifested as both form and function. The
ancient view holds that this energy vibrates at different levels of frequency.
The cosmos above, the elements that surround us, and our body, mind,
emotions and spirit are all qi.

Qigong, or Chi Kung, translated means, "energy skill." It is the art and science of energetic cultivation. Utilizing special methods of posture, breathing,
and creative visualization, Qigong serves to balance and strengthen the body's
energetic system through cleansing, collecting, circulating and storing qi and
it has been used extensively throughout China for thousands of years. It has a
wide variety of benefits including health and healing effects, longevity, physical
prowess, clarity of mind, emotional centeredness, spiritual enlightenment and
personal transformation. In China, Qigong has been shown to be effective
for a wide variety of conditions, particularly for health maintenance, disease
prevention and chronic conditions. Including asthma, arthritis, insomnia,
pain, diabetes, high blood pressure, chronic fatigue and cancer.

Although there are thousands of styles of Qigong, they can be classified into three major schools: Spiritual, Martial and Medical.

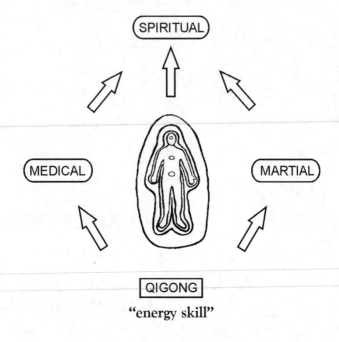

"energy skill"

Spiritual Qigong is the oldest school. Practitioners sought to reach enlightenment and spiritual immortality through various transcendental practices of cultivating subtle energy.

The Taoist path of spiritual cultivation involves an integration of all aspects of being including body, mind, emotions and spirit. Although the potential of enlightenment is always present, this path usually requires a lifetime of practice. The Taoist view is to unify the inner nature, our innate natural potential for self-realization with the outer nature through transcendent integration. Consequently the methods of this path are reflective of the embodiment of nature. Throughout life it is necessary for the practitioner to keep the body pure, clean, healthy and strong. In order to achieve this, it was essential to preserve the vehicle that housed the spirit. Naturally a complete system of holistic medicine evolved from this pursuit and the development of Chinese medicine began.

Qigong was combined with martial arts training to again preserve the vehicle for spiritual cultivation. Some martial arts systems were developed around Qigong utilizing it as a foundation from which fighting and self-defense techniques were created. Three systems in particular, typically referred to as the "internal" martial arts, combined Taoist theories and philosophy with Qigong to form Tai Chi Chuan ("supreme ultimate fist"), Bagua Zhang ("eight trigram palms"), and Xing Yi Quan ("body mind fist"). These arts are physiological manifestations of philosophical concepts that are deeply intertwined extensively throughout Chinese culture. The concept of yin and yang, or the law of opposite but complimentary forces, can be seen in the practice of Tai Chi Chuan which is characterized by the shifting of one's weight distribution between one leg and another, reflecting the ebb and flow of energy. In Bagua Zhang the Eight Trigrams that represent the symbols for change and transformation are reflected in the eight palms and circular movements that are characteristic of this style. Xing Yi Quan expresses itself in the use of five major hand techniques that are a reflection of the five elemental transitions, which emphasize mutual interdependence. These systems are particularly effective for healing, strength development, empowerment and disease prevention. They can be viewed as advanced Qigong systems of internal energetic movement.

Medical Qigong is one of the major branches of Chinese medicine, the others being acupuncture, herbs and nutrition, bodywork and massage. It shares the same theoretical foundation but, like the other branches, has its own unique methods and applications.

Medical Qigong is comprised of two major modalities: Internal and External Modulation.

Internal Modulation, or "self regulation" is the practice of methods taught to the individual in order to accomplish certain objectives on a general and/or specific level correlating to energetic imbalances and dysfunctions found through clinical assessment. These methods consist of a wide variety of techniques that can encompass standing, sitting, walking, lying down and moving postures. Different ways of breathing, which emphasize inhalation and exhalation, are also used. The physical postures and breathing techniques are combined with intention and visualization to achieve certain desired objectives in conducting energy flow. Students may also employ other methods such as self-acupressure, self-massage and the vocalization of special sounds known as toning.

External Modulation, or the emitting of qi, is the second major modality. This is performed by a specially trained practitioner that is able to assess energetic imbalances and dysfunctions in a person, and correct the flow of qi through touching or non-touching qi projection methods. The practitioner should have undergone a comprehensive specialized training program that thoroughly prepares the practitioner for energetic sensitivity pattern identification and the skill of qi projection.

In China there are several interesting tests that are used to evaluate qi projection abilities. One test involves changing the color of red or blue litmus paper. Some practitioners are able to change the blue but not the red litmus paper and vice versa. Furthermore these practitioners have been found to be more effective working with certain diseases but not others. Another test involves emitting qi onto x-ray film to leave a handprint. Yet another test requires the practitioner to manipulate and transform the alcohol content of wine through qi emission skills.

Master Duan Zi Liang, who appears in the widely acclaimed video "Qigong: Ancient Chinese Healing for the 21st Century" by Wuji Productions, is a famous 93-year old master of Chinese medicine, martial and spiritual arts from Beijing. I once witnessed this technique demonstrated by Master Duan. I was having dinner with him and a small group in a restaurant when he ordered some of the strongest wine in the house and poured two full glasses. He pushed one glass aside and placed the second near him, beginning to manipulate the qi by waving his hand in a circular motion over the glass of wine. He also sang and prayed in a gleeful manner. After a few minutes, he then passed the first glass of wine around the table encouraging the guests to take a sip to sample its strength. The second glass quickly followed for all to sip for comparison. Amazingly, the second glass of wine which was altered by hi qi manipulation was significantly weaker than the first! He then took both glasses of wine and again waved his hand over them in the same manner. This time the strength of the wine was transformed to become equal in each glass! The stronger glass of wine was changed to become a little weaker and the weaker glass of wine was changed to become a little stronger. He then joked about how this technique can make good wine bad and bad wine good. Master Duan further explained that these abilities, utilized in a clinical setting, represented increasing and decreasing a patient's qi level through purgation and tonification methods.

In clinical practice the Qigong practitioner needs to be well versed in the Three Regulations of (1) Posture (2) Breath and (3) Mind Intent in order to apply qi emission, teach and monitor the self-regulation formulas given to students. A skilled practitioner should be familiar with the Chinese medical theory in order to differentiate excess and deficient patterns and modulate these patterns accordingly through purgation, tonification or regulation. Furthermore, a practitioner must be able to identify and correct various qi deviations that may occur from incorrect practice or that may already be present from energetic dysfunctions. Just like the herbalist that must learn the healing properties of the many herbs and foods and their various combinations to dispense herbal medicine, the Qigong practitioner must become familiar with the many ways of posturing the body, breathing and focusing the mind. This collection of formulas becomes the Qigong practitioner's "pharmacopoeia" for correcting the many patterns of energetic dysfunction that may be encountered in a clinical practice.

Qigong Oncology

From the Chinese medicine perspective, cancer is viewed as an abnormal growth of tissue or stagnation. This understanding was reflected from a number of sources from ancient times. In the earliest medicine book assembled in China, the *Nei Jing the Yellow Emperor's Classic of Medicine*, there is a chapter that discusses "uncommon diseases" describing how "mass" should be treated by medicine in combination with "Daoyin" (energy regulation exercises). Additional evidence of this understanding was also found among Yin Dynasty ruins in the form of inscriptions of tumors on oracle bones and tortoise shells.

This "mass" is a result of the "pathogenic evils" that enter the body and cause a stagnation of blood, qi, phlegm and fluids. When this excessive accumulation occurs over a long period of time, the cells begin to grow as a reaction to the stagnation. This stagnation can then lead to abnormal, uncontrollable growth resulting in cancer cells. An excessively strained emotional state can also lead to stagnation. The six "pathogenic evils" are: 1) qi stasis 2) blood stasis 3) retention of dampness 4) retention of phlegm 5) toxic invasion, and 6) deficiency of energy. These pathological factors may occur singularly or in combination, creating a debilitating downward cycle draining the person of their vital qi and blood.

With a weakened energetic field the person is overcome by invading "pathogenic evils" and overstrained emotions, causing a "mass" (tumor) to manifest. The strategic approach is to strengthen the energetic field and purge the excess emotions and "pathogenic evils."

The plan for integrating medical Qigong for cancer in one particular hospital in China consists of three major components:

1) A support group and/or therapist sessions that serve to encourage the patients in developing a positive and helpful outlook in dealing with their condition. It is not uncommon for patients to feel sickly or sometimes even feel worse during the initial stages of practicing Medical Qigong. Medical Qigong initiates and facilitates a "peeling away" process of the energetic layers that hold patterns of disharmony. Often times, thoughts, feelings, emotions and or physical pain surrounding past trauma may surface during this period. This is an essential part of natural healing. These support groups or these therapist sessions may allow the individual space for self-regulation and an avenue for expressing and discussing their feelings. In China these groups are often led by cancer survivors who instill hope for patients as they are able to interact with true-life examples.

In the Stanford Complementary Medical Center there are on-going support groups that have proven to be quite effective. One support group for women with breast cancer showed that participants were twice as likely to survive than those did not join the group.

2) Internal modulation or self-practices provides a means or vehicle in which patients can apply methods for themselves and by themselves. This can be very exciting for the individual because of the opportunity for restoring a sense of self-confidence and self-empowerment.

3) External modulation or qi emission allows for the patient to receive an infusion of energy assisting in their healing process at various stages. The effectiveness of self-practice could then be increased.

Internal Modulation Methods

In Qigong there are three internal modulation methods that are used. These are: 1) toning, 2) deep breathing, and 3) walking therapy. For our purposes these methods will only be described to the reader briefly. For further inquiry I encourage seeking more detailed references and/or Qigong practitioners who specialize in these individualized clinical applications. Instead, we will present the reader with some very simple and general practices later in this chapter that can be readily applied.

1. Toning

This practice helps to clear heat and toxins from the body and can be particularly helpful for those undergoing chemo and radiation therapy. This method is used to purge evil pathogenic factors as well as any excessive emotions from the patient's body. There are general sounds that are commonly used in Qigong; however, these particular tones are designed specifically for serious conditions, such as cancer. These tones are performed using rising and dropping tones that are associated with the various organ systems. Along with these respirations, there are certain hand positions and body movements that are performed in unison. Refer to the table below.

	WOOD	FIRE	EARTH	METAL	WATER
Yin Organs	liver	heart	spleen	lung	kidney
Yang Organs	gallbladder	small intestine	stomach	large intestine	bladder
Tissues	tendons	vessels	muscle	skin	bone
High-pitched Tone	guo	zheng	gong	shang	yu

Low-pitched Tone	guo	zheng	gong	shang	yu
Number of Tones	eight	seven	ten	nine	six

2. Deep Breathing

This method increases and strengthens the energetic field of the patient through emphasizing the inhalation and exhalation patterns of breath. The rapid exhalation is especially used to dissolve clots and tumors. Deep, relaxed, slow inhalation can reinforce and build the patient's qi, enhancing immune function and helping to restore health and strengthen the protective or "guardian" qi, which serves to fend off external pathogens.

3. Walking Therapy

This method was made famous by Guo Lin, a famous Qigong Master who was able to put her cancer into remission by developing this special method of walking. This walking method stimulates the energetic field, thereby reinforcing and strengthening the patient's qi. This fast pace stimulates qi and blood flow and helps break up patterns of stagnation within the tissues. This walk is characterized by a coordination of special breathing methods of inhaling and exhaling, arms swinging and hand posturing with patterned stepping. Additionally, there are points that are stimulated by rubbing or pressing the fingertips, palms and toes while walking.

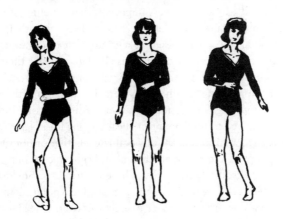

External Modulation or "qi emission" is usually employed to support the above methods and other self-regulation practices. Skilled Qigong practitioners will use a number of different techniques to modulate the qi of the patient through purgation, tonification and regulation. These techniques modulate the energy of the person's organs, meridians, points, centers and overall energetic field and can be categorized as follows:

1) Qigong massage is performed by lightly brushing or touching over the patient's body, utilizing various manipulation techniques

2) Jing point therapy is the application of activating the energetic points on the body through light touching, conducting the qi flow

3) Distance qi emission is performed without touching the patient's body and can be used over various distances ranging from a few inches to several feet or more

4) Invisible needle technique is a unique way of placing "energetic needles" intospecific points for activation.

Qi emission is used often to help rebuild the energetic system for patients undergoing radiation and chemotherapy. Additionally, there are some practitioners that are able to help break up and dissolve cancers, tumors and cysts by projecting a vibrational energy force deep into and throughout the body. Often patients will experience sensations that are similar to ultra sound therapy or an electrical current.

In general, medical Qigong therapy may be employed at various stages of disease. There are several specialized Qigong protocols for many different types of cancer including brain, cervical, breast, uterine, ovarian, liver, lung, prostate, pancreatic, stomach, esophageal and colon cancer. These protocols need to be carefully selected and combined accordingly with other modalities, both Western and Chinese. It is very important that patients have specialists supporting them in as many different areas as needed to treat their condition. I usually encourage people to assemble a group of health care practitioners that work in a complementary manner, as all methods have their strengths and weaknesses. Usually a person's group will consist of a western medical doctor or oncologist, an acupuncturist/herbalist, a massage therapist, and a counselor/support group in addition to a Medical Qigong practitioner. Patients usually need to implement medical Qigong for at least six to eight weeks before the practitioner can fully evaluate whether or not Qigong may be effectively applied as appropriate treatment. Daily practice of their Qigong prescriptions is absolutely necessary. These practice sessions may add up to anywhere between two to five hours per day, incorporating many of the techniques already mentioned. These practices, of course, need to be further supplemented with external Qi emission at least one to two times weekly.

Medical Qigong practitioners are known for their energetic sensitivity abilities and are sometimes able to detect a presence of tumors and cysts.

Here are two incidences where this occurred:

In one case the Medical Qigong practitioner was able to sense the presence of a tumor on one side of a person's chest, confirming the finding of a sonogram scan. Upon further Qigong detection methods, the practitioner sensed that there were several smaller tumors beginning to form on the opposite side of the person's chest and suggested that the person have this checked. An exploratory surgical procedure confirmed the findings of the Qigong practitioner. Another Medical Qigong practitioner was working with a woman that had a uterine fibroid and experienced high levels of pain that could not be alleviated with the Western pain medications that had been prescribed. With the use of external Qi emission, along with self-regulation practices, the pain was greatly diminished and was even totally eliminated at times. After several sessions the practitioner detected a shrinking of the fibroid, which was later verified through ultrasound scan.

Another female suffering from painful fibrocystic breasts was concerned with the short amount of time given to her before her doctor wanted to surgically remove one of her big cysts. With the use of daily herbs, one acupuncture treatment prescribed by my wife, Shasta Tierra-Tayam, L.Ac. (Michael Tierra's daughter), along with Qigong healing sounds and meditation, her cyst progressed from causing severe pain to no pain and was reduced to one half size in four weeks. She eventually was able to avoid surgery completely.

A more extreme example of External Qi Emission involved a middle-aged male afflicted with severe malignant tumors throughout the body and the brain. He was undergoing chemotherapy and radiation treatments. On his first visit he was wheeled into my clinic in a wheel chair and needed to be lifted onto the table. His condition was worsening, as he had been paralyzed for the last four weeks due to the brain tumors, and the prognosis was not good. During his session I applied external Qi emission and taught him a specific daily self regulation routine for at-home practice. He came in the following week and to my surprise he walked in! His Western medical oncologist said "I have never seen that kind of recovery in 25 years of practice. My methods could only account for 30% of your success." Furthermore, he encouraged his patient to continue the Qigong.

I know that there are many miraculous stories regarding disease cures. I don't believe, nor do I promote Qigong to be the "cure-all end-all" medicine. I do believe, however, that Qigong has a place in the broad range of healing possibilities. I know that many students and patients have benefited from Qigong. There are many theories and explanations of how and why it works. What is most important is not the how or why, but for many, that it simply does.

Modern Research

Over the past several years there has been a great amount of data collected in the study and research of Qigong. However, there is a great need for more research data for Qigong efficacy done by the Western scientific community. There is a growing number of people that believe that scientific verification for Qigong is coming from the area of advanced quantum physics. Dr. Ken Sancier, of the Qigong Institute in Palo Alto, California has compiled a database of over 1,000 abstracts that have been presented over the years at the International Qigong Symposiums sponsored by the World Academic Qigong Society. Although many of these studies have been done in China and have been recorded in Chinese, many of these studies have yielded some interesting results in demonstrating the efficacy of Qigong.

One particular study was conducted at Kuangan Men's Hospital in Beijing, China. Two groups of malignant cancer patients were treated, one with a combination of Qigong and drugs and the other with drugs alone. In this study 127 patients were divided into a Qigong group of 97 patients and a control group of 30 patients. All patients received drugs, but the Qigong group practiced Qigong for over two hours a day over a period of three to six months. Improvement could be seen in both groups; however, the Qigong group showed significantly better results as indicated in the following graph:

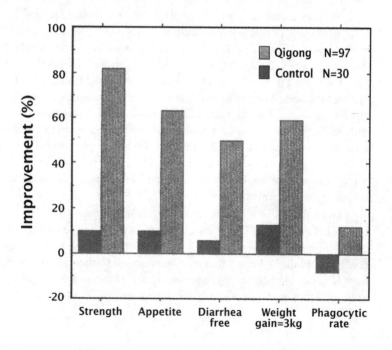

The following portion of this chapter presents several practices that can be learned as a possible introduction to more in depth Qigong practice with a qualified Qigong practitioner/instructor. These practices are for general usage and do not take the place of a licensed or qualified health care practitioner. As always, it is wise to consult with your physician before undergoing any exercise program. Use common sense when practicing and discontinue if any adverse effects are experienced.

Qigong Practice Guidelines

The following is a list of general observations that need to be adhered to when practicing Qigong.

1) Practice in a clean, well-ventilated and undisturbed area. If outside stay away from extreme elements such as wind, cold and heat.

2) Get proper rest and sleep. Qigong practice is not a replacement for either of these.

3) Do regular daily practice (same time, place, and routine). The ideal time for practice is 5-7 a.m. Evening practice must not be too intense or it can cause insomnia.

4) Moderation of sexual activity. The jing, or sexual essence, is the fuel for transformation into qi (energy) and shen (spirit). This is particularly important for men.

5) Women: cease practice during your monthly cycle, or shift your focus to the middle tan tien located in the center of the chest. Qigong practices increase the flow of energy, which can cause a greater loss of energy during the menstrual cycle.

6) Avoid drinks and foods that are ice cold. Coldness in the body can reverse or slow down the benefits of Qigong practice. It is like pouring water on a fire that you are trying to build.

7) Avoid drugs, smoking and alcohol.

8) Avoid practice within 30 to 60 minutes after eating. Eat according to nature (with the seasons and for your constitution).

9) Never try to mix practices from outside sources, or practice without a guided program. Qi deviations may occur from incorrect practice.

Qigong Self-regulations

The following Qigong practices can be utilized on a general level, but at the same time can be individually tailored for specific objectives under the guidance of a qualified instructor. The more advanced practices are not going to be presented here for the simple reason that they must be administered on a one to one basis by a qualified Qigong practitioner in a clinical setting. There is a Complementary/Alternative Modality (CAM) Class being taught at a CAM center that is using Medical Qigong successfully. I teach a 12 week Medical Qigong course that I designed specifically for the Stanford Center for Integrative Medicine, Cancer Supportive Care Program in Palo Alto, CA (www.cancersupportivecare.com). This class has drawn much interest. Recently the Cancer Supportive Care Program submitted an abstract for the Mayo clinic regarding the efficacy of the program. A portion of this abstract regards the Medical Qigong course. Data for a number of quality of life factors (QOL) were measured from Medical Qigong. The following are the results. Data was collected from a sample size of 617 participants between May 2001 and Feb. 2002. This class met once a week for one hour in revolving 12 week classes. Attendees evaluated the class based on a linear scale of QOL parameters including stress level, pain, well-being, energy level, hopefulness, empowerment and restful sleep. The following numbers represent the percentages of respondents indicating a more positive outcome.

Percentage of Positive Outcomes Reported with Medical Qigong at the Stanford Center for Integrative Medicine

Stress	Well-being	Energy	Restful Sleep
↓79%	↑94%	↑56%	↑43%

Cleansing Exercises

The purpose of these exercises is to prepare the body to conduct qi. The energy never flows through a tight, stiff or obstructed area. With these exercises you are also expelling negative emotions, excess thoughts and pathogenic energy. Natural breathing is used throughout these exercises.

Connecting Heaven and Earth

1) Begin by standing naturally with feet pointing straight ahead, knees slightly bent, spine straight.

2) Slowly reach upward with palms pointing to the sky as you inhale. Then, slowly bring down the hands as you exhale, imagine pulling down pure clean energy through the top, front and back of the head simultaneously. Continue to bring the hands downward in front of the face, body and trunk. Imagine this continuous flow of energy from the top of the head washing and pouring down through the internal organs of the body, through the trunk and down through the legs and feet. Envision this

energy cleansing and permeating throughout all of the tissues and cells of the body.

* For consistency, perform 3-5 times

Bouncing

1) Begin by standing naturally with the feet pointing straight-ahead, knees slightly bent and spine straight.

2) Relax your entire body and begin to bounce gently on your toes. As you bounce up and down, begin to feel for areas of tension and tightness, allowing for a release. Guide your feeling attention downward from the top of the head and neck, shoulders and arms down to the fingertips, then chest and upper back, spine, midsection, lower back, trunk, upper legs, lower legs and down through the heels and feet.

3) As you do this, allow for any negative energy, excess thoughts, feelings and emotions to release deep into the earth.

* Perform 3-5 times

Shaking

1) Begin in a natural stance with the feet about shoulder width apart, knees and feet facing forward.

2) Relax your entire body and begin to shake allowing for all the limbs, joints, hips, waist and spine to loosen.

* Perform 3-5 times

Wu Ji Meditation

This natural posture is commonly used to begin and end practice. This posture can be practiced from a sitting or standing position and is representative of the "WU JI" concept, or the embodiment of the "creative nothingness". This practice helps to tonify the immune system. This meditation posture is usually held from 15 – 30 minutes but can be held from 5 minutes to as long as one hour or more.

1) Stand with feet approximately shoulder width apart and facing straight ahead.

2) Knees are slightly bent to allow for proper energetic circulation

3) Pull the tip of the sacrum down as if sitting, allowing the gate of life point to press back. (This point is located on the spine opposite the navel.)

4) Drop the shoulders and spread the back.

5) Tuck the chin and press up the Crown Point at the top of the head.

6) Feel your weight rest through the center of your feet and heels.

7) Place the tip of the tongue on the roof of the mouth, and gently close the anal spinchter.

8) Feel your weight rest through the center of your feet and heels.

9) Breathe slowly, smoothly, evenly and deeply. Inhale and exhale like a balloon through the lower abdominal region.

10) Empty the mind and feel your entire being become calm and centered.

11) Align all three energy centers. The middle of the head, the middle of the chest and the middle of the abdomen.

12) To close, perform "connecting heaven and earth" 2-5 times. Store energy by placing one hand over the other just below the navel. Visualize storing the energy in the lower abdomen with each inhalation. It is important to always perform this last step to safely store the energy and complete any practice session.

Internal Body Scan Meditation

This meditation is designed for a person to get in touch with the different areas of the body. This allows for a person to see within themselves, finding those areas of energetic blockages, stagnation and imbalances.

1) Begin in a sitting position as in the WU JI Meditation. Relax and calm yourself. With each inhalation and exhalation feel yourself sinking deeper and deeper.

2) Connect your mind intent with the third eye point located between the eyebrows in the middle of the forehead. This point is connected with your spiritual intuition and is used to guide the energy through the mind intent.

3) Connect your mind intent with the Crown Point located at the top of the head. This point allows us to access our "higher" healing power.

4) Imagine a gentle beam of light coming in through the crown point and shining down the head, neck, shoulders, arms and hands to the fingertips, illuminating the internal organs then down through the trunk, legs, feet and to the toes, encompassing the tissues throughout the entire body.

5) Use this inner vision to sense any areas of blockage, stagnation and imbalance. Make a mental note of these areas.

Ice, Water, Mist Meditation

This practice is designed to break up energetic stagnation and can be helpful in dissolving tumors and cysts.

1) Continuing from the Internal Body Scan Meditation, use your mind intent to guide the beam of light to the area of blockage, stagnation or imbalance, imagining this area as a thick, dark, heavy, block of ice.

2) As you focus on this area, connect with the energetic state of the tissue.

3) Visualize the beam of light melting the ice to water, then melting the water to mist. Allow for the tissue to energetically dissolve the blockage, stagnation or imbalance.

4) Continue this process as many times as needed to "melt" these areas until they reach the state of balance, clarity and harmony.

5) Conclude with performing the connecting the heaven and earth cleansing exercise several times. Use the storing method as described in WU JI meditation.

6) To close, perform "connecting heaven and earth" 2-5 times. Store energy by placing one hand over the other just below the navel. Visualize storing the energy in the lower abdomen with each inhalation.

Six Healing Sounds

The healing sounds are designed to purge the emotional blockages and negative energies that tend to be attached to the individual organ meridian systems. All of these sounds are done in a seated posture: sit at the edge of a chair with your feet flat, toes pointing straight ahead. Follow the guidelines originally presented in the Wu Ji Meditation.

1) **Kidney Healing Sound:** Place your mind intent on the lower back region, relaxing the lower back, waist, hip and trunk area. Imagine seeing into your kidneys, feeling the size and the shape of the kidneys (they are located on either side of the spine just above waist level opposite the navel) and connecting with the energetic emotional state of the kidneys. Inhale into the kidneys and as you exhale, use the "FFFUUU..." sound. Feel the fear energy release with the breath. With the exhale, imagine any dark heavy energy leaving the kidneys and release with the breath. Allow for the positive quality of gentleness to come forth. As you feel this vibration move through the kidneys, feel as they become lighter and revitalized.

2) **Liver Healing Sound:** Place your mind intent on the right side of your body, through the midsection, under the right ribcage area. Begin to relax the tissues through this region. Imagine seeing into your liver, feeling the size and the shape. Connect with its energetic emotional state. Connect with that which may cause anger within you. Inhale into the liver then exhale, using the "SHHUUU..." sound. Feel any angry, hostile and

impatient energy release with the breath. With the exhalation, imagine the aggressive, negative energy leave the liver. As the vibration moves through the liver, feel the liver being cleansed and rejuvenated, allowing for kindness and forgiveness to exude forth.

3) **Heart Healing Sound:** Bring your mind intent down to the heart region in the middle of the chest. Begin to relax the chest and upper back region. Imagine seeing into your heart and connect with the energetic emotional state of the heart. Get in touch with that which brings over-excitation and uneasiness to you. Inhale into the heart and as you exhale, use the "HHHAAA..." sound. Feel the release of the negative emotions stored there. As you feel the vibration through the heart, allow for the positive qualities of love and compassion to exude forth, feeling clarity and emotional centeredness.

4) **Spleen Healing Sound:** Place your mind intent on the left side of your body, through the midsection, under the right ribcage area. Begin to relax the tissues through this region and imagine seeing into your spleen. Connect with that which causes you worry and anxiety. Inhale into the spleen and as you exhale, use the "HHHUUU..." sound. Feel the negative energies leave the spleen. Guide the vibration down through the spleen and as these negative emotions release, allow for positive qualities of centeredness, balance and fairness to come forth.

5) **Lung Healing Sound:** Place your mind intent on the upper chest and upper back region. Begin to relax through this area. Imagine seeing into your lungs and connect with the energetic emotional state. Get in touch with the negative emotions of grief, sadness and disappointment. Inhale into the lungs, and as you exhale, use the "SSSSS..." sound. Feel the vibration resonate throughout the chest region. Relax through the upper back, feeling the lungs expand, allowing for the negative emotions to leave the lungs. Allow for the positive qualities of courage and confidence to come forth. Feel the energy of the lungs increase, becoming full and abundant.

6) **Triple Heater Healing Sound:** Place your mind intent on the regions of the throat, chest, midsection and lower intestines. Feel the energetic state of these areas and inhale deeply. As you exhale, use the "SHHEEE..." sound. Feel the vibration move downward from the throat all of the way to the lower intestinal region. Feel the vibration as it breaks up and releases the tightness, tension or stagnant negative energies of these areas. Feel a gentle uplifting and harmonization of the energy throughout your entire body.

To conclude, follow the storing method as described in the WU JI meditation.

Trends

As we enter a new millennium, full of exciting possibilities in the area of health and medicine, our need for a complete and effective health care model is of crucial importance. With an aging population, the rising cost of medical care, and the growing need for individuals to reclaim self-empowerment, Qigong presents a simple, effective, low-cost solution. Many Qigong practitioners believe that not only can cancer sufferers benefit but a number of other conditions such as asthma, arthritis, insomnia, pain, diabetes and high blood pressure can be helped.

Qigong is simple to learn, making it very practical. With very little time, space or memorization, and no special equipment, a student can reach a level of practice yielding immediate benefits.

Qigong has shown its effectiveness by being time-tested through many generations over thousands of years. It is the basis, and always has been an integral part of, Chinese medicine. Over the last two decades scientific research, with the use of modern instruments and methods, has produced results that indicate the efficacy of Qigong. The demand for Qigong and other similar approaches is on the rise.

Qigong is easily one of the most inexpensive healing modalities available. With an emphasis on prevention and health maintenance, it is the perfect example of the old saying "an ounce of prevention is worth a pound of cure". With the Qi emission aspect used as support for self-practice, this encourages the individual to become responsible for his/her own health. Additionally, the individual will receive the added benefit of enhancing the effect of acupuncture, herbs, and bodywork and other modalities with Qigong.

With Qigong, one does not only raise their awareness of the nature of healing, but elevate their spiritual consciousness to another dimension. All healing is self-healing and ultimately all self healing is spiritual healing.

Qigong is easily one of the most inexpensive healing modalities available. With an emphasis on prevention and health maintenance, it is the perfect example of the old saying "an ounce of prevention is worth a pound of cure". With the Qi emission aspect used as support for self-practice, this encourages the individual to become responsible for his/her own health. Additionally, the individual will receive the added benefit of enhancing the effect of acupuncture, herbs, and bodywork and other modalities with Qigong.

With Qigong, one does not only raise their awareness of the nature of healing, but elevate their spiritual consciousness to another dimension. All healing is self-healing and ultimately all self healing is spiritual healing.

Bibliography

Chinese Medical Qigong Therapy: A Comprehensive Clinical Text, by Dr. Jerry Alan Johnson

Chinese Qigong Therapy, Compiled by Zhang Mingwu, Sun Xingyuan

The Tao of Nutrition, by Maoshing Ni Ph.D.

References

1. Arnold E. Tayam D.M.Q. (China) (408) 295-5911; www.longevity-center.com

2. *Qi – The Journal of Traditional Eastern Health & Fitness*; www.qi-journal.com

3. The Qigong Institute seeks to improve healthcare by education and research on Qigong (650) 323-1221; www.gigonginstitute.org

4. The National Qigong Association (888) 218-7788; nqa.org

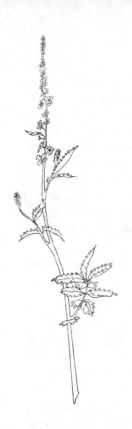

CHAPTER THIRTEEN

PREVENTING CANCER

With 1 in 2 men and 1 in 3 women predicted to develop some form of cancer during their lifetime, prevention should be a primary consideration for all. However, short of enduring direct exposure to radiation or some other toxic substance, many fatalistically view cancer as a matter of heredity. In fact, this is the prevailing belief of some 53% of Americans and undoubtedly has a lot to do with the reasons that many continue to smoke, overeat, consume too much refined and overly processed foods and the plethora of occupations and hazards that are known to significantly increase one's risk of cancer.

In fact, a fascinating study of the health histories of 45,000 twins published in July of 1999 established that such factors as diet and exercise had a far greater influence on subsequent cancer risk than heredity. As a result Dr. David Hunter, M.D. of Harvard Center for Cancer Prevention in Boston said "There's good scientific evidence that more than half of cancer could be prevented if people made certain lifestyle changes." Following is a list of some of the things one should avoid or limit as well as what one should include to prevent cancer:

1. Quit Smoking

With lung cancer ranking second of all cancers worldwide and accounting for 30% of all cancer deaths in the United States, it seems obvious that with the known carcinogenic consequences of smoking tobacco, one of the most obvious things is to quit smoking. While increasing awareness exists in the United States, other countries, especially among the poorest where tobacco is still widely promoted as an acceptable and mature preoccupation, have shown little inclination to diminish smoking. In fact throughout China, Middle Eastern and Eastern block countries and even in more developed countries such as Italy and Greece, tobacco consumption remains endemic. In Italy for instance, it is well known that the "tobaccaio" or tobacco booth is the place to purchase postage stamps.

Besides lung cancer, smoking is linked to cancer of the mouth, larynx, esophagus, bladder, kidney and pancreas.

2. Alcohol Consumption

A Swedish study followed 9,353 diagnosed alcoholics for an average of eight years. It was found that drinkers were 4.1 times more likely to develop cancer of the mouth and pharynx and 6.8 times more likely to develop esophageal cancer than non-drinkers.

The first metabolite of alcohol is acetaldehyde, a substance found to be carcinogenic among laboratory animals. Alcohol also diminishes our reserves of B vitamins, especially folic acid, known to be important in the prevention of several forms of cancer including cancer of the cervix, lungs, rectum, esophagus and brain. Finally, alcohol increases estrogen circulation, which adversely affects hormone-related cancers.

It is estimated that 17% of adult Americans consume two or more alcoholic beverages a day. Limiting oneself to a single drink or beer, wine or even hard liquor each day is not a problem and for those that drink, taking a daily B vitamin supplement would be a wise cancer-preventive measure.

3. Sun Toxicity

Skin cancer is the most common form of cancer in the U.S. and it is usually caused by damage to the skin from ultraviolet (UV) rays resulting from overexposure to the sun. With the now widely acknowledged thinning of the ozone layer, there is a significant increase of skin cancers worldwide. In a study published in 1999 in the *Journal of the American Academy of Dermatology*, from 1973 to 1994 there was a 120.5% increase of malignant melanoma, the deadliest of all forms of skin cancer.

Obviously avoiding over-exposure to the sun is the primary protection against skin cancer. This should be considered even on cloudy or overcast days since it is known that up to 80% of the UV rays of the sun can penetrate the cloud cover. Sitting in the shade, wearing a hat and long-sleeved clothing whenever possible as well as the frequent application of sunscreen all contribute to preventing skin cancer. This despite that there is growing conjectural concerns that sunscreen may not be as effective as previously thought to prevent skin cancer. If this is true, then blocking UV rays alone may not be sufficient.

4. Red Meat Consumption

A year 2001 study published in the International Journal of Cancer found that people who ate red meat seven or more times per week had a 90% risk of developing colon cancer, a 70% risk of developing rectal cancer and a 60% risk of developing stomach cancer over those who ate it three or fewer times a week. Besides these types of cancers, excess red meat consumption is implicated in a higher risk of prostate and breast cancers as well.

One of the factors in this is that cooking red meat at high temperatures produces carcinogens. To support this, I might add that one individual[1] claims to have been able to cure himself and innumerable others not only of a multiplicity of cancers but countless other diseases through an exclusive diet of raw meat and vegetables.

Another reason that meat may contribute to cancer is from the known carcinogens such as bovine growth hormone in non-organically raised meat. For this reason one should select the highest quality meat from free grazing animals raised without growth hormones or antibiotics.

As a result one would be wise to limit oneself to no more than 3 or 4 ounces of red meat three times a week. This is approximately the size of the palm of one's hand. Better yet, substitute anticancer vegetable based proteins such as soy and other legumes or fish.

5. Avoid Sugar and Refined Carbohydrates

By raising blood sugar levels, sugar increases tumor cell metabolism and speeds their growth.[2] It also suppresses the immune system.[3] If one must have sugar, it is best to have it after eating a wholesome meal, especially with sufficient protein.

---

[1] Acajou Vonderplanitz, *We Want To Live*, Carnelian Bay Castle Press, Santa Monica, California.

[2] Rothkopf, 1990

[3] Reviewed in Appleton, 1996

6. Avoid Home and Garden Pesticides

With an estimated 2 billion dollars spent by Americans each year on home and garden pesticides, eliminating these from our lives altogether may be one of the most important things we can do to prevent cancer among children and adults. A German study published in 2000 in the *American Journal of Epidemiology* found a link between household pesticides and childhood cancers. In 1995 the EPA stated unequivocally that common sticky household pest strips emit dichlorvos vapors and people who use them as directed have a 1 in 100 chance of developing cancer over the course of a lifetime. Of course this is only one of the many carcinogenic substances commonly found in home and garden pesticides and defoliants.

Fortunately there are many natural non-toxic alternatives, which despite their inconvenience and diminished efficacy, can nevertheless be substituted to achieve a significant measure of control.

Things To Do or Include to Prevent Cancer

1. Shed Extra Pounds

Individuals who are overweight show an increased risk for certain cancers especially colon and breast cancers. The connection seems to be based on the increased secretion of insulin from the pancreas as a result of higher carbohydrate consumption, especially simple carbohydrates, which in turn cause a secretion of insulin-like growth factors ((IGF's) from the liver. These are considered by Mitchell Gaynor, M.D., director of medical oncology at the Strang Cancer Prevention Center in New York City to be "the most potent tumor-promoters ever identified."

At the Third National Health and Nutrition Examination Survey 33% of Americans are overweight. The Harvard Center for Cancer Prevention found that women who are 40% above their ideal weight have a 55% increased chance of developing cancer of the breast, ovaries, and gallbladder as opposed to their leaner counterparts. Men who are 40% over their ideal weight have a 33% increased chance for developing colon and prostate cancers.

Obviously weight control can play a significant factor in reducing one's risk of cancer.

2. Increase Fiber

Despite current controversy, it is still generally agreed that fiber acts like a broom, binding and eliminating carcinogens from the intestines. However, it is not only the fiber itself that may be anticancer but also the fact that fiber-rich foods such as whole grains, beans, vegetables and fruit are loaded with antioxidants and other cancer-fighting phytonutrients. With an estimate of only 50% of the recommended amount of fiber being consumed daily by Americans, it is obvious that increasing fiber-rich foods such as whole grains, beans, carrots, apples, citrus, oatmeal and organic vegetables should be an important part of our daily diet. To provide a little perspective, the minimum daily requirement of fiber is 20 to 35 grams. A cup of broccoli has 5 grams, one large unpeeled apple has almost 6 grams, and a 1/2 of canned baked beans has 6 grams.

3. Drink Green Tea

Of all the known cancer fighters the primary antioxidant in green tea has 20 times more free-radical fighting power than vitamin E and 200 times more than vitamin C. Furthermore, green tea inhibits cancer growth as well as the COX-2 enzyme that makes carcinogens more active in the body. It is no wonder that Dr. Mitchell Gaynor puts green at the top of all cancer fighters.

One Chinese study published in the *Journal of the National Cancer Institute* found that women who drank 2 to 3 cups of green tea each day diminished their risk of esophageal cancer by 60% while men who drank the same amount reduced their risk by 57%.

The goal is to consume approximately 3 cups of green tea daily. To get the maximum benefit, consume while it is still warm and do not add milk. To make green tea pour two cups of boiling water over 1 teaspoonful of green tea leaves and allow to steep 3 to 5 minutes before drinking.

4. Take a High Quality Multiple Vitamin/Mineral and Antioxidant Supplement

This might be one or as many as three supplements daily. They should not include iron because it may be toxic for some who do not need it. If one has iron-deficient anemia, it is best to take a separate iron supplement.

5. Sleep in Total Darkness

This is to regulate melatonin production. Research suggests that melatonin is a powerful antioxidant and is able to slow tumor growth, but only when it is taken at night.[4]

---

[4] Blask et. Al., 1996; Lissoni et al., 1998

Endnotes

[1] Substantial portions of this chapter were taken from the article "Playing with Fire" by Judy Bass which appeared in the November/December 2000 issues of *Natural Health* magazine.

Reprint with permission. To subscribe to *Natural Health* call 1-800-526-0173

APPENDIX

APPENDIX

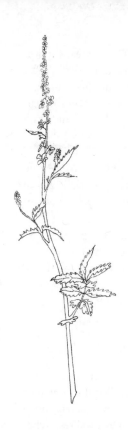

BREAST CANCER
By Camellia C. Pratt, DTCM

The first world conference on breast cancer was held in July 1997, at Kingston Ontario. The chief organizer Janet Collins, a nurse and midwife, had many friends and a sister fall victim to what some say is becoming an epidemic. Breast cancer kills almost one million women worldwide annually, including about 7,000 in Canada in 1997.

As much as cancer has been blamed on genetic quirks or lifestyle factors including smoking and having a high fat diet, about 70% of breast disease causes do not fall into high-risk categories.[1] Now with the high incident rates in the northern New York states and north shore of the Great Lakes second highest only to San Francisco Bay with 18,000 new cases annually, some feel breast cancer could be enduced by environmental pollution. Sandra Stein Graber, a Boston biologist, states 80% of breast cancers are caused by environmental hazards.[2]

Despite the enormous effort to combat breast cancer, the number of new cases increases each year. In spite of the introduction of radiation therapy, chemotherapy, immunotherapy, CT scans, MRI scans and all other new medical technology, life spans for breast cancer patients have remained the same as there hasn't been any significant progress in breast cancer treatment.

Treatment has improved survival only slightly, in fact. The five-year survival rate for breast cancer in 1976 was 75%, in 1983, 77% and in 1989, 78%. Most scientists/physicians are convinced, however, that the slight increase in time of survival is due largely to earlier detection of breast cancer through improved mammography technology. To an oncologist, if the patient lives 5 years + 1 day, that woman survived and is counted as a cure, even if she has died. If, however, she lives one day less than 5 years she is counted as a non-survivor. In 1960 one in 20 women developed breast cancer, in 1974 one in 17. The odds have become worse with each succeeding year. By 1990 the rate rose astronomically to one in 10, and kept increasing in 1991 to one in 9, in 1994 one in eight women developed breast cancer.[3]

In the last two decades the National Cancer Institute has spent over $1 billion on breast cancer alone, touting spectacular progress at the research level with almost no change in reducing mortality or increasing life spans. And that is the primary objective of any treatment – to make the lifespan longer and improve survival. Two advances have come about however:

1. Minimizing pain and suffering
2. Less mutilating surgery to achieve the same survival.

Even though this information is well known to all scientists and physicians, the great majority of all breast cancers are still handled the same way: with modified radical mastectomy rather than lumpectomy, auxiliary node dissection and radiation therapy.[3] Dr. Stephen Narod, a medical researcher from Women's College Hospital in Toronto, concluded "mastectomy before cancer strikes" is the best approach to treating women carrying the genes linked with the disease even though, as some delegates attending the conference in Kingston pointed out, research hasn't proven conclusively that breast removal is an effective prevention strategy.[4]

There is an information gap on the causes, monitoring and prevention of breast cancer because little conclusive research has been done on the subject. However, it is known that 75% of patients survive breast cancer and most breast cancers are present 8 to 10 years before they can be detected as a lump or on a mammogram, according to Dr. Susan Love, M.D., Associate Professor of Clinical Surgery at the University of California, Los Angeles and Director of the Breast Cancer Institute. Dr. Love points out "The problem of the prevention and treatment of breast cancer is the fact that 80% of women who get breast cancer don't have (the traditional) risk factors. A low fat diet may be preventative, but we won't have the results from studies for a good five to ten years. Recent studies, however, have disputed the long-standing belief of that risk factor. The Canadian National Breast Screening study, which examined the diets of almost 57,000 women, claimed that a higher incidence of breast cancer was observed in women consuming the most fat.

They neglected to report that the same high incidence of breast cancer was observed in the women consuming the least amount of fat."

The Nurses Study in the USA found exactly the same pattern. When the data from both studies were compared and evaluated, it was discovered that "The breast cancer rate among these women was virtually the same, whether they ate a lot of fat or very little."[8]

Another study has also recently discounted the high genetic risk factor. Although the risk of breast cancer is doubled among women whose mother or sister contacted breast cancer before the age of 40, the study indicated that within middle-aged women, only 2.5% of breast cancer cases were attributable to family history.[5]

Early detection is currently one of the primary strategies for prevention and successful treatment, which is why the breast self-exam is so important. The benefits of mammography are still a subject of debate. Questions that are still present include whether low-level radiation used in the test can contribute to cancer, whether equivocal results lead to unnecessary surgery, and the accuracy rate of test results.

According to the National Cancer Institute, there is a high rate of missed tumors in women ages 40-49 which results in 40% false negative test results. Breast tissue in younger women is denser, which makes it more difficult to detect tumours, so tumours grow more quickly in younger women, and tumours may develop between screenings. Because there is no reduction in mortality from breast cancer as a direct result of early mammogram, it is recommended that women under fifty avoid screening mammograms although the American Cancer Society still recommends a mammogram every two years for women age 40-49. Dr. Love states, "We know that mammography works and will be a lifesaving tool for at least 30%."[6]

Dr. Norman Boyd, head of the division of epidemiology and statistics at the Ontario Cancer Institute in Toronto, whose research was funded by drug companies,[6] calls dense breast tissue a "major cancer risk," and suggests they should have mammograms "more frequently than other women," also adding that patients should be cautioned to follow a low-fat, high fiber diet and perhaps take specific medication to "block factors that play a role in breast density" and thus cancer. According to the American Academy of Pathology, at least 50% but as many as 80% of North American women suffer some sort of fibrocystic breast disease or density[11] causing a lot of pain and discomfort as well as a great deal of anxiety. Although a benign condition, it can be difficult for both women and their physicians to distinguish a cystic breast lump from a cancerous one. Right now Fibrocystic Breast Disease is a confusing term, or as Dr. Susan Love says, "a wastebasket into which doctors throw every breast problem which isn't cancer" (yet).

Various researchers have suggested a hormonal imbalance, a decreased ratio of progesterone to estrogen in the second half of the menses cycle, an abnormality of prolactin regulation or a hypersensitivity to thyroid stimulating hormones and increased estrogen levels as causes of fibrocystic breast disease.

The following are various treatments of fibrocystic breast disease: Dr. Mauvais Jarvis and his group of French researchers found that breast pain was relieved 95% of the time with a natural progesterone gel rubbed into the breasts.

Dr. John Lee, Clinical instructor at the University of California Department of Family Medicine, has had good success using a 2 oz. jar of 3% natural progesterone cream for the last two weeks of the menstrual cycle for a total of 3-6 months. Maintenance is 1/2 jar a month. Studies have been inconclusive as to whether vitamin supplementation reduces pain or swelling.

Dr. Christine Northrup, an American gynecologist, recommends hot castor oil packs applied to the breast 3 times a week for one hour for 2-3 months with maintenance afterwards of once a week.[12]

Dr. John Myers, a Baltimore gynecologist with a special interest in metabolic disease, is credited as being among the first to recognize the importance of iodine to the breast and ovary. He found he could completely reverse fibrocystic breast disease using iodine orally and vaginally along with trace mineral elements given under the tongue and magnesium given intravenously. Cystic breasts would soften quickly under the regime, sometimes immediately.[11]

In the Canadian Journal of Surgery, Dr. William Ghent, former Professor Emeritus of Surgery at Queen's University in Kingston, Ontario and Dr. Bernard Eskin, Professor of Reproductive Endocrinology and Obstetrics & Gynecology at Medical College of Pennsylvania (who both collaborated on clinical research of iodine deficiency and fibrocystic disease in the 1970's) have speculated that elemental iodine is essential for breast normality, and its absence seems to render the breast ducts more sensitive to estrogen stimulation and subsequent formation of cysts and scar tissue. They theorize that adequate amounts of elemental iodine in breast tissue make them less sensitive to circulating estrogens. As such, the iodine could be classed as a natural anti-estrogen, a sort of natural tamoxifen. Incidentally, during treatment for fibrocystic breast disease, it was noted that some women experienced a marked improvement in their endometriosis. At present this special form of iodine must be taken continuously or the breasts will become cystic again. With Dr. Ghent's research on fibrocystic disease of 3200 women for 12 years, the breast cancer rate of women taking the elemental iodine was 0.00082 women per year, while the projected incidence of breast cancer for Ontarioian women was .0064 women per year.[11]

Sydney Singer, a medical anthropologist, examines the ways in which our lifestyles make us sick, and came up with the theory that "there is no such disease as breast cancer, there is cancer which is manifested in a woman's breast." After conducting a two-year study in which he interviewed over 5000 women regarding their attitude and behavior regarding breasts and bras, he discovered that where there were no brassieres, there was little breast disease. About half of the women had breast cancer, and he discovered that the women with breast cancer had a history of tighter and longer bra wearing than did the women who had not (yet) developed the disease.

The researcher also threw out the challenge that if a woman stopped wearing her bra for two weeks the fibrocystic breast disease would disappear. (I had suffered fibrocystic breast disease for over 35 years, and thought what the heck, I'll give him three weeks. I marked the time off on my calendar and carried on with life as usual. After three weeks, my breast was completely clear of fibrocystic breast disease—from a bag full of marbles to one full of water, what a difference.) Dr. Singer has pointed out that the problem caused by bras is essentially a mechanical interference with the breast lymphatic drainage. However, in today's world we are all exposed to hazardous cancer causing toxins in our food, air, water and medications. Pesticides, herbicides and other chemical contaminants enter our bodies and must be cleared away, along with the damage they cause. This is the basis of the dietary connection with cancer (and environmental pollution). It is through our diets that we are exposed to many toxins, especially the fat-soluble toxins that are found in the fatty part of our foods. High fat diets are associated with cancer not because of the fat itself (which people have been consuming for thousands, if not millions, of years) but because of the toxic content of fats produced in our chemical dependent food production system. Once in our tissues, these toxins must be flushed out via the lymphatics. However, a bra-constricted breast cannot adequately perform this cleansing process, resulting in toxin accumulation in the breasts.

One major reason women wear bras is the myth that bras are needed for "support." This myth assumes that the female body was created with a flaw pertaining to shape. This apparent flaw is a reflection of a fashion image which demands that women have their breasts higher on their chest wall than nature intended and which can be achieved only with the purchase of a product–the brassiere. In fact, bras are creating droopy, weak breasts, the exact opposite of what this myth claims. As the breast relies on the bra for artificial support the body loses its ability to support the breast by itself.[13]

ERT & Cancer: Dr. Alan Gaby, author of *Preventing and Reversing Osteoporosis* explains that at least 28 different studies have evaluated the relationship between estrogen replacement therapy and breast cancer. These analyses suggest that estrogen replacement therapy is associated with an increase in the risk of breast cancer raging from 1-30%.[9]

When suffering stage 3 large C prostate cancer, my husband was prescribed women's hormones to slow the cancer growth. He developed breasts, which produced large tumors. His surgeon wished to operate but we decided against it. Upon chance when visiting an acupuncturist, the DTCM recommended some nightly massage of Zusali (Stomach 36 point) and the tumors went away.

Western Perspective:
Cancer of Breast and Treatment

The value of lymph node removal is increasingly controversial, says Dr. Greg McGregor, head of surgical oncology at the British Columbia Cancer Agency. He is chief investigator in a new trial to see if lymph node conservation affects cancer recurrence or survival.

Dr. Edward Fish, Assistant Surgery Professor at University of Toronto, also questions routine removal of lymph nodes, especially for women with a small lump. An experimental technique is being developed where a dye is injected close to the tumour. The dye then travels to the lymph gland called the senital gland. That gland alone is then removed and if it contains no cancer cells, the lymph nodes can remain safely intact. Dr. Fish studied 100 women who had lumpectomy only. Women over the age 65 with a small non-aggressive tumour had a local recurrence rate of less than five percent and would thus benefit little from radiation.

Recently in Vancouver, B.C., 40 doctors from across North America made a landmark decision to study unconventional cancer treatments.[16] In the question of "preventive" chemotherapy, Steve Austin, a naturopath, says most women have impaired quality of life from chemotherapy, but few benefits. Side effects could include hair loss, nausea, lowered white blood cell count and susceptibility to infection.[17]

Another treatment/preventive used now is Tamoxifen, which was developed about 20 years ago. Researchers discovered it lowered breast cancer rates in animals, and started studying its effects on human breast cancer. The researchers found that Tamoxifen interfered with estrogen in breast tissue by stopping it from binding to particular receptors. Although estrogen promotes the growth of breast cancer cells, it must first bind to these receptors in order to have any effect at all. Tamoxifen blocks these estrogen receptors and helps reduce the chance of a recurrence of breast cancer. Because of this anti-estrogenic effect, the side effects of Tamoxifen mirror that of menopause. The research soon unveiled even more serious side effects of Tamoxifen usage. Even the National Cancer Institute admits that Tamoxifen can cause an increase of uterine cancer. It is also believed to cause liver cancer. Dr. Samuel Epstein, an expert in environmental toxicology has reported Tamoxifen is the most potent liver carcinogen available,[18] while most experts are telling us this is the "most promising anti-cancer drug on the market."[19]

It has been my experience that before cancer can be cured or go into remission, some psychological work must be done. There seems to be a spiritual manifestation of the disease and this must be treated alongside the physical ones. Dr. Louise Hay, an internationally renowned counsellor, teacher and lecturer states "frequently patients with cancer have a deep hurt. Long-standing resentment, a deep secret or grief eating away at self." Carrying hatred, saying 'What's the use?' and then the part of the body involved sometimes shows the person's mind bent. For example, in breast problems perhaps the person had a problem with over-mothering, over-protection or over-bearing attitude, perhaps a refusal to nourish the self, putting everyone else first."[21]

Edward Bach stated that disease is, in essence, the result of conflict between soul and mind and will never be eradicated in the patient except by spiritual and mental effort. We must learn to think, reason, see, hear, speak and pray from the heart, not the head, to be with our soul. "Illness, disharmony and imbalance are often a result of the gap between the inner state and the 'face' that we daily put on to those around us."[22]

Dr. Ron Pratt, Ph.D., F.B.F.S., a social science researcher, has stated that in his experience and observations, cancer, among others, is a disease that not only attacks the physical, it also attacks the spirit. "Such men as Hippocrates with his mighty ideals of healing, Paracelsus with his certainty of the Divinity of Man; and Hahnemann who realized that disease originates in a plane above the physical, Edward Bach with his certainty that the real cause of disease are such defects as pride, cruelty, hate, self-love, ignorance (lack of wisdom), instability of mind (indecision), inconsistency, greed, presumption, pretension, immaturity, deceit, deception, sensuality. What untold misery would have been spared during the last 20 to 25 centuries had the teachings of these great masters and their art been followed. Unfortunately, as in other areas, materialism has appealed too strongly, and for so long a time, that the voices of the detractors and obstructers have risen above the advise of those great masters, who knew the truth."[20]

TCM Perspective

Many people are returning to ancient manuscripts and studying the masters, and now we see the West embracing the 5000 years of documented medicine from the east, commonly known as *Traditional Chinese Medicine.*

The five principles of TCM treatment are:

1. Fu Zheng Qi Xie – promotes, enhances, dispels evil, and strengthens patient's resistance.
2. Huo Xue Qu Yu – eliminates stasis and promotes blood circulation.
3. Qing Re Jie Du – clears and removes evil heat, detoxes, relieves fever and pain.
4. Ruan Jian San Jie – softens, dissolves hard masses.
5. Yi Du Gong Du – combats poisons with poisons.

TCM believes that cancer involves four factors; blood stasis, deficiency, toxicity and phlegm, which all must be present for cancer to develop.

The etiology and pathogenesis of breast cancer is:

Insufficiency of vital Qi – injury of seven emotions.

Stagnation of Liver and Spleen Qi and disorder of Chong and Ren channels leads to disturbance of physiological function of Zang-fu organs and mammary gland, obstruction of the channels and collaterals accumulation of stagnated Qi, blood and phlegm in breast.

1) For stagnation of the Liver Qi

Wishing to relieve the depressed liver and resolve phlegm and masses, use a modified **XIAO YAO SAN**:

Chai hu (Bupleurum falcatum)	10g	*Detoxifies the liver, regulates liver qi*
Bai shao (White peony)	12g	*Tonifies blood, antispasmodic, nourishes ying*
Dang Gui	12g	*Tonifies and moves blood*
Bai Zhu	10g	*Tonifies qi, removes dampness, promotes digestion*
Fu Ling (Poria Cocos)	10g	*Diuretic, drains dampness, purifies the lymphatic system, anticancer*
Tian Nan Xing Arisaema Consanguineum (prepared jack in the pulpit)	10g	*Dissolves and Removes phlegm congestion from the chest, anticancer*

Jiang Ban Xia (Prepared Pinellia ternata)	10g	*Dissolves and removes phlegm from the chest*
Quan Gua Lou (Trichosanthes fruit)	10g	*Clears heat, detoxifies, anticancer, removes phlegm-heat, dissipates nodules (tumors) especially good for the lungs and breast*
Chuan Lian Zi (Meliae Toosendan fruit)	10g	*Moves qi, stops pain, clears heat and detoxifies, anticancer*
Gan Cao (glycyrrhizae uralensis – licorice)	6g	*Harmonizes, tonifies qi, anticancer*

For hypertensive liver fire add:

Mu Dan Pi (tree peony root bark – paeonia suffructicosa)	10g	*Clears heat, moves blood*
Shan Zhi Zi (Gardenia fruit – Gardeniae jasminoides)	10g	*Moves blood, clears heat, detoxifies, anticancer*

2) For disorder of Chong & Ren Channels

Requiring a modified **ER XIAN TANG** (decoction of Curculigo and Epimodium) to regulate the two channels:

Xian Mao (Curculigo orchiodes)	10g	Tonifies kidney yang (adrenals), removes coldness and dampness
Xian Ling Pi (Epimedium grandiflorum)	15g	*Tonifies kidney yang (adrenals), removes damp-cold*
Ba Ji Tan (Morinda officinalis root)	10g	*Strengthens kidney yang (adrenals)*
Dang Gui (Angelica sinensis)	15g	*Tonifies and moves blood*
Lu Jiao Shuang (Cornu cervi degelatinatium)	6g	*This is the dregs after boiling deer antler glue, it is milder than deer antler, but also tonifies qi and blood*

Zi Dan Shen (Red sage root – Salvia miltiorrhizae)	15g	*Moves blood, cools heat, relieves pain, calmative, removes liver qi stagnation, prevents metastasis*
Ban Xia (Prepared pinellia ternata root)	10g	*Dissolves and removes phlegm from the chest*
Bai Jie Zi (mustard seed – brassica alba)	10g	*Promotes digestion, relieves stagnation, anticancer*
Gan Cao (glycyrrhizae uralensis – licorice)	6g	*Harmonizes, tonifies qi, anticancer*

If the breast is hard, painful and complicated with anemia add:

Ezhu (Curcuma zedoaria)	12g	*Moves blood, dissolves stagnation and masses, and relieves pain, anticancer*
Zhi Ru Xiang (Frankincense – Gummi Olibanum)	12g	*Moves blood, dissolves stagnation and masses, and relieves pain*
Zhi Mo Yao (Myrrh – Commiphora myrrha)	12g	*Moves blood, relieves pain, and dissolves masses*

3) Accumulation of noxious fire in the interior

To purge fire, remove toxins, subdue swelling and arrest pain use a modified **LONG DAN XIE GEN TANG**:

Long Dan Cao (Gentiana scabra)	6g	*Clears heat and dampness, relieves inflammation, anticancer*
Shan Zhi Zi (Gardenia fruit – Gardeniae jasminoides)	10g	*Moves blood, clears heat, detoxifies, anticancer*
Huang Qin (Scutellaria baicalensis)	15g	*Clears heat and dampness, detoxifies, anticancer*
Sheng Di (Unprepared Rehmannia glutinosa)	21g	*Clears heat, nourishes the blood and yin*
Che Qian Zi (Plantago asiatica seed)	12g	*Removes dampness, diuretic, clears heat, purifies the lymphatic system*
Ze Xie (Alisma tuber – water plantain)	10g	*Diuretic, clears heat, promotes lymphatic purification*

Mu Tong (Akebia trifoliata)	9g	*Diuretic, antiinflammatory, detoxifies, anticancer*
Dang Gui (Angelica sinensis)	12g	*Tonifies and moves blood*
Chai Hu (Bupleurum falcatum)	10g	*Detoxifies the liver, regulates liver qi*
Zao Xin (Terra flava usta – derived from the center of the ashes from the bottom of a cooking stove where lithospermum has been burned)	30g	*Warms the blood, stops bleeding, warms the stomach, stops vomiting*
Feng Fang (Wasp's nest – Polistes olivaceus)	15g	*Detoxifies, moves blood, anticancer, treats tumors*
Quan Xie (Scorpion – Buthus martensi)	10g	*Detoxifies, regulates qi flow, anticancer*
Long Kei Zi	15g	*Detoxifies*
Sheng Gan Cao (glycyrrhizae uralensis – licorice)	6g	*Harmonizes, tonifies qi, anticancer*

If the fever is severe add:

Jin Yin Hua (Lonicera or honeysuckle flowers)	30g	*Anti-cancer, detoxifies*
Lian Qiao (Forsythia suspensa)	15g	*Detoxifies, clears heat, anticancer, moves blood, dissolves lumps*
Sheng Shi Gao (Gypsum)	30g	*Clears heat*

Alternately, the following could be used for removing heat and toxic material and anti-cancer:

Ban Zhi Lian (Scutellaria barbata)	30g	*Clears heat and dampness, anticancer*
Bai Hua She She Cao (Oldenlandia diffusa)	30g	*Anticancer, clears heat*

4) For deficiency of both Qi and Blood

Where the Breast is like a cauliflower with a continual exudative blood fluid plus other symptoms. Where the practitioner wishes to tonify Qi and Blood, remove toxic material and resolve phlegm a modified **GUI PI TANG** can be used:

Huang Qi (astragalus)	30g	*Tonifies qi, strengthens the immune system, protects the body, anti-cancer*
Dang Shen (codonopsis)	30g	*Tonifies qi*
Bai Zhu (white atractylodes)	12g	*Tonifies Qi, removes dampness, strengthens digestion*
Dang Gui (Angelica sinensis)	10g	*Nourishes and moves blood*
Fu Ling (Poria cocos)	15g	*Diuretic, promotes lymphatic drainage, anticancer*
Chi Shan Yao (red peony root – paeonia rubra)	12g	*Moves blood, breaks up stagnation*
Long Yan Rou (Longan berries – Arillus longus)	30g	*Nourishes blood, mild sedative, tonifies the heart and spleen*
Shuang Hua Teng (Lonicera or honeysuckle vine)	30g	*Anti-cancer, detoxifies*
Ba Jie Zi (mustard seed – brassica alba)	10g	*Promotes digestion, relieves stagnation, anticancer*
Qian Cao Gen (madder root – Rubiae cordifoliae)[23]	15g	*Stops bleeding and yet it promotes blood circulation*

The entire amount is slowly cooked in 6 cups down to 2 or 3, which is consumed three times daily.

Folk Cure

Another folk remedy that has been very successful in dissolving cancer tumours is the use of raw red beetroots; however, when ingested as a juice there is a danger of the patient contracting a high fever because of its incredibly strong ability to quickly break up cancer in the body. The beets can clean up the cancer faster than the liver is capable of processing all of the wastes dumped into it all at once. Reducing the dosage helps.[24]

References

1. *The Vancouver Sun* Monday 14 July 1997

2. Sandra Stein Graber Author of *Living Downstream*

3. *Breast Health Update* - Charles B.Simone, M.D.

4. *The Vancouver Sun* Tue 15 July 1997

5. Colditz, G.A. *"Family History Age & Risk of Breast Cancer, Prospective Data from the Nurses Health Study" Journal of The Amer. Medical Assoc* 270 #3 July 1993

6. *Alternative Medicine* - Burton Goldberg Group

7. *Breast Cancer Scandal* - Rhody Lake; *Alive* / Oct. 1995

8. *Getting Fat & The Myth of the Fat Free Campaign* - Thomas Anderson Ph.D.; Alive/ Oct 1995

9. *Prevention & Reversing Osteoporosis* - Alan Gaby

10. Pizzorio, J.E. & Murray, M.T. *"A Textbook of Natural Medicine"* Seattle, WA, John Bastr College Pubs. 1988-89

11. DeMarco, Carolyn M.D. *Health Counsellor* Aug/Sept 1995

12. Northrup, Christine M.D. Gynaecologist *"Women's Wisdom, Women's Bodies"* Doubleday 1994

13. Singer, Sydney Ross, Medical anthropologist *"Dressed to Kill - the link between Breast Cancer & Bras"*

14. *The Vancouver Sun* Tue 15 July 1997

15. Simone, Charles B. M.D. founder of Simone Cancer Centre *"Breast Health"*- Impakt Communications Ltd.

16. DeMarco, Dr. Carolyn - *The Vancouver Sun* Mon Nov. 18, 1996

17. Austin, Steve author of *"Breast Cancer"* - Prima Press 1994

18. Gazella, Karolyn A. author of *"The Breast Cancer Prevention Trial - Beware of dangerous Science"* Health Counsellor Feb 1995

19. *The Complete Book of Natural & Medical Cures* - Rodale 1994 20. Pratt, Dr. Ph.D. (Psychology) (Humanities) F.B.F.S.

21. Hay, Dr. Louise L. - *"Heal Your Body"*

22. Howard &. Ramsal - *"The Original Writings of Edward Bach"*

23. English Chinese Encyclopaedia of Practical T.C.M. Beijing #10, *Internal Medicine*

24. *Heinemann's Encyclopaedia of Fruits & Vegetables;* John Heinemann - medical anthropologist

Camellia C. Pratt is an East West Herb Course Student and a practitioner. She is developing a wonderful website that describes her clinic. Check it out at www.rainbowclinic.faithweb.com.

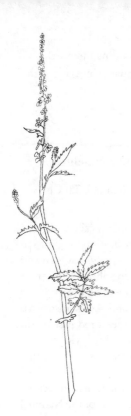

SOURCES & RESOURCES

EAST WEST SCHOOL OF HERBALISM

Michael Tierra O.M.D., L.Ac., founder of the AHG

P.O. Box 275

Ben Lomond, California 95005

Tel: (831) 336-5010 or (800) 717-5010   Fax: (831) 336-4548

This is a 36 lesson distance-learning herb course that includes copious written material, online Internet discussions and a yearly weeklong seminar. It uniquely integrates the study of Western, Chinese and Ayurvedic herbal medicine into a comprehensive system of Planetary Herbalism. More information is available at www.planetherbs.com.

EAST WEST HERB & ACUPUNCTURE CLINIC

912 Center St.

Santa Cruz, California 95060

Tel: (831) 429-8066   Fax: (831) 429-0103

This is the clinic of Dr. Michael Tierra L.A.C., O.M.D., AHG (Founding member) and his wife Lesley Tierra L.A.C., AHG (Founding member).

Telephone and online consultations are also available, check out the website www.planetherbs.com.

THE LONGEVITY CENTER
of CLASSICAL CHINESE MEDICINE
Teaching Qi Gong and Qi Gong massage for cancer patients.

Arnold E. Tayam D.M.Q., Doctor of Medical Qigong (China), Tai Chi/ Bagua Lineage Instructor, Taoist Mentor

With over 20 years experience, Arnold Tayam conducts a Clinical Qigong and Chinese Bodywork practice. He teaches classes and certification programs in Chinese Medical Qigong, Tai Ji Quan (Tai Chi), Bagua Zhang, Yi-Quan and the Taoist arts: chi healing, cultivation, I-Ching, and Feng-Shui. He is senior instructor and top graduate of the International Institute of Medical Qigong system, graduate Haidian University, Co-coordinator and senior instructor for InfiniChi Institute International/College of Tao; featured instructor, and designer for David Carradine's New Chi Kung and Tai Ji video/book series. He has taught for several universities, hospitals and institutes including; Stanford Complementary Medical Clinic, UCSC, Center for Integrated Medicine at O'Connor Hospital, Omega Institute, and the American School of herbalism. Currently he serves as a director board member for the National Qigong Association.

At the Longevity Center he works with his wife, Shasta Tierra-Tayam who practices acupuncture and Chinese herbal medicine.

For information or appointment, please call:

Arnold E. Tayam D.M.Q. and Shasta Tierra-Tayam L.Ac.
P.O. Box 26712
San Jose, CA 95159
Tel: (408) 374-3686 – arnold@longevity-center.com

Programs and Products Available from the Longevity Center
CLASSES
Arnold E. Tayam D.M.Q. teaches the following classes and programs. These classes emphasize energetic skill development and personal healing for health care professionals and lay persons.

Chinese Medical Qigong Certification
Based upon "Chinese Medical Qigong Therapy: A Comprehensive Clinical Text" by Dr. Jerry Alan Johnson, Ph.D., D.T.C.M., D.M.Q.(China).

BASIC 1A/1B: Introduction, theories, 3 regulations, major meridian dilation, cleansing qi emission introduction, clinical skill development, introduction to bodywork.

INTERMEDIATE: Chinese medicine theory and principles, qi emission modalities, power building, intermediate skill development.

ADVANCED: Modulation of common energetic dysfunction's, formulas for internal regulation, advanced external qi emission, case studies, clinical internship, teacher development.

This is a 3 - 4 year residential program.

Infinichi Healing Certification

Based upon the non-religious Taoist teachings of the Integral way from the lineage of 74th generation Master Hua Ching Ni, Infinichi Institute International was founded to cleanse the world of poor health, unhappiness and spiritual devolution. This 3 level program is designed and taught by long-time Taoist mentor Arnold E. Tayam in conjunction with Maoshing Ni Ph.D., L.Ac., D.O.M. Utilizing the teachings of The Integral way and the advanced Traditional Practices as a foundation, this program combines residential intensives and distance learning in a progressive systematic manner that nurtures understanding, facilitates skill development and promotes spiritual self-cultivation.

Internal Martial/Movement Arts

Tai Ji Quan, Bagua Zhang, Yi-Quan are based upon Qigong and Taoist principles. These systems are particularly effective for healing, strength, power, and disease prevention. Training is presented on several different levels, emphasizing structural integration as a foundation for energetic development and martial applications. Classes include exercises that stretch, tone and prepare the body for internal training. Tai Ji short forms and Qigong are taught for beginners leading to the 24 and 48 posture Chen style forms and Bagua Zhang. Instructor certification is available.

VIDEO TAPES

David Carradine's Chi Kung Beginners Workout

In this beginner's workout choreographed by Arnold E. Tayam D.M.Q., Carradine and Tayam guide you through basic chi kung exercises that release pent-up emotions, and improve the flow of chi (or life force) through your body. They will also gently stretch, tone and oxygenate your muscles and help you feel relaxed, rejuvenated and energized. With beautiful music and inspiring nature footage, this 60-minute video is a terrific tool for achieving inner harmony.

David Carradine's Tai Chi Workout for Beginners

In this professionally produced video, Tai Chi instructor Arnold E. Tayam D.M.Q. and Carradine guide you through nine simple and easy-to learn Chen family style Tai Chi movements. The tape starts with stretching exercises and ends with coil and flow of the continuous form. Designed for the beginner, anyone can relax, feel and enjoy the power of Tai Chi. Approximately 60 minutes.

For these and other educational Qi Gong related products email inquiries to: arnold@longevity-center.com

* * *

CHRYSALIS NATURAL MEDICINE CLINIC

Alan Keith Tillotson, PhD, AHG - Medical Herbalist
Naixin Hu Tillotson, OMD, LAc - Chinese Medicine
1008 Milltown Rd., Wilm., DE 19808 USA
(302) 994-0565 Fax: (302) 995-0653
email: AlanT3@aol.com

They offer traditional Chinese, Ayurvedic and up-to-date Western herbal and nutritional services.

WELLSPRINGS CENTER FOR NATURAL HEALING EAST

2226 Black Rock Turnpike
Fairfield, CT 06432
(203) 333-6093

WELLSPRINGS CENTER FOR NATURAL HEALING WEST

1639 Jackson Road
Ashland, OR 97520
(541) 488-3130 Fax: (541) 488-3133

Headed by AHG herbalist Donald Yance, the center specializes in providing lifestyle, nutritional and herbal guidance for cancer patients. He also offers workshops for cancer patients that are of great benefit. Highly recommended.

PRODUCT RESOURCES

Haelen Products
18568 142nd Ave. N.E., Building F
Woodinville, WA USA 98072
1-800-542-3526
Haelen-851 is available from Haelen Products.

Planetary Herb Formulas
P.O. Box 533
Soquel, CA 95073
1-800-606-6226
Available online at www.planetherbs.com

They carry the complete line of Planetary formulas created by Dr. Michael Tierra.

Source Naturals
18 Janis Way
Scotts Valley, CA 95066
1-800-815-2333   (831) 438-1144 or (831) 438-1700
Available online at www.sourcenaturals.com

Source Naturals has a wide range of quality supplements available directly to the consumer. They have just about every supplements mentioned in this book including the following:

Alpha lipoic Acid 200mg, N-Acetyl Cysteine, Beta Glucan, Calcium D-glu-carate, Antioxidant Complex (formerly Plantioxidant—one of the best plant-based antioxidants) to name only a few.

Metagenics health products carry hundreds of quality vitamins, minerals, enzymes, antioxidants. They are either available from a practitioner or from the following:

Doctors Health Supply
2680 Forest Park
Jamul, CA 91935
1-800-578-5939 (619) 445-9306
email: rick@earthtrade.com

Tyler Encapsulations
2204-8 NW Birdsdale
Gresham, OR 97030
Tel: (503) 661-5401   Fax: (503) 66-4913

Wobenzym
4404 E. Elwood
Phoenix, AZ 85040
1-800-899-4499
Website: www.wobenzym.net

Frontier Herbs and Nature's Herbs

P.O. Box 118, Department 34, Q
Norway, IA 52318
1-800-365-4372

Herbalist & Alchemist Inc. (High Quality Extracts)

51 S. Wandling Avenue
Washington, NJ 07882
(908) 689-9020

Herb Pharm

P.O. Box 116
20260 Williams Highway
Williams, OR 97544
(541) 846-6262   Fax: (541) 846-6112

Internatural

P.O. Box 489
Twin Lakes, WI 53181 USA
1-800-643-4221
Tel: (262) 889-8581   Fax: (262) 889-8591
Email: internatural@lotuspress.com
Website: www.internatural.com

Lotus Light Enterprises

P.O. Box 1008
Silver Lake, WI 53170 USA
1-800-548-3824
Tel: (262) 889-8501 (262) 889-8591
Email: lotuslight@lotuspress.com
Website: www.lotuslight.com

MediHerb (High Quality Extracts)

P.O. Box 713
Warwick, Queensland 4370, Australia
(61) 7-4661-0788

Trinity Herb Company
5221 Central, Suite 105
Richmond, CA 94804
1-800-538-1333
An excellent source for bulk organic herbs.

CHINESE HERBS

Bio-Essence/Min Tong
5221 Central, Suite 105
Richmond, CA 94804
1-800-538-1333
A good source for concentrated dried herbal extracts.

Great China Herb Company
857 Washington St.
San Francisco, CA 94108
(415) 982-2195
An excellent source for quality bulk Chinese herbs.

KPC Herb Products, Inc
16 Goddard
Irvine, CA 92618, USA
Tel: (949) 727-4000 Fax: (949) 727-2577
www.kpc.com
A good source for bulk and concentrated dried herbal extracts

Lotus Herbs
1124 North Hacienda Blvd.
La Puente, CA 91744-2021, USA
Tel: (626) 916-1070   Fax: (626) 917-7763
www.lotusherbs.com
A good source for bulk and concentrated dried herbal extracts.

Mayway Corp.
1338 Mandela Parkway
Oakland, CA 94607, USA
Tel: 1-800-2-MAYWAY / (510)-208-3113
Fax: 1-800-909-2828 or (510) 208-3069
A good source for bulk and concentrated dried herbal extracts.

PROFESSIONAL HERBALIST ORGANIZATIONS

American Herbalists Guild (AHG)

1931 Gaddis Rd.
Canton, GA 30115
(770) 751-7548 (home office)
(770) 751-6021 (AHG)
Web: http://www.healthy.net/herbalists

This organization includes individuals who have met strict criteria for professional standards as a clinical herbalist. It has a three-tiered membership including professional clinical herbalists, students and laypersons who are interested and support the goals of herbal evolution in the United States. It has a list of qualified professional herbalists around the United States. You can access these through their website.

National Certification Commission for Acupuncture and Oriental Medicine (NCAAOM)

11 Canal Center Plaza, Suite 300
Alexandria, VA 22314
Phone: 703/548-9004 Fax: 703/548-9079
http://www.nccaom.org

NCAAOM is the leading national organization for professional acupuncturists and Chinese herbalists in the US. They have a national directory where you may find the nearest qualified practitioner.

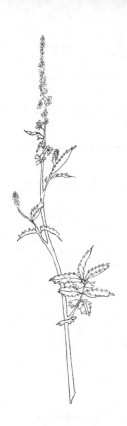

BIBLIOGRAPHY

Books on Cancer

Boik, John, *Cancer and Natural Medicine*, Oregon Medical Press, 2nd edition

Breuse, Rudolf, *The Breuss Cancer Cure*, Alive Books, 1995

Brodie, Douglas, Dr., *Cancer and Common Sense*, Winning Publications, 1997

Diamond, John M.D., Cowden, Lee, M.D., Goldberg, Burton, "An Alternative Medicine Definitive Guide to Cancer," *Future Medicine*, 1997

Frahm, Anne E. and Frahm, David J., *A Cancer Battle Plan*, Tarcher Putnam, 1997

Morra, Marion, Potts, Eve, *Choices*, Avon Books, 1994

Moss, Ralph W. PhD, *Antioxidants Against Cancer*, Equinox Press

Moss, Ralph W. PhD, *The Cancer Industry*, Equinox Press, 1999

Moss, Ralph W. PhD, *Cancer Therapy, The independent Consumer's Guide to Non-Toxic Treatment and Prevention*, Equinox Press, 1997

Moss, Ralph W. PhD, *Questioning Chemotherapy*, Equinox Press, 1995

Pelton, Ross, Overholser, Lee, PhD, *Alternatives in Cancer Therapy*, Fireside, Simon and Schuster, 1994

Spodick, Terry F., Martin-Pitts, Julie, *Diagnosis Cancer, What Can I do Now?* By the Authors living in Santa Cruz, California

Vonderplanitx, Aajonus, *We Want To Live*, Carnelian Bay Castle Press, 1997

Walter, Richard, Options, *The Alternative Cancer Therapy Book*, Avery, 1993

Cancer Salves

Mohs, Frederic E., M.D., *Chemosurgery*, Charles Thomas, 1978

Naiman, Ingrid, *Cancer Salves*, North Atlantic Books, Berkeley, CA, Seventh Ray Press, Santa Fe, New Mexico

Chinese Herbs and Cancer

Hong-Yen Hsu, PhD, "Treating Cancer with Chinese Herbs," Oriental Healing Arts Institute

Jia Kun, *Prevention and Treatment of Carcinoma in Traditional Chinese Medicine*, The Commercial Press, Hong Kong

Lien, Eric J., Wen, Y. Li, "Structure Activity Relationship Analysis of Anticancer Chinese Drugs and Related Plants," Oriental Healing Arts Institute

Mingji, Pan, M.D., *Cancer Treatment with Fu Zheng Pei Ben Principle*, Fujian Science and Technology Publishing house

Minyi, Chang, *Anticancer Medicinal Herbs*, Hunan Science and Technology Publishing House, 1992

Tierra, Michael, *The Way of Chinese Herbs*, Pocket Books, 1998

Zhang Dai-Zhao, *The Treatment of Cancer By Integrated Chinese-Western Medicine*. Blue Poppy Press

Books on Nutrition

Kushi, Michio, *The Cancer Prevention Diet*, St. Martin's Press, 1993

Kushi, Michio, *The Macrobiotic Approach to Cancer*, Avery, 1991

Quillin, Dr. Patrick, *Beating Cancer With Nutrition*, Nutrition Times Press, 1994

Salaman, Maureen, *Nutrition, the Cancer Answer*, Stratford Publishing, 1984

Simone, Charles B., M.D., *Cancer and Nutrition*, Avery, 1992

Western Herbal Medicine

Heinerman, John, *The Treatment of Cancer With Herbs*, Biworld, 1984

Moss, Ralph W. PhD, *Herbs Against Cancer*, Equinox, 1998

Tierra, Lesley, *The Herbs of Life*, Crossing Press

Tierra, Michael, *Planetary Herbology*, Lotus Press

Tierra, Michael, *The Way of Herbs*, Pocket Books, 3rd edition, 1998, Pocket Books

Yance, Donald R., *Herbal Medicine, Healing and Cancer*, Keats, 1999

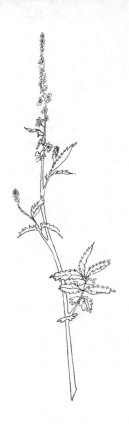

INDEX

A

Asparagus cochinensis 78

Astragalus 18, 76

Astragalus membranicus 78

Atractylodes macrocephela 78

B

B Complex vitamins 322, 328

B-lymphocytes 24

Bagua Zhang 441

Barbat skullcap 94

barberry 18

basic herbal and nutritional
protocol 38

baths 382
epsom salt bath 271

bean soup 308

beans and various legumes 303

Belamcanda chinensis 87

Beta-carotene 299, 330

beverages 304

Bigham, Clark 397

Biotin 327

Bitter melon 91

Black nightshade 95

bladder cancer 18

Bloodroot 94

blood circulation 100

blood moving herbs 102

Boik, John 74

bone cancer 249

bone tumors 104

Bos Taurus Domesticus 88

brain tumors 4

Brandt, Willa 306

brassieres and breast disease 469

breast 91

breast cancer 8, 25, 121, 465

breast cancer (cont'd)
environmental hazards 465
estrogen replacement therapy 469
fat consumption and 467
genetic risk factor 467
odds of contracting 466
spiritual manifestation
of disease 471

Bromelain 18

brown rice 10

Brown Rice and Green Vegetable
Soup 310

Brown sargassum 111

Buckthorne bark 98

Bupleurum chinensis 88

Burdock root (Arctium lappa)
18, 87, 99

Burkitt's lymphoma 19

Burzynski, Stanislaw R. M.D., Ph.D.
367

Buthus martensi 102

Bu Zhong Yi Qi Tang 83

C

Cachexia 292, 365

Caisse, René 99

calcium and phosphorus 335

calcium D-glucarate (CDG) 352

calming spirit and sedative herbs
and therapies 114

calm the mind 115

cancer of the large intestine 90

cancer of the stomach 91

cancer of the stomach,
nasopharynx, lung and cervix 251

cancer staging 20

carbohydrates and cancer 294

carcinogens 23

carcinoma 18

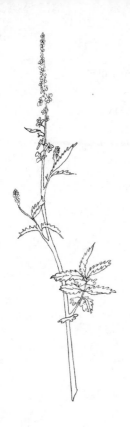

INDEX OF HERBS

Planetary Herbology

by Dr. Michael Tierra

A major work integrating the herbal traditions of the East with those of the West by the bestselling author of "The Way of Herbs". This practical handbook and reference guide is a landmark publication in this field. For unprecedented usefulness in practical applications, the author provides a comprehensive listing of the more than 400 medicinal herbs available in the west, classified according to their chemical constituents, properties and actions, indicated uses and suggested dosages.

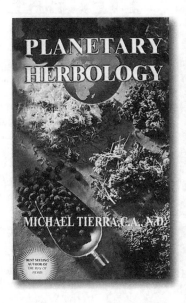

Trade Paper Book   ISBN: 978-0-9415-2427-8   490 pp pb $17.95

Available at bookstores and natural food stores nationwide or order your copy directly by sending $17.95 plus $2.50 shipping/handling ($.75 s/h for each additional copy ordered at the same time) to:

Lotus Press, PO Box 325, Dept. NW, Twin Lakes, WI 53181 USA
toll free order line: 800 824 6396 office phone: 262 889 8561
office fax: 262 889 2461 email: lotuspress@lotuspress.com
web site: www.lotuspress.com

Lotus Press is the publisher of a wide range of books and software in the field of alternative health, including Ayurveda, Chinese medicine, herbology, aromatherapy, Reiki and energetic healing modalities. Request our free book catalog.

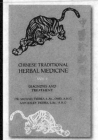
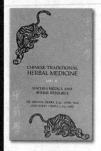

BIOMAGNETIC
and Herbal Therapy
Dr. Michael Tierra

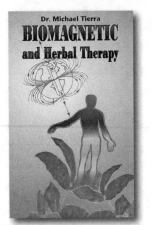

$10.95   **96pp**
5.375" x 8.5" quality trade paper
ISBN: 978-0-9149-5533-7

Magnetic energy is the structural force of the universe.
In this book the respected herbalist, Dr. Michael Tier-
ra, enlightens us on the healing influence of commercially available magnets for
many conditions and describes the sometimes miraculous relief from such problems
as joint pain, skin diseases, acidity, blood pressure, tumors, kidney, liver and thyroid
problems, and more. Magnetizing herbs, teas, water and their usage in conjunction with direct placement of magnets for synergistic effectiveness is presented in a
systematic, succinct and practical manner for the benefit of the professional and lay
person alike. Replete with diagrams and appendices, this is a "how to do" practical
handbook for augmenting health and obtaining relief from pain.

The paradigm of health in the future is based on energy flow. This paradigm reaches
back to the ancient healing arts of the traditional Chinese, the Ayurvedic and the
Native American cultures. It is connected to the work of Hippocrates, the "father"
of Western medicine, in ancient Greek culture, and found its way through the herbal
and homeopathic science that has flourished in Europe over the last few hundred
years.

Dr. Tierra is the author of the all-time best selling herbal *The Way of Herbs* as well as
the synthesizing work *Planetary Herbology*. He is a practicing herbalist and educator
in the field with a background of studies spanning the Chinese and Ayurvedic, the
Native American and the European herbal traditions.

Available at bookstores and natural food stores nationwide or order your copy directly by sending cost of item plus $2.50 ship-
ping/handling ($.75 s/h for each additional copy ordered at the same time) to:

Lotus Press, PO Box 325, Dept. CTM, Twin Lakes, WI 53181 USA
toll free order line: 800 824 6396   office phone: 262 889 8561
office fax: 262 889 2461   email: lotuspress@lotuspress.com
web site: www.lotuspress.com

Lotus Press is the publisher of a wide range of books and software in the field of alternative health, including Ayurveda, Chinese
medicine, herbology, aromatherapy, Reiki and energetic healing modalities. Request our free book catalog.

Planetary Herbology

by Dr. Michael Tierra, C.A., N.D.

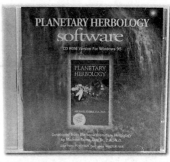